AF689864

GULF WAR and HEALTH

VOLUME 6

PHYSIOLOGIC, PSYCHOLOGIC, AND PSYCHOSOCIAL EFFECTS OF DEPLOYMENT-RELATED STRESS

Committee on Gulf War and Health: Physiologic, Psychologic, and Psychosocial Effects of Deployment-Related Stress

Board on Population Health and Public Health Practice

INSTITUTE OF MEDICINE
OF THE NATIONAL ACADEMIES

THE NATIONAL ACADEMIES PRESS
Washington, D.C.
www.nap.edu

THE NATIONAL ACADEMIES PRESS 500 Fifth Street, NW Washington, DC 20001

NOTICE: The project that is the subject of this report was approved by the Governing Board of the National Research Council, whose members are drawn from the councils of the National Academy of Sciences, the National Academy of Engineering, and the Institute of Medicine. The members of the committee responsible for the report were chosen for their special competences and with regard for appropriate balance.

This study was supported by Contract V101(93)P-2155B between the National Academy of Sciences and the Department of Veterans Affairs. Any opinions, findings, conclusions, or recommendations expressed in this publication are those of the authors and do not necessarily reflect the view of the organizations or agencies that provided support for this project.

International Standard Book Number = 13: 978-0-309-10177-6
International Standard Book Number = 10: 0-309-10177-8
Library of Congress Control Number: 2008920197

Additional copies of this report are available from the National Academies Press, 500 Fifth Street, NW, Lockbox 285, Washington, DC 20055; (800) 624-6242 or (202) 334-3313 (in the Washington metropolitan area); Internet, http://www.nap.edu.

For more information about the Institute of Medicine, visit the IOM home page at **www.iom.edu.**

Copyright 2008 by the National Academy of Sciences. All rights reserved.

Printed in the United States of America.

The serpent has been a symbol of long life, healing, and knowledge among almost all cultures and religions since the beginning of recorded history. The serpent adopted as a logotype by the Institute of Medicine is a relief carving from ancient Greece, now held by the Staatliche Museen in Berlin.

Suggested citation:

IOM (Institute of Medicine). 2008. Gulf War and Health, Volume 6: Physiologic, Psychologic, and Psychosocial Effects of Deployment-Related Stress. Washington, DC: The National Academies Press.

"Knowing is not enough; we must apply.
Willing is not enough; we must do."
—Goethe

INSTITUTE OF MEDICINE
OF THE NATIONAL ACADEMIES

Advising the Nation. Improving Health.

THE NATIONAL ACADEMIES

Advisers to the Nation on Science, Engineering, and Medicine

The **National Academy of Sciences** is a private, nonprofit, self-perpetuating society of distinguished scholars engaged in scientific and engineering research, dedicated to the furtherance of science and technology and to their use for the general welfare. Upon the authority of the charter granted to it by the Congress in 1863, the Academy has a mandate that requires it to advise the federal government on scientific and technical matters. Dr. Ralph J. Cicerone is president of the National Academy of Sciences.

The **National Academy of Engineering** was established in 1964, under the charter of the National Academy of Sciences, as a parallel organization of outstanding engineers. It is autonomous in its administration and in the selection of its members, sharing with the National Academy of Sciences the responsibility for advising the federal government. The National Academy of Engineering also sponsors engineering programs aimed at meeting national needs, encourages education and research, and recognizes the superior achievements of engineers. Dr. Charles M. Vest is president of the National Academy of Engineering.

The **Institute of Medicine** was established in 1970 by the National Academy of Sciences to secure the services of eminent members of appropriate professions in the examination of policy matters pertaining to the health of the public. The Institute acts under the responsibility given to the National Academy of Sciences by its congressional charter to be an adviser to the federal government and, upon its own initiative, to identify issues of medical care, research, and education. Dr. Harvey V. Fineberg is president of the Institute of Medicine.

The **National Research Council** was organized by the National Academy of Sciences in 1916 to associate the broad community of science and technology with the Academy's purposes of furthering knowledge and advising the federal government. Functioning in accordance with general policies determined by the Academy, the Council has become the principal operating agency of both the National Academy of Sciences and the National Academy of Engineering in providing services to the government, the public, and the scientific and engineering communities. The Council is administered jointly by both Academies and the Institute of Medicine. Dr. Ralph J. Cicerone and Dr. Charles M. Vest are chair and vice chair, respectively, of the National Research Council.

www.national-academies.org

COMMITTEE ON GULF WAR AND HEALTH: PHYSIOLOGIC, PSYCHOLOGIC, AND PSYCHOSOCIAL EFFECTS OF DEPLOYMENT-RELATED STRESS

RICHARD MAYEUX, MD, MSc (Chair), Gertrude H. Sergievsky Professor of Neurology, Psychiatry, and Epidemiology, Sergievsky Center, and Codirector, Taub Institute, Columbia University

KATHRYN KARUSAITIS BASHAM, PhD, MSW, Professor, Smith College School for Social Work

EVELYN J. BROMET, PhD, Professor of Psychiatry and Preventive Medicine, State University of New York at Stony Brook

GREGORY L. BURKE, MD, MSc, Professor and Chair, Public Health Sciences, Wake Forest University School of Medicine

DENNIS S. CHARNEY, MD, Dean, Anne and Joel Ehrenkranz Professor, Mount Sinai School of Medicine

MICHAEL DAVIS, PhD, Robert W. Woodruff Professor of Psychiatry, Behavioral Sciences and Psychology, Emory University

DOUGLAS A. DROSSMAN, MD, Professor of Medicine and Psychiatry and Codirector, UNC Center for Functional GI and Motility Disorders, University of North Carolina at Chapel Hill

DWIGHT L. EVANS, MD, Ruth Meltzer Professor and Chair, Psychiatry, and Professor of Psychiatry, Medicine, and Neuroscience, University of Pennsylvania School of Medicine

VINCENT J. FELITTI, MD, Kaiser Permanente Medical Care Program, San Diego, CA

JANICE L. KRUPNICK, PhD, Professor, Department of Psychiatry, Georgetown University School of Medicine

WILLIAM B. MALARKEY, MD, Professor of Internal Medicine and Molecular Virology, Immunology and Medical Genetics and Director, Clinical Research Center, Ohio State University

BRUCE S. MCEWEN, PhD, Alfred E. Mirsky Professor and Head, Harold and Margaret Milliken Hatch Laboratory of Neuroendocrinology, Rockefeller University

THOMAS G. PICKERING, MD, DPhil, Professor of Medicine, Columbia University

JERROLD F. ROSENBAUM, MD, Psychiatrist-in-Chief, Massachusetts General Hospital, and Stanley Cobb Professor of Pyschiatry, Harvard Medical School

B. TIMOTHY WALSH, MD, William and Joy Ruane Professor of Pediatric Psychopharmacology, College of Physicians and Surgeons, Columbia University, and Chief, Division of Clinical Therapeutics, New York State Psychiatric Institute

CONSULTANTS

KERRY L. KNOX, PhD, Associate Professor, Department of Psychiatry and Community and Preventive Medicine, University of Rochester School of Medicine and Department of Veterans Affairs, Director, VISN 2 Center for Excellence at Canandaigua
CAROL NORTH, MD, VA North Texas Health Care System and Department of Psychiatry, University of Texas Southwestern Medical Center at Dallas
MIRIAM DAVIS, Independent Medical Writer, Silver Spring, MD

STAFF

CAROLYN FULCO, Scholar
ROBERTA WEDGE, Senior Program Officer
SANDRA GOODBODY, Senior Program Officer
PETER JAMES, Senior Program Associate
DEEPALI M. PATEL, Senior Program Associate
MICHAEL SCHNEIDER, Senior Program Associate
DAVID J. TOLLERUD, Program Assistant
DANIELLE K. STOLL, Program Assistant
DAMIKA WEBB, Research Assistant
RENEE WLODARCZYK, Senior Program Assistant
NORMAN GROSSBLAT, Senior editor
ROSE MARIE MARTINEZ, Director, Board on Population Health and Public Health Practice
HOPE HARE, Administrative Assistant

REVIEWERS

This report has been reviewed in draft form by persons chosen for their diverse perspectives and technical expertise in accordance with procedures approved by the National Research Council's Report Review Committee. The purpose of this independent review is to provide candid and critical comments that will assist the institution in making its published report as sound as possible and to ensure that the report meets institutional standards of objectivity, evidence, and responsiveness to the study charge. The review comments and draft manuscript remain confidential to protect the integrity of the deliberative process. We wish to thank the following for their review of this report:

Elissa S. Epel, Department of Psychiatry, University of California, San Francisco
Manning Feinleib, Department of Epidemiology, The Johns Hopkins University
Edgar Garcia-Rill, Center for Translational Neuroscience, Department of Neurobiology & Developmental Sciences, University of Arkansas for Medical Sciences
Danny O. Jacobs, Department of Surgery, Duke University Medical Center
Karen A. Matthews, Western Psychiatric Institute & Clinic, University of Pittsburgh School of Medicine
Eric J. Nestler, Department of Psychiatry, The University of Texas Southwestern Medical Center at Dallas
William E. Schlenger, Abt Associates, Inc.
Robert D. Sparks, TASER Foundation
Ezra S. Susser, Department of Epidemiology, Columbia University
Daniel S. Weiss, Department of Psychiatry, University of California, San Francisco
Nancy Fugate Woods, School of Nursing, University of Washington

Although the reviewers listed above have provided many constructive comments and suggestions, they were not asked to endorse the conclusions or recommendations, nor did they see the final draft of the report before its release. The review of this report was overseen by **Dr. Charles E. Phelps,** University of Rochester, and **Dr. Harold C. Sox,** American College of Physicians/*Annals of Internal Medicine*. Appointed by the National Research Council and the Institute of Medicine, they were responsible for making certain that an independent examination of this report was carried out in accordance with institutional procedures and that all review comments were carefully considered. Responsibility for the final content of this report rests entirely with the author committee and the institution.

CONTENTS

Tables

Boxes and Figures

ACRONYMS

ACTH	Adrenocorticotrophic hormone, corticotropin
APA	American Psychiatric Association
ASI	Anxiety sensitivity index
AUDIT	Alcohol use disorder identification test
BIRLS	Beneficiary identification record locator subsystem
BNST	Bed nucleus of the stria terminalis
BSS	Body-system symptom
CAPS	Clinician-Administered PTSD Scale
CCEP	Comprehensive Clinical Evaluation Program
CDC	Centers for Disease Control and Prevention
CES	Combat Exposure Scale
CFS	Chronic fatigue syndrome
CHD	Coronary heart disease
CI	Confidence interval
CIDI	Composite International Diagnostic Interview
CNS	Central nervous system
COPD	Chronic obstructive pulmonary disease
CRH	Corticotropin-releasing hormone
CSF	Cerebrospinal fluid
CSMs	Cerebrospinal malformations
CTS	Conflict Tactics Scale
CVLT	California Verbal Learning Test
DIS	Diagnostic Interview Schedule
DMDC	Defense Manpower Data Center
DoD	Department of Defense
DSM	*Diagnostic and Statistical Manual of Mental Disorders III or IV*
GAD	Generalized anxiety disorder
GI	Gastrointestinal
HDL	High-density lipoprotein
HPA	Hypothalamus-pituitary-adrenal
HU13	Health Utilities Index Mark 3
HVVP	Hawaiian Vietnam Veterans Project
IBS	Irritable bowel syndrome
ICD	*International Statistical Classification of Diseases and Related Health Problems*

IEDs	Improvised explosive devices
IOM	Institute of Medicine
km	Kilometer
MDD	Major depression disorder
MHAT	Mental Health Advisory Team
MHM	Military History Measure
MMPI	Minnesota Multiphasic Personality Inventory
MPI	Martial Problem Index
MRI	Magnetic resonance imaging
MSAs	Metropolitan statistical areas
NART	National Adult Reading Test
NAS	National Academy of Sciences
NCHS	National Center for Health Statistics
NCO	Noncommissioned officer
NCS	National Comorbidity Survey
NHANES	National Health and Nutrition Examination Survey
NHL	Non-Hodgkin's lymphoma
NSVG	National Survey of the Vietnam Generation
NVVRS	National Vietnam Veterans Readjustment Study
OEF	Operation Enduring Freedom
OIF	Operation Iraqi Freedom
OR	Odds ratio
PASAT	Paced Auditory Serial Addition Test
PB	Pyridostigmine bromide
PIR	Proportional incidence rate
PMR	Proportional morbidity ratio
PPI	Parental Problem Index
PTSD	Posttraumatic stress disorder
RR	Relative risk
SCID	Structured Clinical Interview for *DSM-III* or *IV*
SE	Standard error
SF-36	36-Item Medical Outcomes Study Short-Form
T3	Triiodothyronine
T4	Thyroxine
TSH	Thyroid-stimulating hormone
UK	United Kingdom
UN	United Nations
VA	Department of Veterans Affairs

VES	Vietnam Experience Study
VET Registry	Vietnam-Era Twin Registry
vs	Versus
WAIS-R	Wechsler Adult Intelligence Scale-revised
WCST	Wisconsin Card Sorting Test

PREFACE

Deployment to a war zone has a profound impact on the lives of many of the troops who are deployed to foreign soil and on their family members. Needless to say, numerous stressors are associated with deployment, from terrifying concerns about surviving, being taken prisoner, and being tortured to the horrific possibility of seeing friends die, being maimed, and handling dead bodies. Less traumatic but more pervasive stressors include anxiety about home life, such as loss of a job and income, impacts on relationships, and absence from family.

The effects of deployment-related stressors on a veteran's health during and after deployment are numerous. When sudden and life-threatening stressors are encountered, the body will typically react with an acute "flight or fight" response that subsides when the stressor goes away. If the stressor or the acute response persists, the body may react with a more prolonged stress response that can lead to harmful long-term effects on health. The focus of this report, by the Institute of Medicine (IOM) Committee on Gulf War and Health: Physiologic, Psychologic, and Psychosocial Effects of Deployment-Related Stress, is the long-term effects of deployment-related stress. What happens to military personnel when they are subjected to the many stressors that occur in a war zone?

The U.S. Department of Veterans Affairs and Congress have secured the assistance of IOM in evaluating the scientific literature regarding an association between deployment-related stressors and health effects. Congress's request regarding the possible association between illness and exposure to stressors in the Gulf War is similar to its approach after the Vietnam War to exposure to Agent Orange and after the 1991 Persian Gulf War to exposure to numerous biologic and chemical agents. Although seemingly straightforward conceptually, this task has proved to be much more difficult than previous studies. The committee discussed how to define deployment-related stress, the types of stressors encountered, and how they might be assessed or measured.

In this report, the committee equated deployment-related stress with being deployed to a war zone, although it recognized that not everyone deployed to a war zone would respond to stressors in the same way and that not everyone would necessarily find a particular event stressful. The reaction to deployment-related stressors would depend on numerous factors that were present before, during, and after deployment. Stressors that people experienced in childhood, their interactions with friends and family, and whether they were wounded during deployment would all play a role in the nature of the response. The committee also understood that some military personnel would have minor reactions and transient health effects, some would have severe reactions and more chronic health effects, and some would go on to develop posttraumatic stress disorder (PTSD), which could be associated with additional health effects. That approach is detailed in the committee's report.

The committee deliberated for many months and met 14 times. It reviewed all the studies of health effects in veterans deployed to a war zone and found that most studies did not measure the stressors of war (although that was not required for inclusion in the committee's analysis), and that the ones that did measure deployment-related stress were most often related to PTSD. The committee noted that although experimental data from studies in animals indicated numerous health effects associated with various types of stressors, the human literature is much more challenging to interpret.

I am deeply appreciative of the hard work of our committee members: Kathryn Basham, Evelyn Bromet, Gregory Burke, Dennis Charney, Michael Davis, Douglas Drossman, Dwight Evans, Vincent Felitti, Janice Krupnick, William Malarkey, Bruce McEwen, Thomas Pickering, Jerrold Rosenbaum, and Timothy Walsh, and of our expert consultants Carol North, Kerry Knox, and Miriam Davis. The committee would like to thank Jack Gorman for his thoughtful input. Although the committee developed conclusions independently of input from IOM staff, we deeply appreciate their hard work and attention to detail and the extensive research that they conducted to ensure that we had all the information that we needed from the outset. It has been a privilege and a pleasure to work with the IOM staff directed by Roberta Wedge and Carolyn Fulco. Without them, this report would not have been possible. Most of all, our committee appreciates the veterans who have served in this country's wars. It is for them that we do this work, and we hope that this report will inform those who have given so much to our nation.

Richard Mayeux, MD, MSc (*Chair*)
Sergievsky Professor of Neurology, Psychiatry, and Epidemiology
Director, Sergievsky Center; Codirector, Taub Institute
College of Physicians and Surgeons
Columbia University

SUMMARY

On August 2, 1990, Iraq invaded Kuwait, and Operation Desert Storm was launched on January 16, 1991, with an air offensive to liberate Kuwait. On February 24, 1991, the ground war began; by February 28, the war was over, and a ceasefire was signed in April. All U.S. troops who had participated in the ground war had returned home by June 13. About 697,000 U.S. military personnel were deployed to the Persian Gulf during the buildup and the war. Most of them were active-duty military personnel, but 261,871 reservists were called to active duty, and 106,047 of them were deployed to the gulf.

The United States is once again engaged in a military conflict in the Middle East. Operation Enduring Freedom (OEF) began on October 7, 2001, in response to the September 11, 2001, terrorist attacks on the United States. Troops are stationed in and around Afghanistan, Southwest Asia, and other locations for military and humanitarian purposes. Operation Iraqi Freedom (OIF) began on March 19, 2003, when U.S.-led coalition forces invaded Iraq. As of November 4, 2006, about 1.4 million U.S. troops had been deployed to the conflicts in OEF and OIF.

In response to the growing concern about the physical and psychologic health of the Gulf War veterans from the 1990-1991 conflict, Congress passed two laws in 1998: PL 105-277, the Persian Gulf War Veterans Act, and PL 105-368, the Veterans Programs Enhancement Act. Those laws directed the secretary of veterans affairs to enter into a contract with the National Academy of Sciences (NAS) to review and evaluate the scientific and medical literature regarding associations between illness and exposure to toxic agents, environmental or wartime hazards, and preventive medicines or vaccines in members of the armed forces who were exposed to such agents. PL 105-277 also gave NAS permission to identify "other agents, hazards, or medicines or vaccines to which members of the Armed Forces may have been exposed." In 1996, the Presidential Advisory Committee on Gulf War Veterans' Illnesses found that stress was an important contributor to those veterans' illnesses and encouraged the government to continue its research on stress-related disorders. In response to the above laws, the Institute of Medicine (IOM) has had a program to examine health risks posed by specific agents and hazards to which Gulf War veterans might have been exposed during their deployment. Four reports have examined health effects related to depleted uranium, pyridostigmine bromide, sarin, and vaccines; insecticides and solvents; fuels, combustion products, and propellants; and infectious diseases. A fifth report by IOM evaluated the current health status of Gulf War-deployed veterans compared with their nondeployed counterparts.

In recent years, the charge to IOM has been expanded to include not only veterans of the 1990-1991 Gulf War but veterans returning from OEF and OIF. Many of the biologic and chemical exposures and their possible health effects have been considered in previous IOM reports, but the health effects associated with deployment-related stress had yet to be considered.

A recent IOM report, *Gulf War and Health, Volume 4: Health Effects of Serving in the Gulf War*, reviewed the health status of Gulf War-deployed veterans. That report found that veterans of the Gulf War report higher rates of nearly all symptoms than their nondeployed counterparts; a higher prevalence not only of individual symptoms but of chronic multisymptom illnesses was also found among Gulf War-deployed veterans. Multisymptom-based medical conditions reported to occur more frequently among deployed Gulf War veterans include fibromyalgia, chronic fatigue syndrome, and multiple chemical sensitivity. The literature also demonstrates that deployment places veterans at increased risk for symptoms that meet diagnostic criteria for a number of psychiatric illnesses, particularly posttraumatic stress disorder (PTSD), anxiety disorders, depressive disorders, and substance abuse. In light of the 1991 Gulf War and the nature of OEF and OIF, the Department of Veterans Affairs (VA) requested that IOM comprehensively review, evaluate, and summarize the peer-reviewed scientific and medical literature regarding the association between deployment-related stress and long-term adverse health effects in Gulf War veterans. In response to VA's request, IOM appointed the Committee on Gulf War and Health: Physiologic, Psychologic, and Psychosocial Effects of Deployment-Related Stress to conduct the review.

COMMITTEE'S INTERPRETATION OF ITS CHARGE

Given the committee's charge from VA—to assess the long-term health effects of deployment-related stress—the committee began by defining the deployment in question as "deployment to a war zone." Combat is one of the most potent stressors that a person can experience, but as military conflicts have evolved to include more guerilla warfare and insurgent activities, restricting the definition of deployment-related stressors to combat may fail to acknowledge other potent stressors experienced by military personnel in a war zone or in the aftermath of combat. Those stressors include constant vigilance against unexpected attack, the absence of a defined front line, the difficulty of distinguishing enemy combatants from civilians, the ubiquity of improvised explosive devices, caring for the badly injured or dying, duty on the graves registration service, and being responsible for the treatment of prisoners of war. Deployment stressors associated with armed conflict include not only combat stressors but noncombat stressors. Non-combat-related stressors that might be experienced by deployed personnel are separation from family, friends, and colleagues; loss of or reduction in income; and concern over employment status when deployment ends. Therefore, the committee considered that military personnel deployed to a war zone, even if direct combat was not experienced, have the potential for exposure to deployment-related stressors and that the emotional and physical reactions of military personnel to those stressors can vary widely.

COMMITTEE'S APPROACH TO ITS CHARGE

The committee's charge was the comprehensive review, evaluation, and summary of the peer-reviewed scientific and medical literature regarding the association between deployment-related stress and long-term adverse health effects in Gulf War veterans. Specifically, the committee was to study the physiologic, psychologic, and psychosocial effects of stress. Noted in the committee's charge is that the study's findings are applicable not only to veterans of the 1991 Gulf War but to veterans of OEF and OIF.

To evaluate associations between deployment-related stress and adverse effects, the committee considered all studies that identified health effects found in military personnel deployed to a war zone. Deployment to a war zone would be used as a surrogate for deployment-related stress. The potential health effects considered included not only physiologic effects but psychologic effects, such as depression and PTSD, and psychosocial effects, such as marital conflict and incarceration. The committee also considered studies of deployed veterans with combat-related PTSD and associated health effects because PTSD can result only after exposure to a traumatic stressor and a war zone is rife with potentially traumatic events. In conducting its deliberations, the committee considered studies of veterans of World War II, the Korean War, the Vietnam War, the 1991 Gulf War, and OEF and OIF.

The committee sought to characterize and weigh the strengths and limitations of the available evidence regarding the association between deployment to a war zone and specific adverse health effects. The English-language scientific literature was searched to identify health effects in military veterans from World War II to the conflicts in Afghanistan and Iraq. Although most of the literature focused on U.S. military veterans, veterans from other countries were included. Over 3000 potentially relevant references were retrieved and assessed.

The committee used only peer-reviewed published literature as the basis of its conclusions. Committee members read each study critically and considered its relevance and quality. The committee did not collect original data, nor did it perform any secondary data analysis.

The committee also did not address policy issues—such as decisions regarding compensation, potential costs of compensation, or any broader policy implications of its findings—nor did it examine treatment approaches for any health effects.

EVALUATION CRITERIA

When the committee had obtained the studies that met its inclusion criteria, it was necessary to establish which papers would constitute the foundation of its conclusions. In its review of the literature, the committee divided the available studies into two categories: primary and secondary.

Primary Studies

The committee used primary studies as the basis of its evaluation and conclusions. A primary study demonstrates rigorous methods; for example, it includes details of its methods, has an appropriate control or reference group, has a sample size of at least 100, has the statistical power to detect effects, and includes reasonable adjustments for confounders. Ideally, it has information regarding a specific health effect and exposure. To consider a study as primary, the committee insisted that the health effect be diagnosed or confirmed by a clinical evaluation, specific laboratory test, hospital records, or other medical record or, for a psychiatric outcome, by standardized interviews. Primary studies included comparisons of veterans deployed to a war zone with their nondeployed counterparts and studies that evaluated health effects in veterans with deployment-related or combat-related PTSD.

Secondary, or Support, Studies

Secondary studies were less rigorous in their methods; for example, a study might have a small sample, not include a physician's examination or other appropriate evaluation method, or rely only on veterans' self-reports of symptoms or diseases. They might have been population-based surveys of veterans' responses to mailed questionnaires. The committee used those types of studies to support findings based on primary studies.

CATEGORIES OF ASSOCIATION

The committee agreed to base its conclusions on the categories of association that have been used by previous Committees on Gulf War and Health and other IOM committees that evaluated vaccine safety, effects of herbicides used in Vietnam, and indoor pollutants related to asthma. The categories are described below.

Sufficient Evidence of a Causal Relationship

Evidence is sufficient to conclude that there is a causal relationship between deployment to a war zone and a specific health effect in humans, and the evidence is supported by experimental data on humans or animals. The evidence fulfills the guidelines for sufficient evidence of an association (below) and satisfies several of the guidelines used to assess causality: strength of association, dose-response relationship, consistency of association, and temporal relationship.

Sufficient Evidence of an Association

Evidence is sufficient to conclude that there is an association; that is, a consistent association has been observed between deployment to a war zone and a specific health effect in human studies in which chance and bias, including confounding, could be ruled out with reasonable confidence. For example, several high-quality studies report consistent associations, are sufficiently free of bias, and include adequate control for confounding.

Limited but Suggestive Evidence of an Association

Evidence is suggestive of an association between deployment to a war zone and a specific health effect in human studies, but the body of evidence is limited by the inability to rule out chance and bias, including confounding, with confidence. At least one high-quality study reports a positive association that is sufficiently free of bias and includes adequate control for confounding, and other corroborating studies provide support for the association but are not sufficiently free of bias, including confounding. Alternatively, several studies of lower quality might show a consistent association, and the results are probably not due to bias, including confounding.

Inadequate/Insufficient Evidence to Determine Whether an Association Exists

Evidence is of insufficient quantity, quality, or consistency to permit a conclusion regarding the existence of an association between deployment to a war zone and a specific health effect in humans.

Limited/Suggestive Evidence of No Association

Evidence is consistent in not showing a positive association between deployment to a war zone and a specific health effect after exposure of any magnitude. A conclusion of no association is inevitably limited to the conditions, magnitudes of exposure, and length of observation in the available studies. The possibility of a very small increase in risk after exposure cannot be excluded.

LIMITATIONS OF VETERAN STUDIES

Few of the studies reviewed by the committee measured combat exposure or the level of stress experienced by military personnel during deployment to a war zone. Even in the studies that did assess combat exposure, using questionnaires or scales, researchers asked whether an exposure occurred (for example, had a soldier fired on the enemy) rather than the degree to which the veteran may have found the experience to be stressful. Few studies attempted to determine the effects of repeated or combined exposures, such as exposure to extreme heat, to chemical protective gear, and to shooting at an enemy.

Another limitation of many of the studies was their retrospective design, which resulted in an inability to distinguish whether a health effect existed before or was a consequence of deployment. Further limitations include the use of self-report questionnaires to assess health effects and exposure; such questionnaires can lead to recall bias with regard to exposures or to inaccuracies in reporting health effects. For those reasons, the committee weighted more heavily the studies that included an examination by a health professional or other appropriate evaluation method. Similarly, for psychiatric disorders, such as PTSD, some studies relied only on symptom checklists to indicate the presence of the disorders rather than on a proper diagnostic examination by a health professional. Many studies had a selection bias in that health effects were assessed in veterans who were in treatment groups, such as inpatients or outpatients at PTSD clinics, or were selected from registries of veterans established by VA. In addition, sufficient time might not have passed since deployment to detect the development of some health outcomes, for example, cancer or heart disease, particularly in OEF and OIF veterans.

DEPLOYMENT-RELATED STRESSORS

Exposure to combat has been described as one of the most intense stressors that a person can experience; for many people, combat is the most traumatic event of their life.

Deployment stressors in the Persian Gulf War included being in the vicinity of a Scud missile explosion, contact with prisoners of war or dead animals, direct combat duty, witnessing the death of a person, being exposed to dismembered bodies or maimed soldiers, coming under small-arms fire, having artillery close by, and fear of being wounded. It was found that military personnel in the Gulf War were at greatest risk for stress when their work was hazardous and they anticipated exposure to chemical warfare; the risk increased with time spent in the field and exposure to the dead and wounded. Another stressor was the feeling that they were deserting their families at a time of need.

In OEF and OIF, many of the stressors are more reminiscent of the Vietnam War than of the 1991 Gulf War or World War II. With the defeat of the Iraqi Army and later sectarian violence, U.S. troops have been subjected to guerilla warfare and terrorist actions from civilian insurgents and militias, particularly the use of improvised explosive devices. Soldiers must be constantly on guard, and all civilians must be viewed with caution. Department of Defense (DoD) surveys of Army soldiers and Marines stationed in Iraq found that exposure to combat was the critical determinant of a soldier's or Marine's mental health.

THE STRESS RESPONSE

A person exposed to a stressor, deployment-related or not, may experience a stress response. The word *stress* is used in many contexts and has a variety of meanings. It is often used to describe a situation characterized by real or perceived threats, but it is also commonly used to refer to the body's response to such threats. Thus, *stress* has been used both to describe the environmental events (the stressors) that trigger responses and to refer to the resulting changes (stress response) that occur in the brain and the rest of the body.

The stress response is a coordinated set of interactions among multiple organ systems in the body, including the brain, gut, heart, liver, immune system, thyroid, adrenals, pituitary, gonads, bone, and skin. In response to a stressor, the body initiates an acute stress response. Acute stress responses are usually adaptive, preparing the body for "fight or flight." After exposure to the stressor has ended, the acute stress response subsides, and the body returns to its normal state. However, if the body's reactions persist after the stressor has ended, a chronic stress response can develop, which can be maladaptive and result in feelings of anxiety and lack of control and chronic health effects. Stressors can also lead to adverse psychosocial effects—such as marital conflicts and homelessness—concurrently with or after the development of health effects. Whether the stress response leads to adverse health effects either in the short term (hours to days) or in the long term (months to years) is determined by a number of factors, including the intensity and duration of the stressful experience, the effects of previous stressors, and risk factors (such as genetic susceptibility or a history of a psychiatric disorder) and protective factors (such as military training or supportive family and social environment). Thus, each person's response to stress can be modified on the basis of the specific deployment-related stressors, the complex nature of the stress response, and risk and protective factors.

POSTTRAUMATIC STRESS DISORDER

It is widely recognized that soldiers can suffer psychologic consequences during and after combat. After the Vietnam War, research demonstrated that many veterans, particularly those exposed to severe war-related trauma, and such other traumatized populations as Holocaust survivors, suffered from chronic psychologic problems that often resulted in social and occupational dysfunction. The constellation of symptoms that has come to be known as PTSD is an anxiety disorder whose occurrence is precipitated by exposure to a traumatic event. PTSD was formally recognized as a psychiatric diagnosis in the third edition of the *Diagnostic and Statistical Manual of Mental Disorders (DSM-III)*, published in 1980.

Characterized by symptoms of hyperarousal, numbing or avoidance, and re-experiencing of the traumatic event, PTSD may be evident shortly after exposure to a traumatic event or may take years for the veteran to have sufficient symptoms to meet the diagnostic criteria; once developed, the symptoms may persist for many years. PTSD, or symptoms associated with it, has been reported in veterans of World War II, the Korean War, the Vietnam War, the Gulf War, and OEF and OIF. The prevalence of PTSD in veterans increases as combat exposure increases, in some cases showing a dose-response relationship. PTSD is also highly comorbid with other psychiatric disorders, particularly major depression, general anxiety, and substance-use disorders. The presence of comorbid disorders increases the difficulty of diagnosing PTSD. PTSD is also associated with increased reporting of symptoms, medical conditions, and poor health in veterans. The *DSM-IV* requires that a diagnosis of PTSD include "clinically significant distress and/or impairment in social, occupational, and/or other important areas of functioning." Veterans with PTSD report more disability and impaired functioning than those without PTSD.

Although military personnel may be exposed to identical stressors during their deployment to a war zone, their short-term and long-term responses to those stressors will vary. The variation is due to a host of individual risk factors and protective factors that influence the likelihood of long-term health effects after the exposures. The committee found that combat and being physically wounded were among the most significant risk factors for PTSD or other psychiatric disorders. Other important risk factors include childhood maltreatment, the presence of a pre-existing psychiatric disorder, poor social support on returning home, negative coping styles, being a member of a minority group, and lack of hardiness. Protective factors include better education, higher military rank, having a stable family life, and having a sense of control.

HEALTH EFFECTS

The committee reviewed numerous epidemiologic studies to arrive at conclusions about association. It weighed the strengths and limitations of all the epidemiologic studies and reached its conclusions by interpreting the data in the entire body of reviewed literature. It assigned each health outcome being considered to one of the five categories of association according to the specific criteria set forth above. The committee also considered health effects of PTSD. Its findings about the strength of the associations between deployment to a war zone, as a surrogate for deployment-related stress, and various health effects are summarized in Table S-1.

SUMMARY OF CONCLUSIONS

Table S-1 provides a summary of the committee's conclusions for each health effect discussed in the report by category of association. No health effects were found for two categories of association, sufficient evidence of a causal relationship and limited/suggestive evidence of no association. Of all the long-term health effects reviewed, the strongest findings were on psychiatric disorders, including PTSD, anxiety, and depression. Alcohol abuse, suicide and accidental death in the early years after deployment, and marital and family conflict also appear to be adverse sequelae of deployment-related stress.

The committee found limited but suggestive evidence of an association between deployment-related stress and chronic fatigue syndrome, fibromyalgia and chronic widespread pain, gastrointestinal symptoms, skin disorders, incarceration, drug abuse, and increased symptom reporting, unexplained illness, and chronic pain.

Finally, it should be repeated that the committee was charged with reviewing scientific data, not with making recommendations regarding VA policy.

TABLE S-1 Summary of Findings Regarding the Association Between Deployment to a War Zone and Specific Health and Psychosocial Effects

Sufficient Evidence of a Causal Association

Evidence from available studies is sufficient to conclude that there is a causal relationship between deployment to a war zone and a specific health effect in humans. The evidence is supported by experimental data and fulfills the guidelines for sufficient evidence of an association (below). The evidence must be biologically plausible and satisfy several of the guidelines used to assess causality, such as strength of association, dose-response relationship, consistency of association, and temporal relationship.

- No effects.

Sufficient Evidence of an Association

Evidence from available studies is sufficient to conclude that there is a positive association. That is, a consistent positive association has been observed between deployment to a war zone and a specific health effect in human studies in which chance and bias, including confounding, could be ruled out with reasonable confidence. For example, several high-quality studies report consistent positive associations, and the studies are sufficiently free of bias and include adequate control for confounding.

- Psychiatric disorders, including PTSD, other anxiety disorders, and depressive disorders.
- Alcohol abuse.
- Accidental death in the early years after deployment.
- Suicide in the early years after deployment.
- Marital and family conflict.

Limited but Suggestive Evidence of an Association

Evidence from available studies is suggestive of an association between deployment to a war zone and a specific health effect, but the body of evidence is limited by the inability to rule out chance and bias, including confounding, with confidence. For example, at least one high-quality study reports a positive association that is sufficiently free of bias, including adequate control for confounding, and other corroborating studies provide support for the association (corroborating studies might not be sufficiently free of bias, including confounding). Alternatively, several studies of lower quality show consistent positive associations, and the results are probably not due to bias, including confounding.

- Drug abuse.
- Chronic fatigue syndrome.
- Gastrointestinal symptoms consistent with functional gastrointestinal disorders, such as irritable bowel syndrome or functional dyspepsia.
- Skin disorders.
- Fibromyalgia and chronic widespread pain.
- Increased symptom reporting, unexplained illness, and chronic pain.
- Incarceration.

TABLE S-1 Continued

Inadequate/Insufficient Evidence to Determine Whether an Association Exists
Evidence from available studies is of insufficient quantity, quality, or consistency to permit a conclusion regarding the existence of an association between deployment to a war zone and a specific health effect in humans. • Cancer. • Diabetes mellitus. • Thyroid disease. • Neurocognitive and neurobehavioral effects. • Sleep disorders or objective measures of sleep disturbance. • Hypertension. • Coronary heart disease. • Chronic respiratory effects. • Structural gastrointestinal diseases. • Reproductive effects. • Homelessness. • Adverse employment outcomes.
Limited/Suggestive Evidence of No Association
Evidence is consistent in not showing a positive association between deployment to a war zone and a specific health effect after exposure of any magnitude. A conclusion of no association is inevitably limited to the conditions, magnitudes of exposure, and length of observation in the available studies. The possibility of a very small increase in risk after deployment cannot be excluded. • No effects.

RECOMMENDATIONS

The committee recommends that DoD conduct predeployment and postdeployment screening for medical conditions, including psychiatric symptoms and diagnoses, and for psychosocial status to help collect direct evidence about the causal nature of the effects of deployment-related stress. Predeployment screening would also help to identify at-risk personnel who might benefit from targeted intervention programs during deployment and would establish a baseline against which later health and psychosocial effects could be measured after deployment. Postdeployment screening and assessment would provide data that could be analyzed to determine the long-term consequences of deployment-related stress and would allow VA and DoD to implement intervention programs to assist deployed veterans in adjusting to postdeployment life. Such assessments should be made shortly after deployment and should identify those exposures most stressful to the veteran. The assessments should be made at regular intervals thereafter (such as every 5 years) to identify the long-term health and psychosocial effects. The committee further recommends that any longitudinal assessments also be conducted in a representative group of nondeployed veterans to allow appropriate comparisons between deployed and nondeployed veterans regarding health and psychosocial effects.

1

INTRODUCTION

On August 2, 1990, Iraq invaded Kuwait. In response, a coalition of the United States, Canada, the United Kingdom, Australia, and other countries initiated a buildup of military forces called Operation Desert Shield. To liberate Kuwait, Operation Desert Storm was launched on January 16, 1991, with an air offensive; on February 24, the ground war began. By February 28, 1991, the war was over; a ceasefire was signed in April 1991 and all U.S. troops who had participated in the ground war had returned home by June 13, 1991. About 697,000 U.S. military personnel were deployed to the Persian Gulf during the buildup and the war. Most of them were active-duty military personnel, but 261,871 reservists were called to active duty, and 106,047 of them were deployed to the gulf.

In that brief conflict, 148 U.S. personnel died in combat, 145 died outside combat, and 467 were wounded in action. The troops in Iraq experienced uncertainty about possible exposures to chemical and biologic weapons and other contaminants, difficult living conditions, incomplete knowledge of the Iraqi forces they were to engage, and, particularly in the case of reservists, difficulties that accompanied leaving families and jobs. U.S. troops worked and fought in a harsh desert climate far from home and faced an enemy known to have used biologic and chemical weapons. All those factors and others constituted potential physical and psychologic stressors for deployed troops.

The United States is once again engaged in a military conflict in the Middle East. Operation Enduring Freedom (OEF) began on October 7, 2001, in response to the September 11, 2001, terrorist attacks on the United States. Troops are stationed in and around Afghanistan, Southwest Asia, and other locations for military and humanitarian purposes. As of August 8, 2007, in OEF, 419 U.S. military personnel had died (238 as a result of hostile action and 181 as a result of nonhostile action), and 1472 had been wounded in action (DoD 2007).

Operation Iraqi Freedom (OIF) began on March 19, 2003, when U.S.-led coalition forces invaded Iraq. As of August 4, 2007, in OIF, 3672 U.S. military personnel had died (3024 as a result of hostile action and 648 as a result of nonhostile actions) and 27,279 had been wounded in action (DoD 2007). On July 1, 2007, the Department of Defense (DoD) reported that 156,247 U.S. military personnel were deployed in Iraq (Bowman 2007).

OIF can be characterized as a conflict with increasing insurgent attacks. Those attacks include a wide array of tactics, including suicide and car bombs, improvised explosive devices (IEDs), sniper fire, and rocket-propelled grenades. Insurgent attacks are largely unpredictable and often take place in civilian areas, so it is difficult to anticipate and distinguish the enemy. That uncertainty not only increases the risks of being wounded or killed but exacerbates the psychologic stressors experienced by U.S. troops.

In response to the growing concern about the physical and psychologic health of the returning Gulf War veterans from the 1990-1991 conflict, Congress passed two laws in 1998: PL 105-277, the Persian Gulf War Veterans Act, and PL 105-368, the Veterans Programs Enhancement Act. Those laws directed the secretary of veterans affairs to enter into a contract with the National Academy of Sciences (NAS) to review and evaluate the scientific and medical literature regarding associations between illness and exposure to toxic agents, environmental or wartime hazards, and preventive medicines or vaccines in members of the armed forces. PL 105-277 also gave NAS permission to identify "other agents, hazards, or medicines or vaccines to which members of the Armed Forces may have been exposed." In 1996, the Presidential Advisory Committee on Gulf War Veterans' Illnesses (PAC 1996) found that stress was an important contributor to the Gulf War veterans' illnesses and encouraged the government to continue its research on stress-related disorders. In response to the above laws, the Institute of Medicine (IOM) has had a program to examine health risks posed by specific agents and hazards to which Gulf War veterans might have been exposed during their deployment. Four reports have examined health effects related to depleted uranium, pyridostigmine bromide, sarin, and vaccines (IOM 2000); insecticides and solvents (IOM 2003); fuels, combustion products, and propellants (IOM 2005); and infectious diseases (IOM 2007).

In recent years, the charge to IOM has been expanded to include not only veterans of the 1991 Gulf War but veterans returning from OEF and OIF. Many of the biologic and chemical exposures and their possible health effects have been considered in previous IOM reports, but the health effects associated with deployment-related stress have yet to be considered. A recent IOM report, *Gulf War and Health, Volume 4: Health Effects of Serving in the Gulf War* (IOM 2006), reviewed the health status of Gulf War-deployed veterans compared with their nondeployed counterparts. That report found that veterans of the Gulf War report higher rates of nearly all symptoms than their nondeployed counterparts; in addition, a higher prevalence not only of individual symptoms but of chronic multisymptom illnesses was found among Gulf War-deployed veterans. Multisymptom-based medical conditions reported to occur more frequently among deployed Gulf War veterans include fibromyalgia, chronic fatigue syndrome, and multiple chemical sensitivity. The literature also demonstrates that deployment places veterans at increased risk for symptoms that meet diagnostic criteria for a number of psychiatric disorders, particularly posttraumatic stress disorder (PTSD), anxiety disorders, depressive disorders, and substance abuse. Furthermore, comorbidities have been reported, for example, symptoms of both PTSD and depression. Finally, the report noted that Gulf War veterans are at increased risk for amyotrophic lateral sclerosis and that there is weak evidence that Gulf War veterans' offspring might be at risk for some birth defects (IOM 2006).

In light of the 1991 Gulf War and the nature of OEF and OIF, the Department of Veterans Affairs (VA) requested that IOM comprehensively review, evaluate, and summarize the peer-reviewed scientific and medical literature regarding the association between deployment-related stress and long-term adverse health effects in Gulf War veterans. In response to VA's request, IOM appointed the Committee on Gulf War and Health: Physiologic, Psychologic, and Psychosocial Effects of Deployment-Related Stress to conduct the review.

DEMOGRAPHICS

The 1991 Gulf War, OEF, and OIF reflect many changes from previous wars fought by the United States, particularly in the demographic composition of military personnel and the uncertainty of conditions for many reservists. The 1991 Gulf War and, in particular, OEF and OIF have occasioned the increased activation of reserve and National Guard units to supplement the all-volunteer military. Those units and the military in general also have more women serving and have women serving in more occupations than ever before. In the Vietnam War, 3,143,645 men and 7166 women served in the Vietnam theater. The military during the Vietnam era was about 87% white, 11% black, and 5% Hispanic (Kulka et al. 1990). About 75% of those who served in the Vietnam theater were volunteers and 25% were draftees; in World War II, 66% were draftees (MRFA 2007). The average age of a U.S. enlisted soldier was 26 years in World War II and about 21 years in Vietnam (25-27 years for all military personnel serving in Vietnam) (Schlenger 2007). Only very small percentages of the soldiers in World War II and the Vietnam War were in the reserves or National Guard.

Of the nearly 700,000 U.S. troops who fought in Operation Desert Shield and Operation Desert Storm in 1990-1991, almost 7% were women and about 17% were in activated National Guard and reserve units. Military personnel, with a mean age of 28 years, were, overall, older than those who had participated in previous wars. Some 70% of the troops were white, 23% were black, and 6% were Hispanic or other (DoD 1994). As of 2005, 14% of the almost half-million active-duty Army personnel were women, as were 23.2% of Army reserves and 12.8% of Army National Guard. The proportion of Hispanics in the Army increased from about 4% in 1985 to 11% in 2005, and the proportion of blacks decreased in the same period from 27% to 22% (U.S. Army 2007).

COMMITTEE'S INTERPRETATION OF ITS CHARGE

Given the committee's charge from the VA—to assess the long-term health effects of deployment-related stress—the committee began by defining deployment-related stress as deployment to a war zone. Combat is one of the most potent stressors that a person can experience, but as military conflicts have evolved to include more guerilla warfare and insurgent activities, restricting the definition of deployment-related stressors to combat may fail to acknowledge other potent stressors experienced by military personnel in a war zone or in the aftermath of combat (King et al. 2006). Such stressors encompass an enormous array of physical and psychologic events, including constant vigilance against unexpected attack, the absence of a defined front line, the difficulty of distinguishing enemy combatants from civilians, the ubiquity of IEDs, caring for the badly injured or dying, duty on the graves registration service, and being responsible for the treatment of prisoners of war. The deployment stressors associated with any armed conflict also include noncombat stressors. Non-combat-related stressors that might be experienced by deployed personnel are separation from family, friends, and colleagues; loss of or reduction in income; and concern over employment status when deployment ends (O'Toole et al. 1999). Therefore, the committee considered that military personnel deployed to a war zone, even if direct combat was not experienced, have the potential for exposure to deployment-related stressors that might elicit a stress response and that the emotional and physical reactions of military personnel to those stressors can vary widely. The committee recognized that factors other than deployment-related stressors can affect the outcome of exposure to potential stressors, including the stress response itself and individual risk and protective factors.

The stress response is a coordinated set of interactions among multiple organ systems in the body, including the brain, gut, heart, liver, immune system, thyroid, adrenals, pituitary, gonads, bone, and skin. Acute stress responses are usually adaptive, preparing the organism for "fight or flight." When exposure to the stressor has ended, the acute stress response subsides, and the body returns to its normal state. However, if the body's reactions persist after the stressor has ended, a chronic stress response can develop, which can be maladaptive and result in feelings of anxiety and lack of control and chronic health effects. Stressors can also lead to adverse psychosocial effects, such as marital conflicts and homelessness, concurrently with or after the development of health effects.

Whether the *stress response* leads to adverse health effects in either the short term (hours to days) or the long term (months to years) is determined by a number of factors, including the intensity of the stressful experience, the effects of previous stressors, innate and acquired vulnerabilities, and various protective influences. Risk factors, such as genetic susceptibility and prior exposure to stressors, can increase the likelihood of having adverse effects during and after deployment; protective factors, such as military training and a supportive family and social environment, can reduce the likelihood of having adverse effects.

Because of the various deployment-related stressors, the complex nature of the stress response, and risk and protective factors that can potentially modify a person's response to stress, the committee has provided a schematic (Figure 1-1) to indicate how it interpreted its task.

COMMITTEE'S APPROACH TO ITS CHARGE

The committee's charge was to comprehensively review, evaluate, and summarize the peer-reviewed scientific and medical literature regarding the association between deployment-related stress and long-term adverse health effects in Gulf War veterans. Specifically, the committee was to study the physiologic, psychologic, and psychosocial effects of stress. VA requested that the study's findings not be limited to veterans of the 1991 Gulf War but be applicable to veterans of OEF and OIF.

Thus, to evaluate associations between deployment-related stress and adverse effects, the committee considered all studies that identified health effects found in military personnel deployed to a war zone. Potential health effects considered included not only physiologic effects but also psychiatric effects, such as depression and PTSD, and psychosocial effects, such as marital conflict and incarceration. In addition, the committee considered studies of deployed veterans with combat-related PTSD and associated health effects, because PTSD can result only after exposure to a traumatic stressor and a war zone is rife with potentially traumatic events. In conducting its deliberations, the committee considered studies of veterans of World War II, the Korean War, the Vietnam War, the 1991 Gulf War, OEF, and OIF.

Although most of the literature focused on U.S. military veterans, studies of veterans from other countries were included. The possible health effects identified in *Gulf War and Health, Volume 4: Health Effects of Serving in the Gulf War* (IOM 2006) were also considered for this report.

The committee's task was not to judge individual cases of particular diseases or conditions nor did it examine treatment approaches for any health effects. The committee also did not address policy issues, such as decisions regarding compensation, potential costs of compensation, or any broader policy implications of its findings.

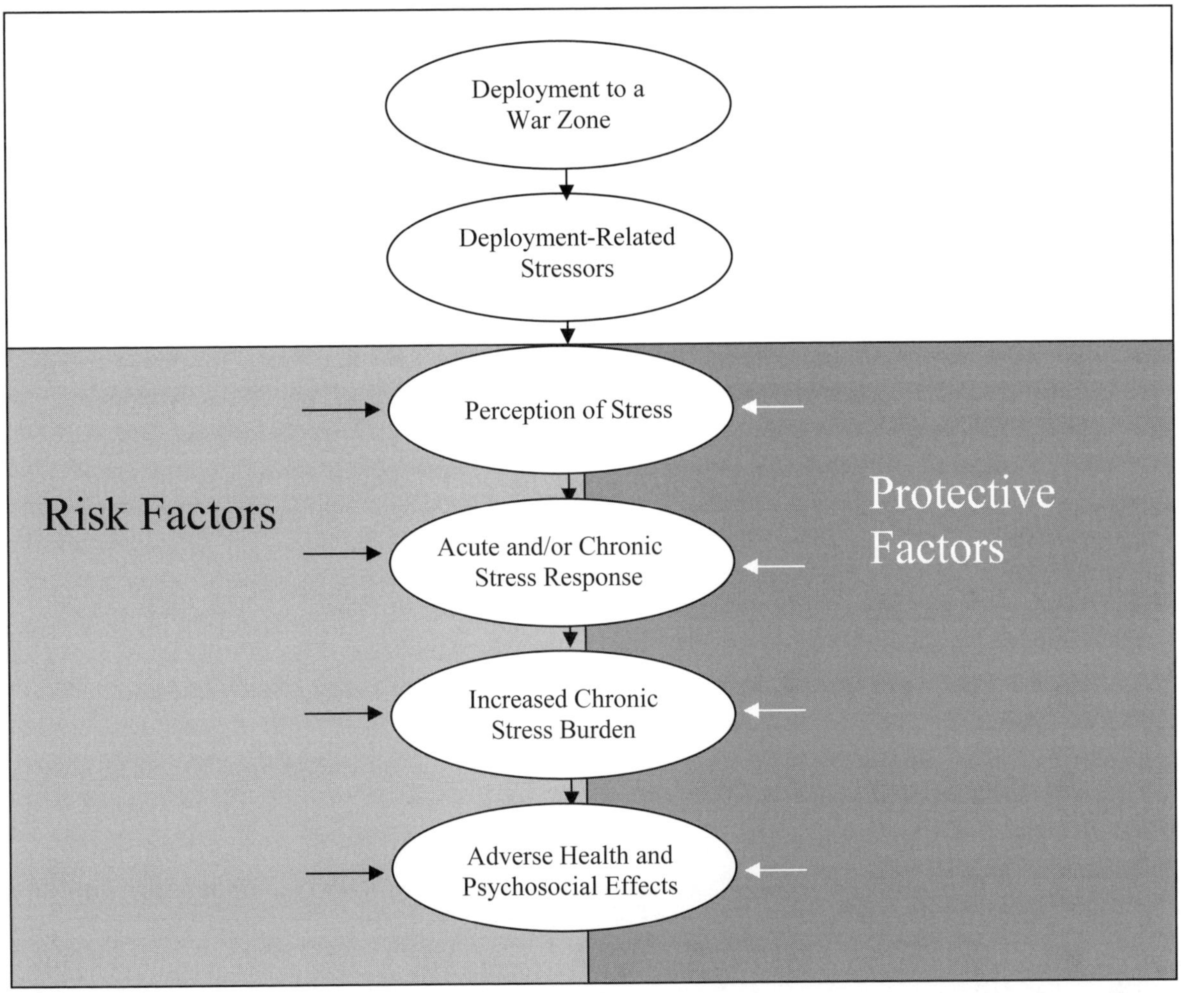

FIGURE 1-1 Schematic depiction of the relationship between deployment to a war zone and adverse health and psychosocial effects. Deployment to a war zone results in exposure to numerous stressors that can lead to acute and chronic stress responses that in turn can have potential long-term consequences, including adverse health and psychosocial effects. The nature of the stress response and the adverse health and psychosocial effects can be modified by a number of risk and protective factors.

ORGANIZATION OF THE REPORT

Chapter 2 presents the types of evidence the committee reviewed, how the committee assessed the strength of the evidence, and the categories of evidence the committee used to summarize its findings. Chapter 3 discusses the many types of stressors to which veterans might be exposed in a war zone. Chapter 4 discusses the biology of the stress response and Chapter 5 the diagnosis, course, prevalence, risk factors, and neurobiology of PTSD. Chapter 6 compiles and summarizes the available data on health effects that might be associated with deployment-related stressors. Psychosocial effects associated with deployment-related stress are discussed in Chapter 7. Finally, Chapter 8 summarizes the committee's conclusions and recommendations.

REFERENCES

Bowman S. 2007. *CRS Report for Congress*. Iraq: U.S. Military Operations. Washington, DC: Congressional Research Service. Order Code RL31701. Updated July 15, 2007.

DoD (Department of Defense). 1994. *Report of the Defense Science Board Task Force on Persian Gulf War Health Effects*. Washington, DC: Office of the Under Secretary of Defense for Acquisition and Technology.

DoD. 2007. *OEF/OIF Casualty Update*. [Online]. Available: www.defenselink.mil/news/casualty.pdf [accessed August 4, 2007].

IOM (Institute of Medicine). 2000. *Gulf War and Health, Volume 1: Depleted Uranium, Pyridostigmine Bromide, Sarin, Vaccines*. Washington, DC: National Academy Press.

IOM. 2003. *Gulf War and Health, Volume 2: Insecticides and Solvents*. Washington, DC: The National Academies Press.

IOM. 2005. *Gulf War and Health, Volume 3: Fuels, Combustion Products, and Propellants*. Washington, DC: The National Academies Press.

IOM. 2006. *Gulf War and Health, Volume 4: Health Effects of Serving in the Gulf War*. Washington, DC: The National Academies Press.

IOM. 2007. *Gulf War and Health, Volume 5: Infectious Diseases*. Washington, DC: The National Academies Press.

King LA, King DW, Vogt DS, Knight J, Samper RE. 2006. Deployment risk and resilience inventory: A collection of measures for studying deployment-related experiences of military personnel and veterans. *Military Psychology* 18(2):89-120.

Kulka RA, Schlenger WE, Fairbank JA, Hough RL, Jordan BK, Marmar CR, Weiss DS. 1990. *Trauma and the Vietnam War Generation: Report of Findings from the National Vietnam Veterans Readjustment Study*. New York: Brunner/Mazel Publishers.

MRFA (Mobile Riverine Force Association). 2007. *Vietnam War Statistics*. [Online]. Available: http://www.mrfa.org/vnstats.htm [accessed July 2, 2007].

O'Toole BI, Marshall RP, Schureck RJ, Dobson M. 1999. Combat, dissociation, and posttraumatic stress disorder in Australian Vietnam veterans. *Journal of Traumatic Stress* 12(4):625-640.

PAC (Presidential Advisory Committee). 1996. *Presidential Advisory Committee on Gulf War Veterans' Illnesses: Final Report*. Washington, DC: U.S. Government Printing Office.

Schlenger WE. 2007. Abt Associates, Inc. Personal Communication.

U.S. Army. 2007. *Demographics*. [Online]. Available: http://www.armyg1.army.mil/hr/demographics.asp [accessed July 2, 2007].

2

CONSIDERATIONS IN IDENTIFYING AND EVALUATING THE LITERATURE

This chapter reviews the approach that the committee took to identify and evaluate the health studies of Gulf War and other veterans. It provides information about the types of evidence the committee reviewed, how the committee assessed the strength of the evidence, and the categories of evidence the committee used to summarize its findings.

The committee began its evaluation by presuming neither the existence nor the absence of associations between deployment-related stress and health effects. It sought to characterize and weigh the strength and limitations of the available evidence. The committee reviewed primarily epidemiologic studies of Gulf War and other veterans to determine the prevalence of diseases and symptoms in deployed vs nondeployed veteran populations, using deployment as a surrogate for deployment-related stress.

In this chapter, the committee describes its approach to enable the reader to assess and interpret its findings and to assist those who may update the committee's conclusions as new information becomes available. It is possible that in the future the literature may suggest other health effects that have an association with deployment-related stress and that merit evaluation of the evidence, or new information may become available that will necessitate revisiting the conclusions presented in this report.

IDENTIFICATION OF THE LITERATURE

The committee's first step was to identify the literature it would review. It began its work by overseeing extensive searches of the English-language, peer-reviewed medical and scientific literature. It identified epidemiologic studies of persistent health effects associated with veterans deployed during World War II, the Korean War, the Vietnam War, the 1991 Gulf War, and Operation Enduring Freedom (OEF) in Afghanistan and Operation Iraqi Freedom (OIF) in Iraq. Although primary consideration was given to studies of U.S. military personnel, studies of veterans of these wars from other countries, such as Australia and the United Kingdom, were also included.

The searches retrieved over 3000 potentially relevant references. January 2007 was the cutoff date for all literature searches. The committee reviewed epidemiologic studies for evidence of an association between deployment and persistent health outcomes in veterans. The committee used its collective judgment in selecting studies thought to reflect the types of stressors that Gulf War and other veterans might have experienced during deployment. Although veterans are exposed to numerous stressors (see Chapter 3), epidemiologic studies are not typically designed to address such types of exposures or the effects associated with specific stressors.

The committee adopted a policy of using only peer-reviewed published literature as the basis of its conclusions. Publications that were not peer-reviewed had no evidentiary value for the committee; that is, they were not used as evidence for arriving at conclusions about the degree of association between deployment to war zone and adverse health effects. The process of peer review by fellow professionals, which is one of the hallmarks of modern science, ensures high standards of quality but does not guarantee the validity of a study or that its results can be generalized, particularly with respect to questions that were not the objective of the original researchers. Accordingly, committee members read each study critically and considered its relevance and quality. In some instances, non-peer-reviewed publications provided background information for the committee and raised issues that required further literature searches. The committee did not collect original data, nor did it perform any secondary data analysis.

The committee chose not to adopt a formal meta-analysis approach because of practical concerns. First, there is a striking amount of heterogeneity in the epidemiologic studies in this report. They vary with respect to the nature, level, and measurement of exposure; the definition and measurement of outcomes; and study design. Further, many studies include multiple odds ratios or relative risk, corresponding to different study groups, control groups, outcomes, exposure measures, statistical models, etc. It is often not possible to choose a single measure from each study in a consistent way, and the meta-analysis would be subject to arbitrary decisions about data extraction. For many health effects the committee found only one or two primary papers and secondary papers. Although the committee used deployment as the exposure of interest for this report, the type, duration, and the nature of the deployment experience varied widely between the studies, again reducing the utility of a meta-analysis. The committee believed that a descriptive analysis would be more comprehensive and accurate given the varying quality and quantity of the studies for each health effect.

With that orientation to the committee's task, the following sections provide a brief discussion of factors influencing the value of epidemiologic studies, the committee's criteria for inclusion of studies in its review, considerations in evaluating the evidence or data provided by the studies, and the categories of association for the conclusions about the strength of the evidence presented in the studies.

TYPES OF EVIDENCE

The committee relied entirely on epidemiologic studies to draw its conclusions about the strength of the evidence for an association between deployment to a war zone (a stressor) and health effects (see Chapter 6). However, animal studies play a critical role in elucidating the mechanisms of the stress response (see Chapter 4) and provide a biological platform for many of the effects seen in humans, including that for posttraumatic stress disorder (PTSD) (see Chapter 5).

Animal Studies

Studies of laboratory animals are essential to understanding mechanisms of action, biologic plausibility, and providing response information about possible health effects when experimental research in humans is not ethically or practically possible (NRC 1991). Such studies permit a stressor to be introduced under conditions controlled by the researcher—such as its intensity and duration—to probe health effects on many body systems. Nonhuman studies are also a valuable complement to human studies of genetic susceptibility.

Animal studies may determine the degree of response to acute (short-term) or chronic (long-term) exposures to stressors. Animal research may focus on the mechanism of action (that is, how a stressor exerts its deleterious effects at the cellular and molecular levels). Mechanism-of-action (or mechanistic) studies encompass a range of laboratory approaches with whole animals and in vitro systems using tissues or cells from humans or animals.

In carrying out its charge, the committee used animal studies to provide a basis for a mechanism of action for the impact of stress on biological functions, including changes in brain structure, hormone concentrations, and neurological activity (see Chapter 4), to help establish biologic plausibility. One of the problems with animal studies, however, is the difficulty of finding animal models to study symptoms that relate to uniquely human attributes, such as cognition, purposive behavior, and the perception of pain. Many symptoms reported by veterans (for example, headache, muscle, or joint pain) are difficult to study in standard neurotoxicological tests in animals (OTA 1990).

For its evaluation and categorization of the degree of association between each exposure and a human health effect, however, the committee only used evidence from human studies. Nevertheless, the committee did use nonhuman studies as the basis for judgments about biologic plausibility, which is one of the criteria for establishing causation (see below).

Epidemiologic Studies

Epidemiologic studies examine the relationship between exposures to agents of interest in a human population and the health effects seen in that population. The challenge of epidemiologic studies is to isolate the risk factors that contribute to health effects in populations that are inherently uncontrollable in the experimental sense; therefore, statistical techniques are used to take into account factors such as bias and confounding. Such studies can be used to generate hypotheses for future study or to test hypotheses posed in advance by investigators.

A principal objective of epidemiology is to understand whether exposures to specific agents are associated with disease or other health effects and, with additional available information, to decide whether such associations are causal. Although they are frequently used synonymously by the general public, the terms “association” and “causation” have distinct meanings (Alpert and Goldberg 2007).

Epidemiologic studies can establish statistical associations between exposures and health effects; associations are generally estimated by using relative risks or odds ratios. To conclude that an association exists, it is necessary for the exposure to be followed by the health effect more frequently than it would be expected to by chance alone. Furthermore, it is almost always necessary to find that the effect occurs consistently in several studies. Epidemiologists seldom consider a single study sufficient to establish an association; rather, it is desirable to replicate the findings in other studies to draw conclusions about the association. Results of separate studies are sometimes conflicting. It is sometimes possible to attribute discordant study results to differences in such characteristics as soundness of study design, quality of execution, and the influence of different forms of bias. Studies that result in a tight confidence interval around a statistically significant relative risk of association suggest that the observed result was unlikely to be due to chance. When the measure of association does not show a statistically significant effect, it is important to consider the size of the sample and whether the study had the power to detect an effect of a given size.

Epidemiologic study designs differ in their ability to provide valid estimates of an association (Ellwood 1998). An important issue is that the studies reviewed by the committee were seldom designed to answer the question in the committee's charge, that is, does exposure to deployment-related stress result in long-term adverse health and psychosocial effects. Cross-sectional studies generally provide a lower level of evidence than cohort and case-control studies. Determining whether a given statistical association rises to the level of causation requires inference (Hill 1965). As discussed by the International Agency for Research on Cancer in the preamble of its monographs evaluating cancer risks (for example, IARC 2004), a strong association is demonstrated by repeated observations in a number of different studies, specificity of effects, and an increased risk of disease with increasing exposure or a decline in risk after cessation of exposure. Those characteristics all strengthen the likelihood that an association seen in epidemiologic studies is a causal effect. Inferences from epidemiologic studies, however, are often limited to population or ecologic associations because of a lack of individual exposure information. Exposures are rarely, if ever, controlled in epidemiologic studies, and in most cases there is large uncertainty in the assessment of exposure. To assess whether explanations other than causality are responsible for an observed association, one must bring together evidence from different studies and apply well-established criteria, which have been refined over more than a century (Evans 1976; Hill 1965; Susser 1973, 1977, 1988, 1991; Wegman et al. 1997). For a review of those criteria, see the 2004 report of the U.S. Surgeon General (Office of the Surgeon General-HHS 2004).

When examining the available epidemiologic studies, the committee addressed the question, "Does the available evidence support a causal relationship or an association between exposure (deployment to a war zone) and a health effect?" Even a causal relationship between deployment and a specific health effect would not mean that deployment invariably results in the health effect or that all cases of the effect are the result of deployment. Such complete correspondence between exposure and disease is the exception in large populations (IOM 1994). The committee evaluated the data and based its conclusions on the strength and coherence of the data in the selected epidemiologic studies that met its inclusion criteria. The major types of epidemiologic studies discussed in this chapter are cohort, case-control, and cross-sectional studies.

Cohort Studies

A cohort, or longitudinal, study follows a defined group, or cohort, over time. It can test hypotheses about whether an exposure to a specific stressor is related to the development of a health effect and can examine multiple health effects that may be associated with exposure to a given stressor. A cohort study starts by classifying study participants according to whether or not they have been exposed to the stressor under study, in this case deployment to a war zone. A cohort study compares health effects in individuals who have been exposed to the stressor in question with those without the exposure. Such a comparison can be used to estimate a risk difference or a relative risk, two statistics that measure association. The risk difference is the rate of disease or health effect in exposed persons minus the rate in unexposed persons. A value greater than zero ($H_0 = 0.0$) implies that extra cases of disease or health effect are associated with the exposure. The relative risk or risk ratio is determined by dividing the rate of developing the disease in the exposed group by the rate in the nonexposed group. A relative risk greater than 1

($H_0 = 1.0$) suggests a positive association between the stressor and the health effect. The higher the relative risk, the stronger is the association.

One major advantage of a cohort study is the ability of the investigator to define the exposure classification of subjects at the beginning of the study. This classification in prospective cohort studies is not influenced by the presence of a health effect because the health effect has yet to occur, which reduces an important source of potential bias known as selection bias (see later discussion). As explained in the section on case-control studies, when it is possible to measure a confounding factor,[1] the investigator can apply statistical methods to minimize its influence on the results. An advantage of a cohort study is that it is possible to calculate absolute rates of disease incidence.[2] A final advantage, especially over cross-sectional studies (discussed below), is that it may be possible to adjust each subject's followup health status for baseline health status so that the person acts as his or her own control vs defining a group as "disease-free"; that may reduce a source of variation and increase the power to detect effects. The disadvantages of cohort studies are high costs as a result of a large study population and prolonged periods of followup (especially if the health effect is rare), attrition of study subjects, and delay in obtaining results.

A prospective cohort study selects subjects on the basis of exposure (or lack of it) and follows the cohort into the future to determine the rate at which the health effect develops. A retrospective (or historical) cohort study differs from a prospective study in terms of temporal direction; the investigator traces back in time to classify past exposures in the cohort and then tracks the cohort forward in time to ascertain the rate of the health effect. They often focus on disease mortality rates because of the relative ease of determining vital status of individuals and the availability of death certificates to determine the cause of death.

For comparison purposes, cohort studies often use general population mortality or morbidity rates (age, sex, race, time, and cause-specific) because it may be difficult to identify a suitable control group of unexposed people. The *observed* number of deaths or illness among a group (from a specific cause such as lung cancer) is compared with the *expected* number of deaths or illness. The ratio of observed to expected deaths produces a standardized mortality ratio. However, for several of the studies cited in Chapter 6, a standardized *morbidity* ratio (SMR) for illness is used instead, as death is not the effect of interest. An SMR greater than 1.0 generally suggests an elevated risk of illness in the exposed group.

The major problem with using general population rates for comparison with military cohorts is the "healthy-warrior effect," which arises when a military population experiences a lower mortality or morbidity rate than the general population, which consists of a mix of healthy and unhealthy people. The military has physical health criteria that personnel must meet when they enter the military and while they are on active duty.

Case-Control Studies

In a case-control study, subjects (cases) are selected on the basis of having a health effect; controls are selected on the basis of not having the health effect. Cases and controls are asked about their exposures to specific agents. Cases and controls can be matched with regard to such

---

[1]A potential confounding factor is a variable that is associated with the health effect and may affect the results of the study because it is distributed differently in the exposed and nonexposed groups.

[2]Incidence is the rate of occurrence of new cases of an illness or disease in a given population during a specified period. Prevalence is the number of cases of an illness or disease existing in a given population at a specific point or period.

characteristics as age, sex, and socioeconomic status to eliminate those characteristics as causes of observed differences, or those variables can be controlled in the analysis. The odds of exposure to the agent among the cases are then compared with the odds of exposure among controls. The comparison generates an odds ratio, which is a statistic that depicts the odds of having a health effect among those exposed to the stressor relative to the odds of having the health effect among an unexposed comparison group. An odds ratio greater than 1 indicates that there is a potential association between exposure to the stressor and the health effect; the greater the odds ratio, the greater the association.

Case-control studies are useful for testing hypotheses about the relationships between exposure to specific stressors and a health effect. They are especially useful and efficient for studying the etiology of rare effects. Case-control studies have the advantages of ease, speed, and relatively low cost. They are also valuable for their ability to probe multiple exposures or risk factors. However, case-control studies are vulnerable to several types of bias, such as recall bias, which can dilute or enhance associations between a health effect and exposure. Other problems include identifying representative groups of cases, choosing suitable controls, and collecting comparable information about exposures on both cases and controls. Those problems might lead to unidentified confounding variables that differentially influence the selection of cases or control subjects or the detection of exposure. For the reasons discussed above, case-control studies are often the first approach to testing a hypothesis about factors contributing to a specific health effect, especially a rare one.

A nested case-control study draws cases and controls from a previously defined cohort. Thus, it is said to be "nested" inside a cohort study. Baseline data are collected at the time that the cohort is identified, which ensures a more uniform set of data on cases and controls. Within the cohort, individuals identified with a health effect serve as cases, and a sample of those who are effect-free serve as controls. Using baseline data, exposure in cases and controls is compared, as in a regular case-control study. Nested case-control studies are efficient in terms of time and cost in reconstructing exposure histories on cases and on only a sample of controls rather than the entire cohort. Additionally, because the cases and controls come from the same previously established cohort, concerns about unmeasured confounders and selection bias are decreased.

Cross-Sectional Studies

The main differentiating feature of a cross-sectional study is that exposure and health effect information is collected at the same time. The selection of people for the study—unlike selection for cohort and case-control studies—is independent of both the exposure to the stressor and health effect characteristics. Cross-sectional studies seek to uncover potential associations between exposure to a specific stressor and development of a health effect. In a cross-sectional study, effect size is measured as relative risk, prevalence ratio, or prevalence odds ratio. It might compare health effect or symptom rates between groups with and without exposure to the specific stressor. Many health studies of Gulf War veterans are cross-sectional studies that compare a sample of veterans who were deployed to the Gulf War with a sample of veterans who served during the same period but were not deployed to the Gulf War.

Cross-sectional studies are easier and less expensive to perform than cohort studies and can identify the prevalence of health effects and exposures in a defined population. They are useful for generating hypotheses, but they are much less useful for determining cause-effect relationships, because effect and exposure data are collected at the same time (Monson 1990). It might also be difficult to determine the temporal sequence of exposures and symptoms or effect.

INCLUSION CRITERIA

The committee's next step, after securing the full text of about 3000 studies, was to determine which studies would be included in the review as primary or support studies. For a study to be included in the committee's review, it had to meet these criteria: methodologic rigor, use of an appropriate control population, specificity of health effect, and an indicator of exposure to the stressor (deployment to a war zone). Studies that met the committee's criteria are referred to as *primary* studies. The committee focused on long-term health effects that persisted after deployment to a war zone ended.

Studies reviewed by the committee that did not necessarily meet all the criteria of a primary study are considered secondary studies. Secondary studies are typically less rigorous in their methods; for example, a study might have a small sample, not include a physician's examination or other appropriate evaluation method, or rely only on veterans' self-reports of symptoms or health effect using a mailed questionnaire. The committee used those types of studies to support its findings based on primary studies.

Methodologic Rigor

The study had to be a published in a peer-reviewed journal, had to include details of its methodology, had to include a control or reference group, had to have a sample size of at least 100, had to have statistical power to detect effects, and had to include reasonable adjustment for confounders. Case studies and case series were generally excluded from the committee's consideration.

Health-Effect Assessment

For a study to be considered primary, it had to have information regarding a specific health effect and exposure information. The committee preferred studies that had an independent assessment of a health effect rather than self-reports of a health effect or self-report of a physician's diagnosis. The health effect must have been diagnosed or confirmed by a clinical evaluation, a specific laboratory test, hospital record, or other medical record; for psychiatric outcomes, standardized interviews were necessary, such as the Structured Clinical Interview for the *Diagnostic and Statistical Manual of Mental Disorders* (*DSM*)-*IV-TR*, the Diagnostic Interview Schedule, and the Composite International Diagnostic Interview; for psychosocial effects, the effect needed to be obtained through the use of a validated or well-recognized instrument or the data obtained from databases maintained by a government agency or other appropriate organization. Primary studies are studies of veterans deployed to a war zone compared with their nondeployed counterparts or studies that evaluated health effects of veterans with deployment-related or combat-related PTSD.

Furthermore, a study had to examine long-term rather than immediate or transitory outcomes. For example, the committee considered veterans with PTSD but not with acute stress disorder for which symptoms of disturbance last no longer than a month (APA 2000).

ADDITIONAL CONSIDERATIONS

In addition to determining the primary and secondary literature that would be used to draw conclusions, the committee considered other characteristics of the studies related to the methods used by researchers in their design and conduct.

Bias

Bias refers to systematic, or nonrandom, error. Bias causes an observed value to deviate from the true value, and could weaken an association or generate a spurious association. Because all studies are susceptible to bias, a goal of the research design is to minimize bias or to adjust the observed value of an association by correcting for bias. There are different types of bias, such as selection bias and information bias.

Selection bias occurs when systematic error in obtaining study participants results in a potential distortion of the true association between exposure and outcome. Information bias results from the manner in which data are collected and can result from measurement errors, imprecise measurement, and misdiagnosis. Those types of errors might be uniform in an entire study population or might affect some parts of the population more than others. Information bias might result from misclassification of study subjects with respect to the outcome variable or from misclassification of exposure. Other common sources of information bias are the inability of study subjects to recall the circumstances of their exposure accurately (recall bias) and the likelihood that one group more frequently reports what it remembers than another group (reporting bias). Information bias is especially harmful in interpreting study results when it affects one comparison group more than another.

Confounding

Confounding occurs when a variable or characteristic otherwise known to be predictive of an effect and associated with the exposure (and not on the causal pathway) can account for part or all of an apparent association. A confounding variable is an uncontrolled variable that influences the outcome of a study to an unknown extent, and makes precise evaluation of its effects impossible. Examples of confounders are age, sex, smoking, and pre-existing illness. Carefully applied statistical adjustments can often control for or reduce the influence of a confounder.

Random Error

A false positive (type-one error) occurs when routine statistical variation leads to an apparent association between an exposure to a stressor and a health effect when no association is present. This happens when the observed result of a study falls in the tail of the probability distribution hypothesized to describe the process being studied. Standard statistical methods, such as p-values and confidence intervals, allow one to assess the likelihood that random error due to sampling is responsible for positive findings. Replication of a positive finding in additional studies demonstrates that it is not simply a false positive, but does not guard against the same biases and confounders distorting the results if the studies' designs are the same. Consistent results in multiple studies with different designs, and hence vulnerabilities to different confounders and sources of bias, increases confidence that the observed relationship is real and helps to rule out the possibility that the positive results are due to random error, bias, or confounders.

CONSIDERATIONS IN ASSESSING THE STRENGTH OF EVIDENCE

The committee's process of reaching conclusions about deployment to a war zone and its potential for adverse health effects was collective and interactive. Once a study was included in this review because it met the committee's criteria, there were several considerations in assessing the strength of associations. They were patterned after those introduced by Hill (1971) and include presence of a temporal relationship, strength of the estimated association, presence of a dose-response relationship, consistency of the association, and biologic plausibility.

Temporal Relationship

If an observed association is real, exposure must precede the onset of disease by at least the duration of health effect induction. The committee considered whether a health effect occurred within a period after deployment that was consistent with current understanding of the natural history of the health effect. The committee interpreted the lack of an appropriate time sequence as evidence against association but recognized that insufficient knowledge about the natural history and pathogenesis of many of the health effects under review limited the utility of this consideration. Without a temporal relationship being established between exposure and outcome, other evidence to support the association becomes useless.

Strength of an Association

The strength of an association is usually expressed as the magnitude of the measure of effect, for example, relative risk or odds ratio. Generally, the higher the relative risk, the greater the likelihood that the exposure-effect association is causal and the lower the likelihood that it is due to undetected error, bias, or confounding (discussed above). Measures of statistical significance, such as p-values, are not indicators of the strength of an association.

Small increases in relative risks that are consistent among studies, however, might be evidence of an association, whereas some forms of extreme bias or confounding can produce a high relative risk. The statistical power of a study was important for it had to be able to detect effects of an unspecified magnitude, especially important for negative results. This factor explains the committee's inclusion criteria regarding statistical power.

Dose-Response Relationship

The existence of a dose-response relationship—that is, an increased strength of association with increasing intensity or duration of exposure or other appropriate relation—strengthens an inference that an association is real. However, the lack of an apparent dose-response relationship does not rule out an association. If the *relative* degree of exposure among several studies can be determined, indirect evidence of a dose-response relationship may exist. For example, if studies of presumably low-exposure cohorts show only mild increases in risk whereas studies of presumably high-exposure cohorts show larger increases in risk, the pattern would be consistent with a dose-response relationship.

Consistency of Association

A consistent association requires that the association be found regularly in a variety of studies, for example, in more than one study population and with different study methods. However, consistency alone is not sufficient evidence of an association. The committee considered findings that were consistent in direction among studies of different designs to be supportive of an association. It did not require exactly the same magnitude of association in different populations to conclude that there was a consistent association. A consistent association could occur when the results of most studies were positive and the variations in measured effects were within the range expected on the basis of sampling error, selection bias, and confounding.

Thus, for a health effect to be considered associated with deployment there had to be corroboration, that is, replication of findings among studies and populations. The degree to which an effect could be consistently reproduced gave the committee confidence that they were observing a true effect.

Specificity of Association

Specificity of association is the degree to which exposure to a given stressor predicts a particular outcome. A positive finding is more convincing of causality when the association between the exposure and the health effect is specific to one or both than when the association is nonspecific to the exposure and the health effect. The committee recognized, however, that one-to-one specificity is not to be expected, given the multifactorial etiology of many of the health effects under examination.

Biologic Plausibility

Biologic plausibility reflects knowledge of the biologic mechanism(s) by which an agent could lead to a health outcome. That knowledge comes through mechanism-of-action or other studies in pharmacology, physiology, and other fields—typically in studies of animals. A biologically plausible mechanism may not be known when an association is first documented. Biologic plausibility was required by the committee only in drawing a conclusion of "sufficient evidence of a causal association" (see below); for the other categories of association, it was not necessary to demonstrate a biologically plausible mechanism.

CATEGORIES OF ASSOCIATION

The committee attempted to express its judgment about the available data as clearly and precisely as possible. The committee agreed to use the categories of association that have been established and used by previous Committees on Gulf War and Health and other Institute of Medicine (IOM) committees that have evaluated vaccine safety, effects of herbicides used in Vietnam, and indoor pollutants related to asthma (IOM 2000, 2003, 2005, 2006, 2007). These categories of association have gained wide acceptance over more than a decade by Congress, government agencies (particularly the Department of Veterans Affairs [VA]), researchers, and veterans groups.

The five categories below describe different levels of association and sound a recurring theme: the validity of an association is likely to vary to the extent to which common sources of error—chance variation and bias, including confounding—could be ruled out as the reason for the observed association. Accordingly, the criteria for each category express a degree of confidence based on the extent to which sources of error were reduced. The committee discussed the evidence and reached consensus on the categorization of that evidence for each health and psychosocial effect in Chapters 6 and 7, respectively. The committee was conservative in its judgment of the evidence as the quantity and quality of studies used for the determination of association for each health effect varied considerably, but in each case, the minimum requirements for the specific category of association were met.

Sufficient Evidence of a Causal Relationship

Evidence is sufficient to conclude that there is a causal relationship between exposure to deployment-related stress and a specific health effect in humans, and the evidence is supported by experimental data on humans or animals. The evidence fulfills the guidelines for sufficient evidence of an association (below) and satisfies several of the guidelines used to assess causality: strength of association, dose-response relationship, consistency of association, and a temporal relationship.

Sufficient Evidence of an Association

Evidence is sufficient to conclude that there is an association; that is, a consistent association has been observed between exposure to deployment-related stress and a specific health effect in human studies in which chance and bias, including confounding, could be ruled out with reasonable confidence as an explanation for the observed association. For example, several high-quality studies report consistent associations, and the studies are sufficiently free of bias, including adequate control for confounding.

Limited but Suggestive Evidence of an Association

Evidence is suggestive of an association between exposure to deployment-related stress and a specific health effect in human studies, but the body of evidence is limited by the inability to rule out chance and bias, including confounding, with confidence. At least one high-quality[3] study reports a positive association that is sufficiently free of bias, including adequate control for confounding, and corroborating studies provide support for the association but are not sufficiently free of bias, including confounding. Alternatively, several studies of lower quality might show a consistent association with results that are probably not due to bias, including confounding.[4]

Inadequate/Insufficient Evidence to Determine Whether an Association Exists

Evidence is of insufficient quantity, quality, or consistency to permit a conclusion regarding the existence of an association between exposure to a specific agent and a specific health effect in humans.

---

[3]Factors used to characterize high-quality studies include the statistical stability of the association, whether a dose-response relationship or other trend was demonstrated, and the quality of the assessments of exposure and effect.
[4]Factors used to make this judgment include the data on the relationship between potential confounders and related health effects in a given study, information on subject selection, and classification of exposure.

Limited/Suggestive Evidence of No Association

Evidence from well-conducted studies is consistent in not showing a positive association between exposure to a specific agent and a specific health effect after exposure of any magnitude. A conclusion of no association is inevitably limited to the conditions, magnitudes of exposure, and length of observation in the available studies. The possibility of a very small increase in risk after exposure studied cannot be excluded.

LIMITATIONS OF VETERAN STUDIES

A major limitation of the studies reviewed by the committee is that few of them measured combat exposure. Even in the studies that did assess combat exposure with questionnaires or scales, the researchers usually asked only whether the exposure occurred rather than attempting to determine the degree to which the veteran may have found the experience stressful. Furthermore, few studies attempted to determine the effects of repeated or combined exposures, for example, exposure to extreme heat, wearing of chemical protective gear, and shooting at the enemy.

Another limitation in many of the studies was their retrospective design, which resulted in an inability to distinguish whether health effects existed before or were consequences of deployment. Some studies used self-reports from questionnaires to assess health effects, exposure, and the presence of risk or protective factors. Such questionnaires can lead to recall bias with regard to exposures or inaccuracies in reporting health effects. For those reasons, the committee weighted more heavily studies that included an examination by a health professional or other appropriate evaluation method. Similarly, for psychiatric disorders, such as PTSD, those studies that relied on symptom checklists to indicate the presence of disorders were weighted less heavily than those that involved a diagnostic interview by a health professional. Many studies had a selection bias in that health effects were assessed in veterans who were in treatment groups, such as inpatients or outpatients at PTSD clinics, or were selected from registries of veterans established by VA. In addition, sufficient time might not have passed since deployment to detect the development of some health outcomes, for example, cancer or heart disease particularly in Gulf War, OEF, and OIF veterans.

SUMMARY

The committee reviewed and evaluated studies from the scientific and medical literature that were identified with searches of bibliographic databases and other methods. The committee adopted a policy of using only peer-reviewed published literature as the basis of its conclusions. Publications that were not peer-reviewed were given no evidentiary value by the committee. The committee came to its conclusions using the categories of association used by previous IOM committees and widely accepted by Congress, the VA, and veterans' service organizations.

Committee members read each article critically. In some instances, non-peer-reviewed publications provided background information for the committee and raised issues that required further research. The committee, however, did not collect original data, nor did it perform any secondary data analysis. In its evaluation of the peer-reviewed literature, the committee considered several important issues, including quality and relevance; error, bias, and confounding; and the diverse nature of the evidence and the research.

REFERENCES

Alpert JS, Goldberg RJ. 2007. Dear patient: Association is not synonymous with causality. *American Journal of Medicine* 120(8):649-650.

APA (American Psychiatric Association). 2000. *Diagnostic and Statistical Manual of Mental Disorders, 4th Edition, Text Revision*. Washington, DC: American Psychiatric Publishing Association.

Ellwood JM. 1998. *Critical Appraisal of Epidemiological Studies and Clinical Trials, 2nd Edition*. Oxford, UK: Oxford University Press.

Evans AS. 1976. Causation and disease: The Henle-Koch postulates revisited. *Yale Journal of Biology and Medicine* 49(2):175-195.

Hill AB. 1965. The environment and disease: Association or causation? *Proceedings of the Royal Society of Medicine* 58:295-300.

Hill AB. 1971. *Principles of Medical Statistics*. New York: Oxford University Press.

IARC (International Agency for Research Cancer). 2004. *Tobacco Smoke and Involuntary Smoking. IARC Monographs on the Evaluation of Carcinogenic Risks to Humans*. Lyon, France: International Agency for Research on Cancer.

IOM (Institute of Medicine). 1994. *Veterans and Agent Orange: Health Effects of Herbicides Used in Vietnam*. Washington, DC: National Academy Press.

IOM. 2000. *Gulf War and Health, Volume 1: Depleted Uranium, Pyridostigmine Bromide, Sarin, Vaccines*. Washington, DC: National Academy Press.

IOM. 2003. *Gulf War and Health, Volume 2: Insecticides and Solvents*. Washington, DC: The National Academies Press.

IOM. 2005. *Gulf War and Health, Volume 3: Fuels, Combustion Products, and Propellants*. Washington, DC: The National Academies Press.

IOM. 2006. *Gulf War and Health, Volume 4: Health Effects of Serving in the Gulf War*. Washington, DC: The National Academies Press.

IOM. 2007. *Gulf War and Health, Volume 5: Infectious Diseases*. Washington, DC: The National Academies Press.

Monson R. 1990. *Occupational Epidemiology, 2nd Edition*. Boca Raton, FL: CRC Press.

NRC (National Research Council). 1991. *Animals as Sentinels of Environmental Health Hazards*. Washington, DC: National Academy Press.

Office of the Surgeon General-HHS. 2004. *The Health Consequences of Smoking: A Report of the Surgeon General*. [Online]. Available: http://www.surgeongeneral.gov/library/smokingconsequences [accessed October 26, 2004].

OTA (Office of Technology Assessment). 1990. *Neurotoxicity: Identifying and Controlling Poisons of the Nervous System*. Washington, DC: U.S. Government Printing Office.

Susser M. 1973. *Casual Thinking in the Health Sciences: Concepts and Strategies of Epidemiology*. New York: Oxford University Press.

Susser M. 1977. Judgment and causal inference: Criteria in epidemiologic studies. *American Journal of Epidemiology* 105(1):1-15.

Susser M. 1988. Falsification, verification, and causal inference in epidemiology: Reconsideration in the light of Sir Karl Popper's philosophy. Rothman KJ, editor. *Causal Inference*. Chesnut Hill, MA: Epidemiology Resources. Pp. 33-58.

Susser M. 1991. What is a cause and how do we know one? A grammar for pragmatic epidemiology. *American Journal of Epidemiology* 133(7):635-648.

Wegman DH, Woods NF, Bailar JC. 1997. Invited commentary: How would we know a Gulf War syndrome if we saw one? *American Journal of Epidemiology* 146(9):704-711.

3

DEPLOYMENT-RELATED STRESSORS

The U.S. military has participated in numerous wars on both U.S. and foreign soil and, regardless of the conflict, many of the deployment-related stressors to which military personnel can be exposed are the same: possible death or injury to oneself, killing or injuring others, poor living conditions, and harsh physical environment. Military personnel may be exposed to multiple deployment-related stressors and have multiple exposures to a single stressor, all of which may adversely affect their physical and mental health. The psychiatric sequelae of war are well documented (Hotopf et al. 2006), and a recent Institute of Medicine (IOM) report notes that depression, substance abuse or dependence, and anxiety disorders, especially posttraumatic stress disorder (PTSD), were increased in Gulf War veterans after deployment, and that symptom severity was associated with the level of war stress (IOM 2006).

The 1980s saw the beginning of studies on the psychologic effects of combat on veterans. Numerous studies (Goldberg et al. 1990; Kang et al. 2003; Kulka et al. 1990; O'Toole et al. 1998) found that the feature of combat that was uniformly traumatic in three wars—the Vietnam War, the Korean War, and World War II—was being an "agent" of killing the enemy (rather than just being a "target"). Some researchers interpreted that finding as signifying that responsibility for killing someone may be the "most pervasive" trauma of war (Fontana and Rosenheck 1994).

A 2002 Department of Defense (DoD) (Bray 2003) survey of mental-health issues among all branches of the military found that in the 12,756 active-duty personnel who responded to the questionnaire the most frequently reported sources of stress were being away from family and deployment. DoD has periodically surveyed soldiers and Marines deployed to Iraq during Operation Iraqi Freedom (OIF) to assess their need for behavioral-health care and to determine what effect, if any, multiple deployments have had on their mental health (MHAT 2006a,b). Four such surveys have been conducted: September-October 2003 (OIF I), September-October 2004 (OIF II), October-November 2005 (OIF 04-06), and August-October 2006 (OIF 05-07). In the last two surveys, both active-duty troops and reservists reported that the most important noncombat stressors were deployment length and family separation; deployment length was of even greater concern for soldiers who had been deployed more than once. Increased deployment length was also related to increased mental-health problems and marital problems (MHAT 2006a,b). Those findings are particularly important because in April 2007, the length of active-duty U.S. Army deployments to Iraq and Afghanistan was extended from 12 to 15 months (Tyson and White 2007). The 2006 survey found that the level of combat experienced by a soldier or Marine was the most important determinant of their mental health (MHAT 2006b).

Specific deployment-related stressors include all those experienced during actual combat, the anticipation of deployment to a war zone, noncombat stressors, military sexual harassment and assault, poor living conditions, and exposure to environmental and chemical stressors. Some stressors are specific to reserve and National Guard troops, peacekeepers, and women.

STRESSORS DURING COMBAT

Exposure to combat has been described as one of the most intense stressors that a person can experience (Grinker and Spiegel 1945), and for many people who experience combat, it is the most traumatic experience of their life (Kulka et al. 1990). Combat may encompass many threatening situations. Among those reported most frequently by all U.S. combat veterans are killing or attempting to kill the enemy; being shot at by others; exposure to dead and wounded comrades, enemy combatants, and civilians; and being injured.

Deployment stressors in the Persian Gulf War included being in the vicinity of a Scud missile explosion, contact with prisoners of war or dead animals, direct combat duty, witnessing the death of a person, forced sexual relations or a sexual assault, being exposed to dismembered bodies or maimed soldiers, coming under small-arms fire, having artillery close by, and having a combat-related injury (Kang et al. 2000; Unwin et al. 1999). Hobfoll et al. (1991) noted that military personnel in the Gulf War were at greatest risk for stress when their work was hazardous and they anticipated exposure to chemical warfare; the risk increased with more time spent in the field and more exposure to the dead and wounded. Another stressor was the feeling that they were deserting their families at a time of need.

Sutker et al. (1993) asked 215 Gulf War veterans about their perception of injury and death, preparedness for deployment and combat, unit cohesiveness, harshness of the physical environment, perceived level of national support for the war, and stress attributable to nonmilitary events. Respondents were also asked to describe the three most stressful events they had experienced during their deployment. The stressful events cited most frequently were hardships associated with separation of home and family (18%), fear of Scud missile and other military attacks (15%), and discomfort with the physical environment (13%). Other stressors included loss of control, uncertainty, and fear of the unknown (8%); lack of leadership (7%); protracted delays in returning home after cessation of hostilities (5%); inadequacy of supplies and equipment (5%); prolonged truck transport through the desert (4%); lack of information (4%); and financial difficulties (3%).

In one of the few studies to determine not only stressful exposures but the level of stress experienced by the veterans, Stretch et al. (1996a) conducted a survey of 1524 veterans deployed to the Persian Gulf during Operation Desert Shield and Operation Desert Storm. The veterans, about half of whom were reservists, were asked to indicate what stressors they had experienced and how stressful each was. Of the stressors associated with combat exposures, 80% of the veterans indicated that threats of Scud missile, terrorist, or chemical attacks were stressful; 59-69% of the veterans rated the stress as moderate or greater. Such events as being in danger of being killed or wounded or being fired on by the enemy were stressors for almost half the veterans. Almost 83% of the veterans reported lack of contact with their families to be stressful; 68% of those surveyed found it to be moderately stressful or worse. In a study of Pennsylvania and Hawaii active-duty and reserve or National Guard soldiers who had been deployed to the Gulf War (Stretch et al. 1996b), the stressors that were most closely associated with PTSD were those related to combat, such as exposure to the killing or wounding of American soldiers by friendly fire, having a buddy killed or wounded in action, and exposure to dead or dying people. Other significant stressors for PTSD included concern about exposure to oil-well fires in Kuwait, crowding in base camps, long duty days, being fired on by the enemy, and noise from guns and artillery.

Kulka et al. (1990) asked Vietnam veterans about both war-zone stressors and traumatic events for the National Vietnam Veterans Readjustment Study (NVVRS). They distinguished between the two with the understanding that exposure to war-zone stress, such as being on frequent long-range patrols in hostile enemy territory, could increase the risk of exposure to a traumatic event, such as being in an ambush in which their colleagues were killed or wounded. Male veterans were asked 94 questions about war-zone stress exposures: 48 items about exposure to combat, 24 items about exposure to abusive violence and related conflicts, 12 items about deprivation, 9 items about loss of meaning and control, and 1 item about ever having been a prisoner of war in Vietnam. They found that 75% of veterans with high levels of war-zone stress also had exposure to at least one traumatic event during the war, and one-third of theater veterans with low war-zone stress described at least one traumatic experience. When war-zone combat exposure based on military records was compared with self-reports of combat exposure, Dohrenwend et al. (2006) found that 96.5% of Vietnam veterans who were classified as having low combat exposure on the basis of their military records reported having low or moderate exposure, and 72.1% of those classified as having very high combat exposure reported high exposure.

Fontana and Rosenheck (1999) used NVVRS data to identify important war-zone stressors. Primary stressors are killing or injuring others and insufficiency (inadequate food, inadequate water, inadequate weapons or munitions, inadequate equipment or supplies, loss of freedom of movement, and lack of privacy)—part of what King et al. (1995) called a malevolent environment. Other studies of Vietnam veterans indicate that participating in or witnessing atrocities against the enemy or civilians, both dead and alive, can be an important stressor (Fontana and Rosenheck 1999; King et al. 1995).

Schlenger et al. (1992) sought to develop a comprehensive exposure measure that would capture the array of war-zone stressors. They used principal-component analysis of the 100 interview items on the National Survey of the Vietnam Generation (part of the NVVRS) to develop a list of major stressors for men and women. For men, the stressors were exposure to combat (such as frequency of receiving enemy small-arms fire), abusive violence and related conflict (such as involvement in mutilation of bodies), deprivation (such as lack of shelter from weather), and loss of meaning and control (such as a sense of purposelessness). For women, the stressors were exposure to dead and wounded (such as frequency of giving care to people who later died), exposure to enemy fire (such as frequency of being under enemy fire), direct combat involvement (such as frequency of firing a weapon in a combat situation), exposure to abusive violence (such as seeing or hearing of Americans who had been tortured), deprivation (such as frequency of fatigue or exhaustion), and loss of meaning and control (such as feeling out of touch with the world).

In Operation Enduring Freedom (OEF) and OIF, many of the stressors are more reminiscent of the Vietnam War than of the 1991 Gulf War or World War II. With the defeat of the Iraqi Army and later sectarian violence, U.S. troops have been subjected to guerilla warfare and terrorist actions from civilian insurgents and militias; soldiers must be constantly on guard against snipers, improvised explosive devices (IEDs), and suicide bombers; and all civilians must be viewed with caution.

In 2003, Hoge et al. (2004) surveyed 2856 Army and 815 Marine combat infantry troops before and several months after their deployment to Iraq and Afghanistan for the Army units and to Iraq only for the Marines. The postdeployment surveys indicated that during deployment in Iraq, on the average, 92% of the soldiers and Marines were attacked or ambushed; 95% were shot at or received small-arms fire; 94% saw dead bodies or human remains; 89% received incoming artillery, rocket, or mortar fire; and 86% reported knowing someone who was seriously injured or killed. Over 81% of the soldiers and Marines reported shooting or directing fire at the enemy, 57% reported being responsible for the death of an enemy combatant, and 21% reported being responsible for the death of a noncombatant. Soldiers deployed to Afghanistan reported far fewer combat experiences than those deployed to Iraq (see Table 3-1).

TABLE 3-1 Combat Experiences Reported by Members of the U.S. Army and Marine Corps After Deployment to Iraq or Afghanistan

	Army Groups		Marine Group
Experience	**% in Afghanistan (n = 1962)**	**% in Iraq (n = 894)**	**% in Iraq (n = 815)**
Being attacked or ambushed	58	89	95
Receiving incoming artillery, rocket, or mortar fire	84	86	92
Being shot at or receiving small-arms fire	66	93	97
Shooting or directing fire at the enemy	27	77	87
Being responsible for the death of an enemy combatant	12	48	65
Being responsible for the death of a noncombatant	1	14	28
Seeing dead bodies or human remains	39	95	94
Handling or uncovering human remains	12	50	57
Seeing dead or seriously injured Americans	30	65	75
Knowing someone who was seriously injured or killed	43	86	87
Participating in demining operations	16	38	34
Seeing ill or injured women or children and being unable to help them	46	69	83
Being wounded or injured	5	14	9
Having a close call, being shot or hit, but being saved by protective gear	Not asked	8	10
Having a buddy shot or hit nearby	Not asked	22	26
Clearing or searching homes or buildings	57	80	86
Engaging in hand-to-hand combat	3	22	9
Saving the life of a soldier or civilian	6	21	19

SOURCE: Adapted with permission from Hoge et al. (2004).

In the 2006 DoD Soldier and Marine Well-Being Survey of 1767 active-duty personnel stationed in Iraq, the troops reported being unable to respond to threats from Iraqis, such as having concrete blocks dropped on their vehicles from overpasses, by the rules of engagement. An important combat stressor that has increased during OIF is sniper attacks. Almost two-thirds of the soldiers and Marines reported having a member of their unit killed or injured (MHAT 2006b).

Graves registration, the handling and retrieving of dead bodies or body parts, can also be stressful for military personnel. McCarroll and colleagues found that regardless of age, sex, previous experience with handling remains, or volunteer status, veterans who handled remains or even saw body transfers had more PTSD symptoms than veterans with other military occupations (McCarroll et al. 2001) and a higher rate of diagnosis of PTSD (Sutker et al. 1994). Mere anticipation of working in the mortuary with exposure to mass deaths was stressful to many of the military personnel, although those who had more mortuary experience and those who had volunteered for the duty found it less stressful than those who did not (McCarroll et al. 1993, 1995). Stressors associated with mortuary work included handling bodies, working with x-rays, handling personal effects, and observing bodies being moved from transfer cases.

NONCOMBAT STRESSORS

Uncertainty about the duration of deployment was a continuing concern for U.S. troops during the Gulf War, particularly during the early phases of the buildup (Wright et al. 1996). A large epidemiologic study of Gulf War veterans (Fiedler et al. 2006) found that veterans who had had other deployments, such as in Vietnam or Bosnia, in addition to their deployment to the gulf did not have an increased risk of major depression or generalized anxiety disorder or any anxiety disorder, including PTSD. However, additional deployments were associated with a two-fold increase in substance dependence. A study of nearly 60,000 military and civilian peacekeepers deployed on a NATO mission to Bosnia (Huffman et al. 1999) found that prior deployment was associated with lower rates of depression symptoms (measured with the Self-Rating Depression Scale) and PTSD (determined with the PTSD Checklist). Neither study queried veterans regarding the length of their deployment.

DoD Mental Health Advisory Team surveys of both active-duty troops and reserve and National Guard soldiers deployed to Iraq during OIF in 2005 and 2006 found that the most important noncombat stressors were deployment length and family separation; deployment length was of even higher concern to soldiers who had been deployed more than once (MHAT 2006a,b). Furthermore, the number of soldiers who were anxious about uncertain redeployment dates rose from 35% in 2005 to 40% in 2006. DoD noted that the 5% increase may have been due to the survey's inclusion of soldiers from a brigade combat team that had had its tour extended beyond 12 months and had learned of the extension only from their spouses, who, in turn, had learned of the extension from the garrison leadership. Morale was particularly low among enlisted men who had had multiple deployments to Iraq. The committee notes that in April 2007 the length of deployment of active-duty Army personnel in Iraq was extended from 12 to 15 months and that 13,000 National Guard troops were expecting to be called up for second tours to Iraq. Marines have shorter deployments than Army soldiers, generally 9 months compared with 12 months.

About one-third of the soldiers in the 2006 DoD survey reported finding their work boring and repetitive. Of particular concern to many soldiers and Marines was a perceived inequity in access to base amenities, such as recreational equipment and communication equipment, for personnel who had missions outside the base camp (MHAT 2006b). Those concerns contributed to the low morale of the troops.

ANTICIPATION OF DEPLOYMENT TO A WAR ZONE

Human and animal studies show that the anticipation or perception of exposure to a severe stressor in the absence of actual exposure can be as powerful as the actual exposure in eliciting the stress response (see Chapter 4). Several of the questionnaires developed after the Gulf War (for example, Sutker et al. 1995; Ikin et al. 2004, 2005) to identify war-zone stressors include anticipated or perceived exposure to chemical weapons in addition to actual combat exposure. Before deployment, most stressors are associated with fear of unknown or expected enemy tactics. In a survey of 1400 U.S. troops just before the January 15, 1991, deadline for the withdrawal of Iraqi troops from Kuwait, researchers found that the fear of Iraqi use of chemical or biologic weapons was the greatest stressor (Norwood et al. 1996). Kang et al. (2003) defined veterans as having been "combat-exposed" if they were "wearing chemical protective gear" or "hearing chemical alarms sounding." Stretch et al. (1996a), in a survey of over 1500 Gulf War veterans, found that waiting for deployment to the gulf was moderately to extremely stressful for 67% of them.

Predeployment anticipation of an event might be more stressful than its occurrence during deployment. Before the January 1991 gulf air war, Gifford et al. (2006) conducted interviews of Gulf War troops in Saudi Arabia to identify potential stressors and then followed up 6-9 months after the troops returned to the United States. They found that the stressors changed as the soldiers adapted to the new environment in the gulf, the infrastructure was modified with new equipment and facilities, and communication to and from families, the public, and top military and political figures improved (see Table 3-2). However, some stressors persisted throughout the war; for example, soldiers had been told by senior military personnel to expect large numbers of casualties, and this anticipation existed until virtually the end of the war.

Australian Navy Gulf War veterans were surveyed to identify stressors in military units that were not actively engaged in combat or that had little direct combat exposure—those troops served in blockade efforts or provided transport, supplies, or medical support (Ikin et al. 2004, 2005; McKenzie et al. 2004). Of the 1232 respondents, 81% indicated that they had been on a ship or aircraft passing through hostile water or airspace; 71% had been in fear of artillery, missile, Scud rocket, or bomb attack; 71% had been on formal alert or in fear of nuclear, biologic, or chemical attack; 67% felt cut off from family or significant others; and 54% felt that while on board a ship they feared death, injury, or being trapped as a result of a missile attack or hitting a sea mine. For Australian Gulf War-era veterans who had been deployed to areas other than the gulf and for veterans who had not been deployed, the greatest stressor was feeling cut off from family members and significant others. Similarly, a study of the entire cohort of 3000 Gulf War veterans from Canada found that although the vast majority served at sea, they frequently saw Scud missiles overhead, and that resulted in stress because they feared that the missiles contained chemical-warfare agents (Goss Gilroy Inc. 1998).

When United Kingdom (UK) Gulf War-deployed troops were compared with UK troops deployed to Bosnia or not deployed, the Gulf War-deployed troops reported more exposure to all stressors except dead animals and exhaust from heaters or generators (Unwin et al. 1999). Anticipation of attack with chemical or biologic agents was the most common predeployment fear among the UK troops.

TABLE 3-2 Stressors Experienced by U.S. Forces in the Gulf War

Deployment Phase	Stressors
Early	Uncertainty of tour length, no projected date of return
	Lack of communication (slow mail and poor telephone availability)
	Information deprivation and resulting rumors
	Ambiguous demands (precombat vs garrison environment)
	Austere, crowded living conditions
	Harsh desert conditions (heat and sand)
	Lack of respite—always in chain of command
	Lack of recreational or entertainment opportunities
	Lack of amenities, such as hot meals
	Cultural isolation, restriction of behavior, and ambivalent perceptions of rules
	Uncertainty about public support
Buildup	Lack of companionship of opposite sex
	Lack of contact with family
	Lack of private time
	Leaders around too much of the time
	Not being allowed to "act like Americans"
	Lack of adequate morale, welfare, and recreation equipment
	Lack of alcoholic drinks
	Fatigue and lack of sleep
	Flies
Anticipation of combat	Threat of attack with chemical or biological weapons
	Expectation of massive casualties
	Possibility of friend getting killed or wounded
	Possibility of self getting killed or wounded
	Fear of not getting adequate medical care if hit
	Possibility of losing a leader

SOURCE: Adapted with permission from Gifford et al. (2006).

MILITARY SEXUAL ASSAULT AND HARASSMENT

Sexual assault and harassment[1] are widely acknowledged stressors in the general population and are severe stressors when incurred in a war zone. In the military environment with its overwhelmingly male population, sexual victimization is more likely to be experienced

[1]The U.S. Army defines *sexual assault* as "intentional sexual contact, characterized by use of force, physical threat or abuse of authority or when the victim does not or cannot consent. Sexual assault includes rape, nonconsensual sodomy, indecent assault (unwanted, inappropriate sexual contact or fondling), or attempts to commit these acts." The Army defines *sexual harassment* as "a form of gender discrimination that involves unwelcome sexual advances, requests for sexual favors, and other verbal or physical conduct of a sexual nature" (U.S. Army 2005).

by women, regardless of their military occupation and background (Wolfe et al. 1993a). The rate of reported sexual assault was about 70 per 100,000 uniformed service members in 2002-2003 for all duty stations; 9% of the victims were men (DoD 2004). Reported rates of sexual harassment of women in the military were about 46% and 24% in 1995 and 2002, respectively, and of men 8% and 3%. The female-to-male ratio for being a victim of sexual assault in the Gulf War was 16.5:1 and for sexual harassment 25:1 (Kang et al. 2005).

The 1995 National Health Survey of Gulf War Era Veterans and Their Families, conducted by the Department of Veterans Affairs (VA), found that of the 11,441 Gulf War veterans who responded (4202 women and 7239 men), 24% of the women reported having been subject to sexual harassment, and 3.3% reported sexual assault; only 0.6% of the men reported experiencing sexual harassment, and even fewer (0.2%) reported a sexual assault (Kang et al. 2005). Wolfe et al. (1998) interviewed 160 Army women on their return from the Gulf War and 18-24 months later; the women reported rates of sexual assault of 7.3%, physical sexual harassment 33.1%, and verbal sexual harassment 66.2%—all higher rates than those found in peacetime military and civilian population. Goldzweig et al. (2006) reported rates of sexual harassment in veterans and active-duty military that ranged from 55% to 79%, with sexual assault ranging from 4.2 to 7.3% in active-duty women and 11 to 48% in female veterans.

LIVING CONDITIONS

During the buildup to the 1991 Gulf War, combat troops were crowded into warehouses and tents on arrival in the Persian Gulf region and then often moved to isolated desert locations. Most troops lived in tents and slept on cots lined up side-by-side, affording virtually no privacy or quiet. Sanitation was often primitive, with communal washing facilities and shortages of latrines. Hot showers were infrequent, the interval between launderings of uniforms was sometimes long, and desert flies, scorpions, and snakes were a constant nuisance. Military personnel worked long hours and had narrowly restricted outlets for relaxation. Troops were ordered not to fraternize with local people, and alcoholic drinks were prohibited in deference to religious beliefs in the host countries. The diet of most of the military units consisted mostly of packaged foods and bottled water. In a 2006 survey of 1767 soldiers and Marines stationed in Iraq for OIF, over one-third reported the lack of privacy and personal space to be a stressor (MHAT 2006b).

Temperature extremes are also a source of stress. In the first 2 months of troop deployment (August and September 1990) to the Persian Gulf region, the weather was extremely hot and humid, with air temperatures as high as 115°F and sand temperatures reaching 150°F. Troops had to drink large quantities of water to prevent dehydration. In some of the areas of Iraq that U.S. troops patrol in OIF, the temperature can reach 140°F.

Although the summers in the Middle East are hot and dry, temperatures in winter (December-March) are low, and wind-chill temperatures at night can drop to well below freezing. Wind and blowing sand make protection of skin and eyes imperative. Goggles and sunglasses help somewhat, but visibility is often poor, and contact lenses were prohibited in the Gulf War (Ursano and Norwood 1996).

In a survey of 1576 Gulf War veterans, 62-85% experienced the chronic stressors associated with living and working in the gulf, including crowding, lack of privacy, working in the desert, long hours, and boredom; 35-61% of the veterans found the conditions to be at least moderately stressful (Stretch et al. 1996a).

ENVIRONMENTAL AND CHEMICAL STRESSORS

The exposure of Gulf War troops to numerous environmental and chemical agents has been addressed in previous volumes of the *Gulf War and Health* series, and such exposures will not be considered here except to note that many troops may have found such exposures—anticipated, known, or suspected—to be psychologically stressful and physiologically challenging. Troops in the 1991 Gulf War were exposed to environmental and chemical agents, possibly including chemical-warfare agents. Some exposures were the result of living and working conditions at camp or in the field, such as exposures to petroleum-based combustion products, including those of kerosene, diesel, and leaded gasoline used in unventilated tent heaters, cooking stoves, and portable generators. Some troops were exposed to the smoke from more than 750 oil-well fires. Pesticides, including dog flea collars, were widely used by troops in the Persian Gulf to combat the region's ubiquitous insect and rodent populations. Exposure of U.S. personnel to depleted uranium occurred as the result of "friendly-fire" incidents, cleanup operations, and accidents (including accidental fires).

U.S. troops in the gulf had been warned that they might be exposed to biologic and chemical weapons. Iraq previously had used such weapons in fighting Iran and in attacks on the Kurdish minority in Iraq. U.S. military leaders feared that the use of such weapons in the gulf could result in the deaths of tens of thousands of Americans. Therefore, in addition to the standard predeployment immunizations, the anthrax and botulinum toxoid vaccine were also provided to some military personnel. Troops were also given blister packs of 21 tablets of pyridostigmine bromide (PB) to protect against nerve gas. Troops were to take PB on the orders of a commanding officer when a chemical-warfare attack was believed to be imminent. Alarms sounded often, and troops responded by donning the confining protective gear and ingesting PB as an antidote to nerve gas. DoD has estimated that about 250,000 personnel took PB at some time during the Gulf War (IOM 2006). The sounding of the alarms, the reports of dead animals, and rumors that other units had been hit by chemical-warfare agents caused the troops to be concerned that they would be or had been exposed to such agents.

Despite the relatively small numbers of U.S. personnel injured or killed during combat in the Gulf War, the troops, as in any war, faced the fear of death, injury, capture by the enemy, and, in the case of the demolition of a munitions-storage complex at Khamisiyah, Iraq, possible exposure to the nerve agents sarin and cyclosarin.

RESERVE AND NATIONAL GUARD TROOPS

The Gulf War was the first since World War II in which reserve and National Guard units were activated and deployed. The greater participation of reserve and National Guard troops in the Gulf War has now been surpassed by OEF and OIF (Table 3-3). As of February 14, 2007, almost 85,000 reserve and National Guard personnel have been mobilized to serve in OEF and OIF.

Reservists and National Guard troops may encounter more stressors going to a war zone than those faced by active-duty military personnel; many of the additional stressors were unanticipated at the time the reservists and National Guard troops signed up for service. The stressors experienced by reservists and National Guard troops might include financial concerns, such as significant loss of income due to leaving more lucrative civilian jobs for lower military

TABLE 3-3 Percentage of Active-Duty vs Reserve and National Guard Troops, by War

Military Status	War	Percentage of Troops
Active duty	Vietnam War	> 99%
	Gulf War	83%
	OEF and OIF	80%
Reserves and National Guard	Vietnam War	< 1%
	Gulf War	17%
	OEF and OIF	20%

SOURCE: DoD (2007); Joseph (1997); Kapp (2006).

wages; logistic issues, such as having to make arrangements for the care of children, elderly parents, or other family members; and arranging legal and financial matters. Over 13,000 of the 265,322 reservists mobilized for the 1991 Gulf War were single parents (Ursano and Norwood 1996). Employment was also a concern; although some employers kept the reservists' jobs open until their return, this was not always the case. For business owners and self-employed people, there were issues associated with delegating work responsibilities, ensuring continuity, or handling obligations to clients or others. Uncertainty about the length of the deployment, the destination of the unit if and when deployed, and the short notice given before deployment (generally 2-9 days) contributed to the stress of activation and deployment on the reservists and their families (Ursano and Norwood 1996). Gulf War reservists also experienced stress resulting from rapid, unexpected activation and deployment to a combat zone and then rapid demobilization from the combat zone, perceived and actual threats to their safety, lack of confidence about equipment and training, poor communication and leadership, and loss of prestige and income when disbanded (Malone et al. 1996).

PEACEKEEPERS

U.S. troops are often deployed around the world as part of United Nations (UN) peacekeeping forces and have performed this function in Lebanon, Sinai, Bosnia, and Somalia. The inherent conflict between being trained for active combat duty and acting in a peacekeeping capacity can lead to stress in military peacekeepers particularly if they are involved in maintaining an established peace as opposed to a more traditional combat role of establishing peace among warring parties (Litz et al. 1997). Researchers at VA interviewed 3461 U.S. troops deployed to Somalia after their return from the peacekeeping mission. They found that the psychologic stressors faced by U.S. peacekeepers on dangerous missions like that in Somalia included frustration with the rules of engagement, such as exercising restraint in dangerous situations; demoralization; hostility and anger; and witnessing death and violence. Potentially traumatic events included sniper attacks, contact with land mines, witnessing starvation, and violence.

Maguen et al. (2004) surveyed 203 U.S. military peacekeepers before and after deployment to Kosovo about possible stressors. The most frustrating stressors were being overseas during special events (74%), being separated from family and friends (71%), being bored (54%), knowing that many of the war criminals were not arrested (73%), seeing children who were victims of war (67%), and seeing civilians in despair (58%). About 88% of the soldiers also reported fear of having their unit fired on (of whom 28% found this fear moderately to extremely negative), 85% had gone on patrols or performed other dangerous duties (22% found this to be moderately to extremely negative), 83% had patrolled in areas where there were mines (33%), and 76% reported potential for being ambushed or attacked (21%). Other significant stressors experienced by the soldiers included risk of being taken hostage (67%), needing to manage civilians in chaotic conditions (62%), witnessing violence (61%), and patrolling through the zone of separation (61%). Similarly stressful conditions have been described in other peacekeeping populations and missions, for example, in the Norwegian UN peacekeepers in Lebanon (Mehlum and Weisaeth 2002).

Bartone et al. (1998) described similar findings among a group of 300 U.S. Army personnel deployed from Germany to serve as medical support to the UN peacekeeping mission in Croatia in 1993. Personnel identified stressors at predeployment and at three times during the 6-month deployment. Stressors changed during the deployment phases; in the predeployment phase, the major stressors were uncertainty about who was going to be deployed, when and for how long deployment would last, the introduction of new unit members with disparate field experiences, the amount of time required for unit training and preparation that conflicted with family preparations, and uncertainty about possible base closures during deployment. Other stressors associated with getting ready to deploy were changes in unit leadership and having to move families back to the United States (units were stationed in Germany with families). During the middle deployment phase, the primary stressors were associated with missing a spouse and not knowing where the unit would be based at the end of deployment; Army base closures, uncertainty about where the family would live, and boredom associated with lack of meaningful work were also stressors. In the late phase of deployment, the primary stressor continued to be missing a spouse, followed by Army drawdown, lack of ready access to transportation, and boredom.

Research on Danish military units sent to northern Iraq as peacekeepers after the 1991 Gulf War also indicated the stressful nature of this duty. Self-reported exposures included witnessing direct war actions such as shootings, grenade attacks, and bomb explosions; witnessing assaults on civilians; seeing severely wounded or dead people; being threatened with arms; watching colleagues or friends being threatened with arms or shot at; being shot at; pointing a gun at or shooting someone; and being exposed to threats from the local population (Suadicani et al. 1999).

WOMEN

The role of women in the military has changed over the last century. In World War II, almost 350,000 women served in the armed forces in a variety of health-related, clerical, and other noncombat roles. In the Korean War, 48,700 women served in support roles; and during the Vietnam War, over 7000 women served in the Vietnam Theater, most as nurses. In 1973, at the end of the Vietnam War, 55,000 women were in the active-duty military, making up 2.5% of the armed forces. But it was only with the Gulf War that the number and responsibilities of military women dramatically increased. By late February 1991, 37,000 military women were in the Persian Gulf, making up 6.8% of the U.S. military forces. Women served in all the services, although they were excluded from some combat specialties; they were administrators, air-traffic controllers, logisticians, engineering-equipment mechanics, ammunition technicians, ordnance specialists, communicators, radio operators, drivers, law-enforcement specialists, and guards. Many female truck drivers hauled supplies and equipment into Kuwait. Some took enemy prisoners of war to holding facilities, and others flew helicopters and reconnaissance aircraft. Still others served on hospital, supply, oiler, and ammunition ships or served as public-affairs officers and chaplains. Several women commanded units the size of brigades, battalions, companies, and platoons in the combat service-support areas (DoD 2004). By September 30, 2004, the number of women on active duty in all branches of the military was more than 212,000—nearly 15% of the active-duty armed forces. As the number of women in the military has grown, so has the number of female veterans. In 1990, female veterans numbered an estimated 1.2 million; that number had increased to 1.6 million by 2000 and to 1.7 million by the end of 2004. The number is expected to rise to about 1.9 million in 2020 (Klein 2005).

As greater numbers of women serve in more combat-support occupations, they are exposed to many of the same war-zone stressors as are men. Schlenger et al. (1992) found that for female Vietnam veterans, the primary stressors were exposure to dead and wounded (for example, giving care to people who later died), exposure to enemy fire, direct combat involvement (for example, firing a weapon in a combat situation), exposure to abusive violence (for example, seeing or hearing of Americans tortured), deprivation (for example, being fatigued or exhausted), and loss of meaning and control (for example, feeling out of touch with the world).

Vogt et al. (2005) queried 317 Gulf War veterans (including 83 females) about combat experiences, the aftermath of battle (such as handling human remains and dealing with prisoners of war), perceived threats, difficult living and working environments, concerns about family and relationship disruptions, lack of deployment social support, and sexual harassment. There were no sex differences for most of the stressor measures; however, women reported more exposure to interpersonal stressors, such as incidents of sexual harassment, and reported that they received less postdeployment social support than men. In contrast, men reported more mission-related stressors, such as combat experiences.

These findings were supported by Wolfe et al. (1993b), who also found that immediately after their Gulf War deployment, men (n = 2136) and women (n = 208) reported similar deployment experiences, that is, 74% of men and 78% of women had been on alert for chemical and biologic attack, 74% of men and 70% of women received incoming fire from large arms, and 50% of men and 45% of women had seen death or disfigurement of enemy troops. However, when the participants generated and ranked their own lists of stressors, there were significant differences between the men and the women. Almost half of the women (48%) reported combat exposure as their most significant stressor compared with 38% of men. Almost equal percentages of women (24%) and men (28%) reported a war-zone but noncombat event (such as a unit member's being injured or killed in nonmission activities or nearness to a prisoner-of-war riot) as their most significant stressor, and 20% of women and 25% of men reported that a personal or domestic stressor was the most stressful event during deployment. Only 7% of women and 9% of the men did not report a stressful event. In a similar study of the Iowa Gulf War cohort, Carney et al. (2003) asked men and women who were deployed to the Gulf War theater (Saudi Arabia, Bahrain, Persian Gulf, Iraq, Kuwait, or other country) about exposure to nine combat-related stressors. Among 129 women and 1767 men in the study, the most frequently reported stressors for both sexes were seeing dead bodies or severely maimed or injured people, having a Scud missile explode within 1 mile, and having explosions other than Scuds within 1 mile; the men, however, had significantly more exposure to combat. In all, with the exception of combat exposure and sexual threat, women and men had similar deployment exposures.

Although men and women may experience many of the same deployment-related stressors, women may have different reactions to those stressors. Just being female may put some women veterans at greater risk for adverse mental-health effects when exposed to a deployment-related stressor. One study attempted to distinguish between men's and women's reactions to combat stressors. Fontana et al. (2000) found that men and women had similar responses to many of the stressors experienced while on a peacekeeping mission in Somalia. Both men and women became more frightened as their exposure to combat and to witnessing Somalis dying increased. For men, being frightened, being sexually harassed as a result of showing fear in a combat situation, and witnessing Somalis dying were all associated with PTSD. The same stressors were associated with PTSD in women; however, just being female was sufficient for a woman to be subjected to sexual harassment, regardless of whether or not she had shown fear in a combat situation. In another study of Navy health-care providers deployed to the Persian Gulf on a hospital ship days before the Gulf War, there was anticipation of large numbers of casualties and concerns for safety. Women were more likely to report having depression; however, when training and experience were factored into the analysis with fear of injury and the stress of work demands, the sex difference for depression disappeared (Slusarcick et al. 2001).

CONCLUSIONS

The many stressors associated with being deployed to a war zone are not limited to the actual period of deployment, but extend into the pre- and postdeployment periods. Among the most serious are combat stressors which include killing someone, seeing comrades killed or injured, being threatened or fired on, and seeing and handling dead bodies. In OEF and OIF, stressors inherent in guerilla warfare are also present, such as not recognizing the enemy, being constantly on guard for the presence of IEDs, and balancing military activities with humanitarian services. Others stressors are associated with being deployed to an unfamiliar location, concern about financial obligations, and being away from family and loved ones. The committee notes that most of the studies discussed in this chapter queried veterans about a prescribed list of stressors or exposures that the investigators thought the veterans would find stressful. With the exception of Sutker et al. (1993), the studies did not ask open-ended questions about what stressors, exposures, or conditions the veterans found most stressful. Furthermore, many studies asked veterans to indicate only whether they had experienced a particular situation and not the degree to which the veterans found the exposure to be stressful. Therefore, the findings must be interpreted with the knowledge that, by and large, veterans could respond only to what they were asked and that their responses may not reflect the whole spectrum of stressors to which they were exposed and the level of stress that such exposures elicited. An understanding of deployment-related stressors, their frequency, and their magnitude is critical for interpreting the epidemiologic studies that are evaluated in Chapters 6 and 7.

REFERENCES

Bartone PT, Adler AB, Vaitkus MA. 1998. Dimensions of psychological stress in peacekeeping operations. *Military Medicine* 163(9):587-593.

Bray RM. 2003. *2002 Department of Defense Survey of Health Related Behaviors Among Military Personnel*. Research Triangle Park, NC: RTI International.

Carney CP, Sampson TR, Voelker M, Woolson R, Thorne P, Doebbeling BN. 2003. Women in the Gulf War: Combat experience, exposures, and subsequent health care use. *Military Medicine* 168(8):654-661.

DoD (Department of Defense). 2004. *Task Force Report on Care for Victims of Sexual Assault.* Washington, DC.

DoD. 2007. *U.S. Department of Defense News Releases.* [Online]. Available: http://www.defenselink.mil/Releases/ [accessed July 18, 2007].

Dohrenwend B, Turner J, Turse N, Adams B, Koenen K, Marshal R. 2006. The pychological risks of Vietnam for U.S. veterans: A revisit with new data and methods. *Science* 313(5789):979-982.

Fiedler N, Ozakinci G, Hallman W, Wartenberg D, Brewer NT, Barrett DH, Kipen HM. 2006. Military deployment to the Gulf War as a risk factor for psychiatric illness among U.S. troops. *British Journal of Psychiatry* 188:453-459.

Fontana A, Rosenheck R. 1994. Traumatic war stressors and psychiatric symptoms among World War II, Korean, and Vietnam War veterans. *Psychology and Aging* 9(1):27-33.

Fontana A, Rosenheck R. 1999. A model of war zone stressors and posttraumatic stress disorder. *Journal of Traumatic Stress* 12(1):111-126.

Fontana A, Litz B, Rosenheck R. 2000. Impact of combat and sexual harassment on the severity of posttraumatic stress disorder among men and women peacekeepers in Somalia. *Journal of Nervous and Mental Disease* 188(3):163-169.

Gifford RK, Ursano RJ, Stuart JA, Engel CC. 2006. Stress and stressors of the early phases of the Persian Gulf War. *Philosophical Transactions of the Royal Society of London—Series B: Biological Sciences* 361(1468):585-591.

Goldberg J, True WR, Eisen SA, Henderson WG. 1990. A twin study of the effects of the Vietnam War on posttraumatic stress disorder. *Journal of the American Medical Association* 263(9):1227-1232.

Goldzweig CL, Balekian TM, Rolon C, Yano EM, Shekelle PG. 2006. The state of women veterans' health research: Results of a systematic literature review. *Journal of General Internal Medicine* 21(Suppl 3):S82-S92.

Goss Gilroy Inc. 1998. *Health Study of Canadian Forces Personnel Involved in the 1991 Conflict in the Persian Gulf.* Ottawa, Canada: Goss Gilroy Inc. Department of National Defence.

Grinker RR, Spiegel JP. 1945. *Men Under Stress.* Philadelphia, PA: Blakiston.

Hobfoll SE, Spielberger CD, Breznitz S, Figley C, Folkman S, Lepper-Green B, Meichenbaum D, Milgram NA, Sandler I, Sarason I. 1991. War-related stress. Addressing the stress of war and other traumatic events. *American Psychologist* 46(8):848-855.

Hoge CW, Castro CA, Messer SC, McGurk D, Cotting DI, Koffman RL. 2004. Combat duty in Iraq and Afghanistan, mental health problems, and barriers to care. *New England Journal of Medicine* 351(1):13-22.

Hotopf M, Hull L, Fear NT, Browne T, Horn O, Iversen A, Jones M, Murphy D, Bland D, Earnshaw M, Greenberg N, Hughes JH, Tate AR, Dandeker C, Rona R, Wessely S. 2006. The health of UK military personnel who deployed to the 2003 Iraq war: A cohort study. *Lancet* 367(9524):1731-1741.

Huffman AH, Adler AB, Castro CA. 1999. *Impact of Deployment History on the Well-Being of Military Personnel*. Army Medical Research Unit, Europe.

Ikin JF, Sim MR, Creamer MC, Forbes AB, McKenzie DP, Kelsall HL, Glass DC, McFarlane AC, Abramson MJ, Ittak P, Dwyer T, Blizzard L, Delaney KR, Horsley KW, Harrex WK, Schwarz H. 2004. War-related psychological stressors and risk of psychological disorders in Australian veterans of the 1991 Gulf War. *British Journal of Psychiatry* 185:116-126.

Ikin JF, McKenzie DP, Creamer MC, McFarlane AC, Kelsall HL, Glass DC, Forbes AB, Horsley KWA, Harrex WK, Sim MR. 2005. War zone stress without direct combat: The Australian naval experience of the Gulf War. *Journal of Traumatic Stress* 18(3):193-204.

IOM (Institute of Medicine). 2006. *Gulf War and Health, Volume 4: Health Effects of Serving in the Gulf War*. Washington, DC: The National Academies Press.

Joseph SC. 1997. A comprehensive clinical evaluation of 20,000 Persian Gulf War veterans. *Military Medicine* 162(3):149-155.

Kang H, Dalager N, Mahan C, Ishii E. 2005. The role of sexual assault on the risk of PTSD among Gulf War veterans. *Annals of Epidemiology* 15(3):191-195.

Kang HK, Mahan CM, Lee KY, Magee CA, Murphy FM. 2000. Illnesses among United States veterans of the Gulf War: A population-based survey of 30,000 veterans. *Journal of Occupational and Environmental Medicine* 42(5):491-501.

Kang HK, Natelson BH, Mahan CM, Lee KY, Murphy FM. 2003. Post-traumatic stress disorder and chronic fatigue syndrome-like illness among Gulf War veterans: A population-based survey of 30,000 veterans. *American Journal of Epidemiology* 157(2):141-148.

Kapp L. 2006. *CRS Report for Congress: Reserve component personnel issues: Questions and answers*. Washington, DC: Congressional Research Service, The Library of Congress.

King DW, King LA, Gudanowski DM, Vreven DL. 1995. Alternative representations of war zone stressors: Relationships to posttraumatic stress disorder in male and female Vietnam veterans. *Journal of Abnormal Psychology* 104(1):184-195.

Klein RE. 2005. *Women Veterans: Past, Present and Future*. Washington, DC: U.S. Department of Veterans Affairs.

Kulka RA, Schlenger WE, Fairbank JA, Hough RL, Jordan BK, Marmar CR, Weiss DS. 1990. *Trauma and the Vietnam War Generation: Report of Findings from the National Vietnam Veterans Readjustment Study*. New York: Brunner/Mazel Publishers.

Litz BT, Orsillo SM, Friedman M, Ehlich P, Batres A. 1997. Posttraumatic stress disorder associated with peacekeeping duty in Somalia for U.S. military personnel. *American Journal of Psychiatry* 154(2):178-184.

Maguen S, Litz BT, Wang JL, Cook M. 2004. The stressors and demands of peacekeeping in Kosovo: Predictors of mental health response. *Military Medicine* 169(3):198-206.

Malone JD, Paige-Dobson B, Ohl C, DiGiovanni C, Cunnion S, Roy MJ. 1996. Possibilities for unexplained chronic illnesses among reserve units deployed in Operation Desert Shield/Desert Storm. *Southern Medical Journal* 89(12):1147-1155.

McCarroll JE, Ursano RJ, Fullerton CS, Lundy A. 1993. Traumatic stress of a wartime mortuary. Anticipation of exposure to mass death. *Journal of Nervous and Mental Disease* 181(9):545-551.

McCarroll JE, Ursano RJ, Fullerton CS, Lundy A. 1995. Anticipatory stress of handling human remains from the Persian Gulf War. Predictors of intrusion and avoidance. *Journal of Nervous and Mental Disease* 183(11):698-703.

McCarroll JE, Ursano RJ, Fullerton CS, Liu X, Lundy A. 2001. Effects of exposure to death in a war mortuary on posttraumatic stress disorder symptoms of intrusion and avoidance. *Journal of Nervous and Mental Disease* 189(1):44-48.

McKenzie DP, Ikin JF, McFarlane AC, Creamer M, Forbes AB, Kelsall HL, Glass DC, Ittak P, Sim MR. 2004. Psychological health of Australian veterans of the 1991 Gulf War: An assessment using the SF-12, GHQ-12 and PCL-S. *Psychological Medicine* 34(8):1419-1430.

Mehlum L, Weisaeth L. 2002. Predictors of posttraumatic stress reactions in Norwegian U.N. peacekeepers 7 years after service. *Journal of Traumatic Stress* 15(1):17-26.

MHAT (Mental Health Advisory Team). 2006a. *Mental Health Advisory Team (MHAT) III Operation Iraqi Freedom 04-06: Final Report.* [Washington, DC]: Office of the Surgeon Multinational Force-Iraq and Office of the Surgeon General United States Army Medical Command. 29 May 2006. [Online]. Available: http://www.armymedicine.army.mil/news/mhat/mhat_iii/mhat-iii.cfm.

MHAT. 2006b. *Mental Health Advisory Team (MHAT) IV Operation Iraqi Freedom 05-07: Final Report.* [Washington, DC]: Office of the Surgeon Multinational Force-Iraq and Office of the Surgeon General United States Army Medical Command. 17 November 2006. [Online]. Available: http://www.armymedicine.army.mil/news/mhat/mhat_iv/MHAT_IV_Report_17NOV06.pdf.

Norwood AE, Fullerton CS, Hagen KP. 1996. Those left behind: Military families. In: Ursano RJ, Norwood AE, editors. *Emotional Aftermath of the Persian Gulf War: Veterans, Families, Communities, and Nations.* Washington, DC: American Psychiatric Association. Pp. 163-196.

O'Toole BI, Marshall RP, Schureck RJ, Dobson M. 1998. Posttraumatic stress disorder and comorbidity in Australian Vietnam veterans: Risk factors, chronicity and combat. *Australian and New Zealand Journal of Psychiatry* 32(1):32-42.

Schlenger WE, Kulka RA, Fairbank JA, Hough RL. 1992. The prevalence of post-traumatic stress disorder in the Vietnam generation: A multimethod, multisource assessment of psychiatric disorder. *Journal of Traumatic Stress* 5(3):333-363.

Slusarcick AL, Ursano RJ, Dinneen MP, Fullerton CS. 2001. Factors associated with depression on a hospital ship deployed during the Persian Gulf War. *Military Medicine* 166(3):248-252.

Stretch RH, Bliese PD, Marlowe DH, Wright KM, Knudson KH, Hoover CH. 1996a. Psychological health of Gulf War-era military personnel. *Military Medicine* 161(5):257-261.

Stretch RH, Marlowe DH, Wright KM, Bliese PD, Knudson KH, Hoover CH. 1996b. Post-traumatic stress disorder symptoms among Gulf War veterans. *Military Medicine* 161(7):407-410.

Suadicani P, Ishoy T, Guldager B, Appleyard M, Gyntelberg F. 1999. Determinants of long-term neuropsychological symptoms. The Danish Gulf War Study. *Danish Medical Bulletin* 46(5):423-427.

Sutker PB, Uddo M, Brailey K, Allain AN. 1993. War-zone trauma and stress-related symptoms in Operation Desert Shield/Storm (ODS) returnees. *Journal of Social Issues* 49(4):33-50.

Sutker PB, Uddo M, Brailey K, Vasterling JJ, Errera P. 1994. Psychopathology in war-zone deployed and nondeployed Operation Desert Storm troops assigned graves registration duties. *Journal of Abnormal Psychology* 103(2):383-390.

Sutker PB, Davis JM, Uddo M, Ditta SR. 1995. Assessment of psychological distress in Persian Gulf troops: Ethnicity and gender comparisons. *Journal of Personality Assessment* 64(3):415-427.

Tyson AS, White J. 12 April 2007. Strained army extends tours to 15 months: Move is needed for Iraq troop increase. *Washington Post* A:1.

Unwin C, Blatchley N, Coker W, Ferry S, Hotopf M, Hull L, Ismail K, Palmer I, David A, Wessely S. 1999. Health of UK servicemen who served in Persian Gulf War. *Lancet* 353(9148):169-178.

Ursano RJ, Norwood AE. 1996. *Emotional Aftermath of the Persian Gulf War: Veterans, Families, Communities, and Nations*. Washington, DC: American Psychiatric Association.

U.S. Army. 2005. *U.S. Army Sexual Assault and Prevention Program*. [Online]. Available: http://www.sexualassault.army.mil/content/faqs.cfm [accessed July 18, 2007].

Vogt DS, Pless AP, King LA, King DW. 2005. Deployment stressors, gender, and mental health outcomes among Gulf War I veterans. *Journal of Traumatic Stress* 18(2):115-127.

Wolfe J, Brown PJ, Furey J, Levin KB. 1993a. Development of a wartime stressor scale for women. *Psychological Assessment* 5(3):330-335.

Wolfe J, Brown PJ, Kelley JM. 1993b. Reassessing war stress: Exposure and the Persian Gulf War. *Journal of Social Issues* 49(4):15-31.

Wolfe J, Sharkansky EJ, Read JP, Dawson R, Martin JA, Ouimette PC. 1998. Sexual harassment and assault as predictors of PTSD symptomatology among U.S. female Persian Gulf War military personnel. *Journal of Interpersonal Violence* 13(1):40-57.

Wright KM, Marlowe DH, Gifford RK. 1996. Deployment stress and Operation Desert Shield: Preparation for the war. In: Ursano RJ, Norwood AE, editors. *Emotional Aftermath of the Persian Gulf War: Veterans, Families, Communities, and Nations*. Washington, DC: American Psychiatric Association. Pp. 283-314.

4

THE STRESS RESPONSE

In considering whether being deployed to a war zone may result in long-term health effects in veterans, it is important to ask whether the stressors experienced by the veterans during their deployment could produce the stress response. If they could, might that response lead to physiologic changes that could eventually be manifested as long-term health effects? Those questions address the issue of biologic plausibility as discussed in Chapter 2: Are there biologic mechanisms by which exposure to deployment-related stress could lead to adverse health effects? This chapter explores the research being done on why and how people and animals respond to stress. It describes the stress response, including its basic biology and physiology, and its modifiers. The chapter also surveys some of the potential adverse consequences of the stress response that can occur in organ systems after exposure to chronic stressors. The implications of the stress response for long-term health effects in humans are described in Chapters 6 and 7.

The word *stress* is used in many contexts and has a variety of meanings. It is often used to describe a situation characterized by real or perceived threats to a person, but it is also commonly used to refer to the body's response to such threats. Thus, *stress* has been used both to describe the environmental events (the stressors) that trigger responses and to refer to the resulting changes (stress responses) that occur in the brain and the rest of the body.

The stress response enables humans and other organisms to survive unsafe and life-threatening conditions through "fight or flight," as the response is widely called. As described below, it is a cascade of physiologic changes that is activated rapidly in emergencies. Some of the changes occur immediately, within minutes to hours; others emerge after days to weeks (Box 4-1), depending on the stressor's severity. The repertoire of responses is similar across human cultures and other species.

One of the earliest steps in the stress response is the brain's perception that an event is threatening, which determines how an organism responds physiologically, emotionally, and behaviorally to the stressor. Possible responses include aggression, escape, anxiety, and executive function (a complex set of behaviors). The response to the stressor—for example, the sound of a gun—is dictated by the split-second appraisal of whether it poses a genuine threat. A feature that is most refined in humans is the capacity to learn from stressful experiences, to think abstractly, and to draw on lessons when coping with harm in the future (McEwen and Lasley 2002). The lessons learned are often etched into the brain through measurable structural and functional alterations in nerve cells and networks. Human stressors are not only external; they can be internal, such as worry, guilt, or rumination about past or future events. Internal and external stressors both contribute to allostatic overload, a concept for explaining in physiologic terms the effects of chronic or cumulative stress (McEwen 2007).

BOX 4-1 Physiologic Changes During the Stress Response

Early Phase of the Stress Response (Duration: Minutes to Hours)

- Increased heart rate and blood pressure
- Increased respiration
- Mobilization of energy from liver and body fat
- Sharpening of attention and cognition
- Increased fear conditioning (learning)
- Blunting of pain
- Altered intestinal motility

Later Phases of the Stress Response (Duration: Days to Weeks)

- Enhanced immune system
- Suppression of appetite and digestion
- Suppression of growth
- Suppression of reproduction
- Persistence of increased heart rate and blood pressure in some cases
- Persistence of increased cortisol in some cases
- Release of stress hormones

When a stressor is eliminated, the stress response may shut off quite slowly or not at all (McEwen and Lasley 2002). It is the long-term activation of the stress response—long after the threat has ceased—that poses the greatest risk to human health. Paradoxically, the human stress response is life-saving in the short term (and is adaptive) when immediate stressors are confronted, but it can lead to illness or disease when stressors are severe, recurrent, or persistent in the long term (and is maladaptive).

Although many veterans consider deployment, particularly combat, to be highly stressful and even traumatic, there are many periods during deployment when stressors are not traumatic but are severe and persistent (for example, separation from family and worry about home or work). Prolonged exposure to such stressors, whether in military or civilian life, can overwhelm otherwise healthy people and can lead to health-damaging behaviors, such as smoking and excessive drinking, in an attempt to alleviate the stress.

CENTRAL ROLE OF THE BRAIN

Once the brain interprets a situation as threatening, it assumes immediate control over the endocrine, cardiovascular, immune, and digestive system. The brain relies on an elaborate communication network that includes hormones, neurotransmitters, chemicals associated with the immune system, and other molecular signals. This section discusses the various regions of the brain involved in the body's response to stress, the effects of the brain on other organ systems that play roles in the stress response, and the feedback mechanisms that occur in response to acute and chronic stress.

The stress response is spearheaded by the hypothalamus-pituitary-adrenal (HPA) axis in the peripheral stress-response pathway and by the sympathetic nervous system in the central stress-response pathway. The sympathetic system activates internal organs (such as heart, lungs, and liver) and mobilizes energy to respond to stressors. The parasympathetic nervous system does the opposite, preserving energy, putting a brake on the heart rate, increasing intestinal activity, relaxing muscles in the gastrointestinal system, and decreasing inflammation. Those functions have earned the parasympathetic system the nickname "rest and digest," compared with the "fight or flight" of the sympathetic system. The stress response is adaptive (it promotes survival), but it is maladaptive if it is chronically activated over a long time. Long-term activation of the stress response can cause abnormalities in the brain or in other parts of the body.

Reticular Activating System

In response to any stimulus, including stimuli that are novel or potentially threatening, a primary brain system that is activated is the reticular activating system (RAS). Without activation of the RAS there would be no stress response or waking behavior; indeed, loss of RAS function results in a persistent vegetative state. The RAS works closely with the cholinergic, noradrenergic, and serotonergic systems of the brainstem and influences other brain areas, such as the cerebral cortex, hypothalamus, amygdala, and cerebellum. Novel and potentially threatening stimuli, such as a loud sound, induce a massive output from the RAS that does three things: it activates the pontine reticular formation to potentiate the startle response, which is part of a general protective system (the eyes close, flexion in humans lowers the head from danger, and muscles tighten in preparation for attack from an enemy); it activates the thalamus to trigger synchronization of fast rhythms between the thalamus and cortex that "awaken" the cortex, placing it in a "ready" position; and it participates with forebrain structures in activating the hypothalamus to trigger the HPA axis and the surge of epinephrine from the adrenal medulla. The "fight or flight" response is therefore a brainwide and bodywide response to novelty and threat that involves activation of the RAS with other coordinated brain systems.

The RAS is dysregulated in anxiety disorders and depression. In fact, some of the first symptoms of posttraumatic stress disorder (PTSD) and depression are sleep-wake problems (see Chapter 5). Both disorders are marked by increased vigilance and increased REM-sleep drive, which can result in vivid dreaming and REM-sleep intrusion into waking, for example, hallucinations (Pfaff 2005). In some cases, the RAS can be activated directly by inputs to the brainstem from the periphery, such as a loud sound, pain, touch, or signals from the gut via the vagus nerve. For the other senses, the sensory information reaches the RAS via the amygdala, which also can respond directly to a stimulus, such as a loud sound, pain, or touch.

Importance of the Amygdala

The stress response begins with sensory information about a stressor—its visual images, sounds, smells, touch, or other sensations (Figure 4-1). Information from sensory nerve cells in peripheral tissues is relayed to several regions of the brain, including the hypothalamus, thalamus, somatosensory cortex, nucleus of the solitary tract, ventral lateral medulla, and the parabrachial nucleus and insular cortex. Each of those regions sends signals to the amygdala (in the temporal lobes of the cerebrum) which integrates all the incoming sensory signals (Bonne et al. 2004) and to the hypothalamus. The amygdala consists of collections of cell types (nuclei) that form the "extended amygdala." The extended amygdala consists of the central and basolateral nucleus of the amygdala, and the lateral bed nucleus of the stria terminalis (BNST) (Alheid and Heimer 1988; Davis and Whalen 2001). The BNST also receives input from the hippocampus (a part of the brain in the medial temporal lobe). Both the central nucleus of the amygdala and the lateral BNST, when activated, transmit impulses to several other regions of the brain, including the locus coeruleus, which uses norepinephrine (also called noradrenalin) to send signals to numerous other parts of the brain. Several parts of the hypothalamus and many of the same brainstem nuclei activate the sympathetic nervous system, which with the locus coeruleus forms part of the "central stress response," preparing for fight or flight. The hypothalamus is especially important for regulating the sympathetic nervous system because it receives sensory input from virtually the entire body, including the amygdala and BNST.

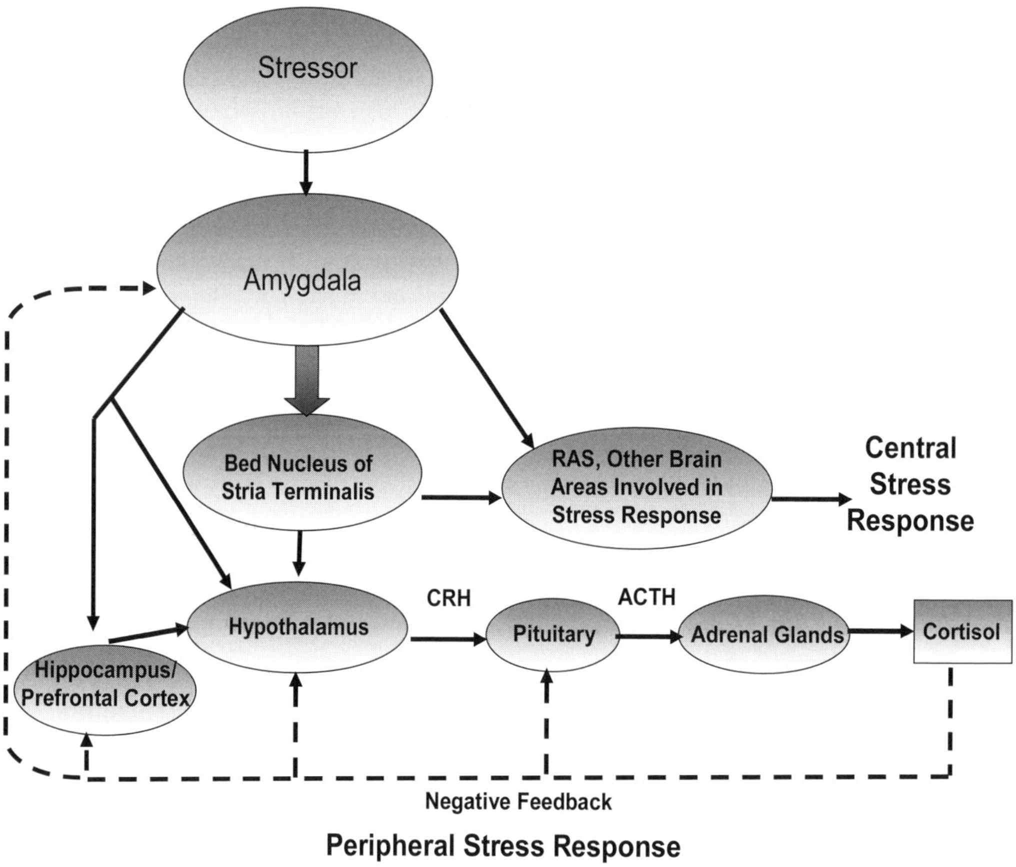

FIGURE 4-1 Stress-response pathways. NOTE: ACTH = adrenocorticotrophic hormone, CRH = corticotropin-releasing hormone, RAS = reticular activating system.

The sympathetic nervous system uses epinephrine to stimulate the inner region of the adrenal gland to secrete large amounts of epinephrine and other catecholamines[1] into the circulation. The surge of epinephrine floods the brain and peripheral tissues, thereby producing the full-fledged fight or flight response: faster heartbeat, greater energy, more blood flow to skeletal and cardiac muscle, dilation of the pupils and airways, and higher blood glucose concentration and so on. With chronic stress, however, the sympathetic nervous system may

[1]Catecholamines are a class of hormones and neurotransmitters that includes epinephrine and dopamine.

remain reactive and produce catecholamines for many years. That is commonly seen in people with anxiety disorders who have increased heart rates and blood pressure. Long-term increase in catecholamines can produce chronic inflammation, as discussed later in the chapter.

The Hypothalamus-Pituitary-Adrenal Axis

In the peripheral stress pathway, the hypothalamus secretes corticotropin-releasing hormone (CRH), which acts on the pituitary to secrete corticotropin (also known as adrenocorticotropic hormone). Corticotropin enters the bloodstream and acts on the adrenal cortex to induce release of the glucocorticoid hormone cortisol. This pathway is known as the HPA axis or peripheral stress response (Chrousos and Gold 1992; Selye 1956).

Cortisol is distributed to body tissues where it serves several functions, such as replenishing energy lost to the epinephrine surge, increasing cardiovascular tone; enhancing memory for avoiding danger in the future; preserving energy; and, if necessary, activating immune-cell migration to areas of the body where there is infection or injury (McEwen and Lasley 2002). Cortisol also has key functions in the brain: it acts to increase arousal, vigilance, attention, and formation of memories (Charney 2004). It can also act in the amygdala and BNST to increase production and release of CRH from the hypothalamus. Cortisol also facilitates fear conditioning (Roozendaal et al. 2006). However, if the cortisol surge is large and prolonged, it can suppress growth, tissue repair, reproduction, digestion, and inflammation (Sapolsky 2003).

When cortisol reaches the brain it exerts a negative feedback on the HPA axis. First, it binds to glucocorticoid receptors in the hippocampus (McEwen et al. 1968), which projects into the hypothalamus, and binds to glucocorticoid receptors in the hypothalamus. Cortisol binding in both the hippocampus and the hypothalamus acts to turn off CRH production and release by the hypothalamus (Herman et al. 1989; McEwen et al. 1992). The net effect is that high cortisol concentrations reaching the brain inhibit the HPA axis (McEwen 2002b; Vermetten and Bremner 2002). Thus, glucocorticoids, such as cortisol, enhance CRH in the amygdala and help to turn on the HPA axis when activated by stress, and a feedback mechanism turns the HPA axis off at the level of the hypothalamus and pituitary (see Figure 4-1). It is the balance between activation via the amygdala and inhibition via the hypothalamus, prefrontal cortex, and hippocampus that determines HPA activity and how rapidly it is turned on and off.

The hippocampus plays a key role in shaping memories; it forms explicit memory, which is the ability to recollect an event consciously and to assemble its pieces to form a coherent memory of the whole event. The opposite, nondeclarative memory, refers to memories not consciously recalled, for example, such skills as playing the piano and reading. For fearful memories, the hippocampus works with the amygdala and the prefrontal cortex of the brain. The prefrontal cortex modulates the actions of the amygdala, usually through inhibition, and thus can control cortisol secretion and activation of the parasympathetic and sympathetic nervous systems (Radley et al. 2006; Thayer and Brosschot 2005). The prefrontal cortex also participates in attention, decision making and sense of control, working memory, extinction of fear memories, and other aspects of cognitive flexibility (Hariri et al. 2006; McDougall et al. 2004).

The effects of cortisol (peripheral pathway) and epinephrine (central pathway) are not restricted to the central nervous system (CNS). Many other tissues respond to cortisol and communicate with the CNS in a bidirectional manner. Of particular concern for the stress response is the immune system. In the acute phase of the stress response, the immune system fights infection and repairs wounds by boosting immunity. Some immune cells (such as leukocytes, white blood cells) are rapidly deployed from the circulation to the skin, where they protect wounds against viruses, bacteria, and fungi. They are summoned there by cytokines, which are released at the wound site (Dhabhar 2000). Cytokines are small proteins that are secreted most typically by immune cells and signal or activate other immune cells. Functioning somewhat as hormones do, they regulate the immune response to infection and injury.

The communication link between the HPA axis and the immune system is strong: lymphocytes and macrophages (types of white blood cells) have receptors for cortisol, and some immune-related cells in the brain have receptors for cytokines (Reiche et al. 2004) and are activated by cortisol. In response to chronic stress, a long-term increase of glucocorticoids, such as cortisol, can dysregulate and suppress immune function, as discussed later.

Allostasis

The classic fight or flight response entails activation of epinephrine and cortisol with resulting increases in immune function, energy mobilization (in the form of glucose), and enhancement of memory, which helps to avoid the threat in the future. To maintain homeostasis, the brain regulates the stress response by inducing the body to release chemical mediators—including neurotransmitters, immune-system messengers, and hormones, including cortisol and epinephrine, a process called allostasis (McEwen 1998, 2005, 2007; McEwen and Wingfield 2003). Homeostasis refers to stability in various physiologic characteristics, such as body temperature, pH, and oxygen tension, which are tightly regulated within narrow ranges that promote survival.

The chemical mediators of allostasis are released from the sympathetic and parasympathetic branches of the nervous system but are also released from the immune, cardiovascular, and metabolic systems. Their interactions occur through a nonlinear network, that is, mediators from each system regulate the production of others in a series of checks and balances.

Corresponding to multiple mediators of the stress response, there are multiple pathways by which they regulate it. In the sympathetic system, for example, greater activity of proinflammatory cytokines, signaling molecules used by the immune system, elicits greater activity of anti-inflammatory cytokines—that is, negative feedback—and negative regulation by the parasympathetic and glucocorticoid pathways. Parasympathetic activity working through the acetylcholine receptors on immune cells reduces production of proinflammatory cytokines (Tracey 2002). In other words, as the activity of proinflammatory cytokines increases, other systems can produce the opposing activity. That example shows how homeostasis can be achieved through numerous routes using a common set of interacting mediators (McEwen 2007).

Allostatic Load and Overload

Allostatic load refers to the burden of chronic stress and altered personal behaviors ("lifestyle") that results from effects of overuse and dysregulation of the mediators of allostasis (Figure 4-2; McEwen 1998). Allostatic load is often manifested by fatigue, anger, frustration, and feeling out of control. Those feelings can lead to sleep loss (McEwen 2006, 2007), anxiety,

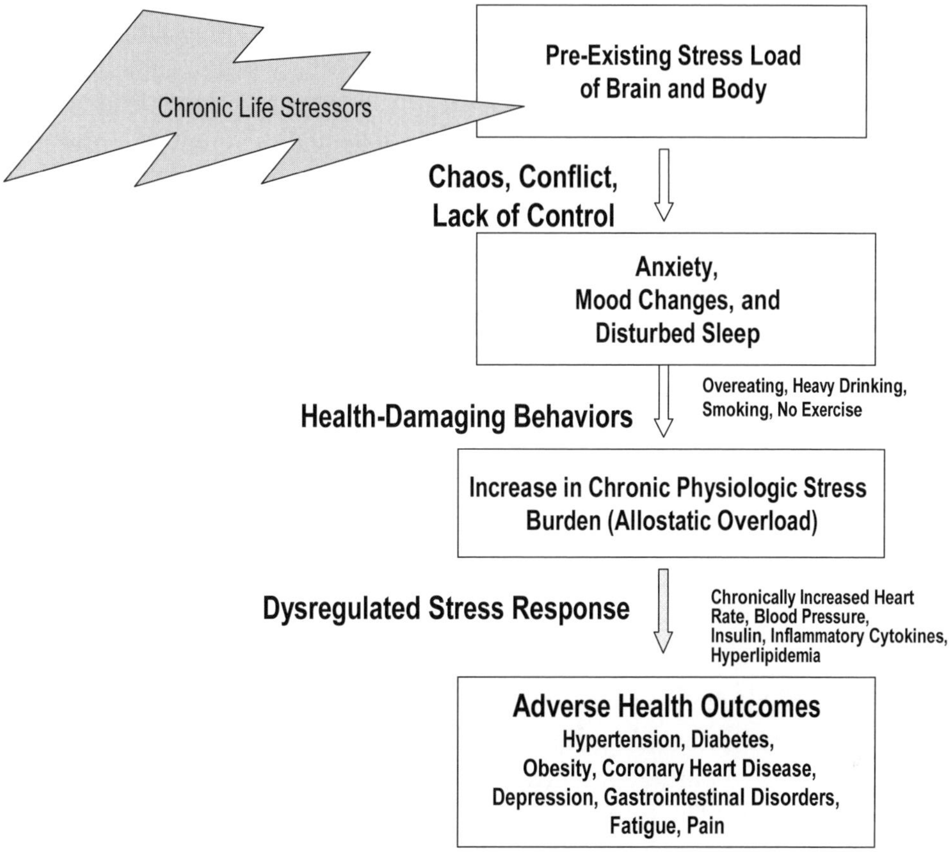

FIGURE 4-2 How chronic stress can affect behavior and health. All people have some pre-existing load of stressful experiences reflected in brain and body. Chronic life stressors (such as interpersonal conflicts, care-giving, pressure at work, and crowded and noisy living and working conditions) can affect people by creating a sense of chaos, conflict, and a lack of control. The result of the chronic stressors will often be chronic anxiety and depressed mood with poor-quality sleep. Anxiety, mood changes, and inadequate sleep can lead to self-medication through eating "comfort foods," excessive alcohol drinking, smoking, and neglecting regular exercise. Together with the anxiety, depressed mood, and poor sleep, these behaviors dysregulate the normal physiological activities and create a chronic stress burden (allostatic overload). The dysregulated stress response involves increased cortisol, insulin, and inflammatory cytokines at night; along with increased heart rate and blood pressure; and reduced parasympathetic tone. If this abnormal dysregulated state persists for months and years, there are likely to be adverse health outcomes, such as hypertension, coronary heart disease, stroke, obesity, diabetes, arthritis, major depression, gastrointestinal disorders, chronic pain, and chronic fatigue.

depression, and such health-damaging behaviors as overeating (Dallman et al. 2003), smoking, and excessive drinking (Anda et al. 1990; Dube et al. 2002). Those behaviors, in turn, increase and dysregulate the body's mediators normally involved in allostasis. When one mediator, such as cortisol, is present in excessive or insufficient amounts, other mediators are also changed. Over the course of days, weeks, and longer, allostatic load eventually can disrupt health, a condition called allostatic overload or toxic chronic stress response. Allostatic overload is maladaptive: it serves no useful purpose and predisposes the body to disease.

Allostatic load and allostatic overload are points on a continuum. The pattern, frequency, and duration of stressors are important determinants of the severity of the outcome, as are a person's response to the stressors. Four types of physiologic responses lead to allostatic load and overload (Figure 4-3). Two of them are related to individual differences in the stress response: prolonged response (B) and inadequate response (C). The other two are related to chronic stressor characteristics: repeated exposure (D in the figure) and lack of adaptation (E). Initially, the health consequences of allostatic load or overload are early indicators of possible later disease, such as hypertension, obesity, increased cholesterol, bone mineral loss, muscle protein loss, memory impairment, and increased anxiety.

MODIFIERS OF THE STRESS RESPONSE

Many factors may alter a person's response to stress, including genetic makeup, early-life history, and the degree to which the stressor can be controlled. Research is under way on all those, primarily in animal models. Each is discussed below.

Genes

Many aspects of the stress response—such as learned and innate fear (see, for example, Shumyatsky et al. 2005), reward, social behavior, and resilience (Charney 2004)—are likely to be under the influence of particular genes. Genes determine which proteins will be made and where they will be made. The same gene might have slightly different sequences (alleles) that alter the protein production. An example of allelic variation occurs in the gene that codes for the serotonin-transporter protein. That protein removes serotonin—a chemical messenger in the brain that affects emotions, mood, behavior, and thought—from the synaptic cleft between nerve cells after it is released by a presynaptic cell. A short allele makes less of this protein than the long allele found in most people, thus altering serotonin transmission (Hariri et al. 2006). In some studies, people with the short allele are prone to more anxiety and more likely to acquire conditioned fear responses (Hariri et al. 2006). Furthermore, they are more likely to develop depression but only if they were maltreated in childhood (Caspi et al. 2002). Thus, just having the short allele does not necessarily lead to depression, but combined with early life stress it can increase the risk of depression. Conversely, people with the longer allele (and higher levels of serotonin transporter) were less likely to develop depression even if they had been maltreated in childhood; the longer allele protected them. That is an example of gene-environment interactions in which a medical condition cannot be predicted only by a gene or only by a serious life event but requires a combination of a genetic factor and an environmental event for the outcome to occur.

Researchers have investigated the mechanisms that might explain such gene-environment interactions. For example, Ichise et al. (2006) examined the same interactions between a short serotonin-transporter allele and exposure to early-life stress in rhesus monkeys. Monkeys reared by peers rather than by their mothers—a stressful condition—showed a decrease in serotonin

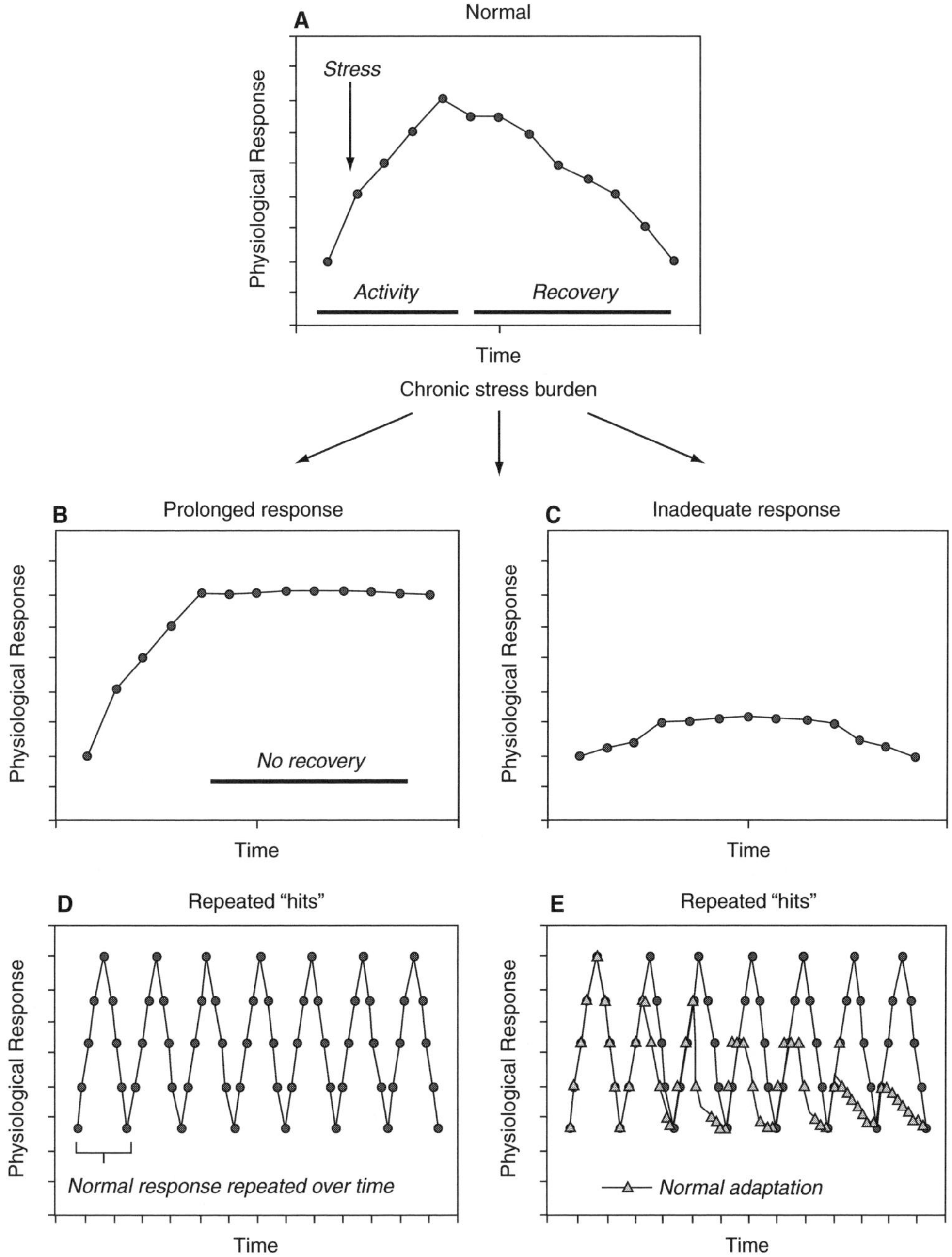

FIGURE 4-3 Chronicity of stressors. Top panel (A) shows a normal stress response that is turned on by the stressor and shut off when the stressor is terminated. Individual stress responses may be prolonged (B) or inadequate for the situation (C). The repetition of stressful events (D) and lack of adaptation to similar stressors (E) can lead to toxic stress and a chronic stress burden. SOURCE: Adapted with permission from McEwen (1998).

binding in several regions of the brain involved in the stress response (for example, the amygdala, hypothalamus, hippocampus, and raphe nucleus). The authors suggested that early-life stress affects the development of the serotonin system and that it might account for some of the behavioral abnormalities—including greater alcohol consumption, aggressiveness, and impaired impulse control—seen in the peer-reared monkeys (Barr et al. 2004). Such studies may elucidate the neural circuits governing the stress response and how they interact with the environment and on some of the variation in response to stress.

Early-Life Stress

In the 1950s, Harlow found that lack of maternal care and handling is a severe form of early-life stress. Rhesus monkeys that had been "raised" by artificial mothers (made of bare wires) were stricken with terror when they were placed in novel situations (Harlow 1974), and those raised by their peers showed more anxiety and hyperarousal than monkeys raised by their biologic mothers (Mineka and Suomi 1978).

Early-life stress has been associated with increases in cortisol and other markers of increased HPA-axis activity (Levine 1962). In rats, normal maternal handling during infancy leads to a life-long increase in the number of glucocorticoid receptors in the hippocampus, whereas a lack of maternal handling decreases the number of glucocorticoid receptors in the stressed animals, and the decreases persist into adulthood and old age (Meaney et al. 1985, 1988). A greater density of glucocorticoid receptors after normal handling would be expected to increase negative feedback between the hippocampus and the HPA (see Figure 4-1) and result in greater inhibition of the HPA axis after a stressful event, which in turn would lead to a less reactive HPA axis, lower cortisol concentrations, and more rapid initiation of the stress response. But the lower density of receptors in the heavily stressed offspring would be expected to reduce negative feedback and lead to greater reactivity of the HPA axis, higher cortisol concentrations, and more prolonged stress response. Higher cortisol concentrations, which persisted from youth through old age, were indeed found in nonhandled (stressed) animals. At greater ages, the excess secretion of cortisol was associated with structural changes in the hippocampus and with deficits in spatial memory (Meaney et al. 1988). Normal maternal care led to lower concentrations of corticotropin and cortisol, indications of a less reactive HPA axis (Liu et al. 1997; Meaney et al. 1985; Sapolsky et al. 1986).

Evidence that early-life stress results in an overreactive HPA axis has come also from studies of CRH. As described earlier, CRH is released by the hypothalamus under the regulatory influence of the hippocampus, prefrontal cortex, and amygdala, and it signals the pituitary gland to release corticotropin, which leads to a release of cortisol by the adrenal gland (see Figure 4-1). Primates reared under conditions of early-life stress (unpredictable conditions for the mother to find food) displayed persistent increases of CRH throughout adulthood (Coplan et al. 1996). The timing of exposure to the stressor was important: CRH decreased when the stressful condition occurred later in infancy (Mathew et al. 2002). Those studies have helped to establish that early-life stress has permanent effects on the regulation of the HPA axis.

Human studies have demonstrated associations that appear to be consistent with the findings on early-life stress in animal studies. In a study of the effects of childhood abuse in New Zealanders followed from birth until their 30s, an association was found between childhood abuse and chronic inflammation in adulthood. The inflammatory marker C-reactive protein—a better marker for myocardial infarction than cholesterol concentrations—was found to be above normal in many of the young adults known to have been abused. A dose-response relationship was seen between the level of abuse and the concentration of C-reactive protein (Danese et al. 2007).

Controllability

One important modifier of the stress response is the degree to which a stressor is perceived as controllable (Maier and Watkins 2005). Animal studies have indicated that a sense of control is an important aspect of hardiness. Experiments have shown that animals with control over the amount of shock they received fared much better those deprived of control (Maier et al. 1969; Seligman and Maier 1967; Weiss 1968). Rats that lacked control of the shock they received ate less, lost more weight, developed more ulcers, had higher resting blood pressure and higher plasma cortisol, displayed less aggression in the face of an intruder, were less responsive on standard measures of pain sensitivity and reactivity, and had more immunosuppression (Maier and Watkins 1998); they also had changes in epinephrine in the locus coeruleus and hypothalamus (Weiss et al. 1981). Similar experiments in dogs (Chourbaji et al. 2005; Overmier and Seligman 1967; Vollmayr and Henn 2001) found that those given inescapable shocks failed to avoid later shocks even when they were able to, a behavior called learned helplessness.

The biologic mechanism that underlies how uncontrollable stress might lead to deficits in escape appears to be abnormal activation of two brainstem nuclei: the dorsal raphe nucleus and the locus coeruleus (Maier et al. 1995). Activation of neurons there leads to the release of the neurotransmitters serotonin and norepinephrine into almost all parts of the brain, where they modify cellular activity. However, the mechanism by which those primitive brainstem nuclei mediate the complex cognitive process required to judge the uncontrollability of a stressor has been unclear. It has recently been shown in rats that stress always activates the brainstem nuclei, but activation is inhibited by the prefrontal cortex, a brain structure that appears to be dysregulated in people with PTSD (see Chapter 5) (Amat et al. 2005). Thus, a dysfunctional prefrontal cortex in PTSD could perhaps exacerbate a feeling of being out of control. Animal studies illustrate the potential role of perception of control in the stress-response process.

CHRONIC STRESS AND HEALTH

Activation of the stress response ensures survival in the short term, but is maladaptive when its activation persists as a result of chronic, severe, or repeated stress. Chronic stress can lead to adverse health outcomes that affect multiple body systems such as the CNS and the endocrine, immune, gastrointestinal, and cardiovascular systems. Stress-induced abnormalities are due to dysregulation of a common set of mediators: cortisol, epinephrine, and immune-system cytokines. The model of stress-related illness is built on evidence of interrelationships between stress hormones and other systems, including the endocrine and immune systems. Stress hormones can trigger interactions between the endocrine and immune systems that culminate in a state of chronic inflammation. Stress-induced chronic inflammation appears to be a driving force behind wide-ranging conditions linked to stress, such as obesity, heart disease, diabetes, and chronic pain (Black and Garbutt 2002; Black et al. 2006; Malarkey and Mills 2007). Research on the role of inflammation with the CNS is focusing on interrelationships between immune cells, cytokines, and nearby neurons situated in regions of the brain implicated in stress-related disorders (MacPherson et al. 2005).

This section reviews some of those adverse health effects; in many cases, they are markers of disease or symptoms rather than specific diseases.

Brain Function

In the brain, there is evidence of structural and functional changes resulting directly from chronic or severe stress. The changes are associated with alterations of the most profound functions of the brain: memory and decision making. They also are associated with symptoms of fear and anxiety, and they might sensitize the brain to substances of abuse and increase the risk of substance-use disorders (Brady and Sinha 2005; Will et al. 1998). The impact of chronic stress on those brain functions is discussed below.

Memory and Cognition

Memory and cognition have been studied extensively in three regions of the brain: the hippocampus, the prefrontal cortex, and the amygdala. The hippocampus, the center of explicit memory, appears be especially vulnerable to chronic stress. Repeated stress, according to animal models, changes the structure of and connections between neurons in the hippocampus devoted to receiving signals from other nerve cells (McEwen 1999b; Sapolsky 2003). When hippocampal neurons are remodeled by glucocorticoids working together with some neurochemicals, they lose their plasticity. Plasticity is vital for encoding memories and learning from them, and its loss leads to impairment of essential cognitive functions of the brain. Cognitive dysfunction is seen in people who use glucocorticoids chronically as treatment for autoimmune or inflammatory disorders, in people who secrete cortisol excessively, and in healthy volunteers given glucocorticoids (Sapolsky 2003).

Plasticity in the hippocampus is thought to depend in part on the production of new nerve cells by proliferation and differentiation of stem cells or progenitor cells in a process known as neurogenesis. In animal models, chronic stress inhibits neurogenesis in the hippocampus and can reduce the number of neurons (Pham et al. 2003). Increases in glucocorticoids, endogenous opioids, and excitatory amino-acid transmitters play a role in this inhibition (Eisch and Harburg 2006; Mirescu and Gould 2006). The inhibition of neurogenesis might also be mediated in part by proinflammatory cytokines (Kempermann and Neumann 2003) that direct neuron stem cells to mature into non-nerve cells in the brain at the expense of generating new nerve cells. That effect can be blocked by anti-inflammatory agents (Monje et al. 2003).

As discussed earlier, the prefrontal cortex integrates such information as whether a sudden noise poses a threat and modulates activity of the HPA axis (McDougall et al. 2004; Radley and Morrison 2005). Repeated stress causes structural remodeling of the neurons in the axis that reduce their ability to receive signals from other neurons. As explicated by McEwen et al. (1999a) in connection with structural remodeling in the hippocampus, changes in the prefrontal cortex are most likely driven by increased concentrations of glucocorticoids and by other neurochemicals in the brain that are increased by repeated exposure to stressors (Radley and Morrison 2005); those changes impair cognitive flexibility (Liston et al. 2006).

The amygdala undergoes structural changes that are the opposite of those seen in the hippocampus and prefrontal cortex. In animal models, the changes are accompanied by an increase in fear conditioning and anxiety-like behaviors (Vyas et al. 2002). That also appears to be the case in humans; veterans with PTSD evaluated with brain-imaging techniques (see Chapter 5) show activation of the amygdala after being exposed to traumatic images (for example, Shin et al. 2004).

Memories formed in association with stressful life events can be indelible and can be triggered, even years later, by cues associated with the original event. The memories can be triggered by stimuli associated with the original traumatic event (flashbacks) and in some people are so intrusive that normal functioning is no longer possible. Those strong traumatic memories are often expressed in the form of intrusive recollections, flashbacks, and repetitive nightmares (McGaugh et al. 1992).

Anxiety and Fear

Epinephrine plays a critical role in the encoding of memory for events and stimuli that are arousing, stressful, or fear provoking. In animal models, it has been implicated in memory consolidation, and the effect appears to be time-dependent (Gold and Van Buskirk 1975). As discussed earlier, the acute stress response activates the fast pathway in which the locus coeruleus releases epinephrine in response to signals from the amygdala and BNST. Most nerve projections from the locus coeruleus are excitatory in function and activate, for example, the sympathetic nervous system, amygdala, and HPA axis. However, some of the projections are inhibitory and act on the prefrontal cortex and the parasympathetic nervous system, the systems that normally keep the sympathetic nervous system in check. Inhibiting the prefrontal cortex favors instinctual responses at the expense of more complex thinking and planning (Charney 2004). Chronic stress also increases the activity of the locus coeruleus with the same effects as acute stress but over longer periods, thereby contributing to chronic anxiety, fear, and intrusive memories (Charney 2004). As previously discussed, chronic stress also goes on to increase concentrations of epinephrine outside the brain that can affect other organ systems.

Endocrine System

During the acute stress response, epinephrine mobilizes the body's energy for fight or flight. The energy comes from stored fats and from glycogen in the liver. When mobilized by epinephrine during the acute stress response, the liver breaks down fats into fatty acids and glycerol and breaks down glycogen into glucose and releases them into the circulation. Circulating glucose, fatty acids, and glycerol are distributed to each cell in the body, particularly muscles (during the acute stress response) where they are oxidized for energy. With the cessation of acute stress, cortisol acts to replenish energy supplies in the liver and adipose tissue. Many of the basic metabolic functions related to food intake, storage, and conversion to energy are altered by excess concentrations of cortisol and epinephrine in chronic stress (McEwen and Lasley 2002). The endocrine system can respond to chronic stress with an array of effects that are often overlapping and interactive; some of these are described below.

Obesity

Chronic stress has long been associated with obesity in humans and animal models (McEwen 2002a; Rosmond et al. 1996). Cortisol enhances pathways that lead to increased deposition of fat (adipose tissue) in the abdominal area. An increase in abdominal fat, as opposed to that in the hips and buttocks, is an important risk factor associated with hypertension, diabetes, and cardiovascular diseases (Black and Garbutt 2002).

Obesity is also caused by higher food intake, which commonly occurs with chronic stress, either as a coping strategy (Dallman et al. 2003) or because of sleep deprivation. Sleep deprivation appears to increase hunger through its association with lower concentrations of an appetite-suppressing hormone (leptin) and higher concentrations of an appetite-enhancing hormone (ghrelin) (Spiegel et al. 2004). An association has been found between body-mass index (BMI) and sleep duration; people getting less than 8 hours of sleep each night exhibited increased BMI (Taheri et al. 2004).

Obesity has serious consequences for the development of diabetes and heart disease because it causes or contributes to insulin resistance (Reaven et al. 2004). Fat is now considered to be the largest endocrine organ in the body, and it is the source of numerous cytokines involved in inflammation and insulin resistance.

Insulin Resistance and Glucose Intolerance

Insulin resistance refers to a cell's inability to use blood glucose because of poor uptake of insulin and is a major risk factor for diabetes (Brindley 1995). Insulin is produced by the pancreas and acts on cells throughout the body to stimulate the uptake, use, and storage of glucose. It also stimulates the liver to store glucose in the form of glycogen and promotes the synthesis of fatty acids in the liver. Normally, insulin binds to insulin receptors on the cell surface, but insulin resistance occurs when there is a decrease in the number or function of insulin receptors, and higher concentrations of insulin are needed to keep glucose within the normal range. The higher insulin concentrations can also lead to increased fat deposition, which in turn aggravates insulin resistance that may eventually lead to glucose intolerance and diabetes mellitus.

Immune and Inflammatory Responses

There are close interactions between the endocrine and immune systems. Pituitary and adrenal hormones, normally parts of the endocrine system, can be synthesized and released by immune cells in lymphatic organs (Wu et al. 1996). Conversely, the adrenal gland and other endocrine organs can produce cytokines (Judd et al. 2000), typically released by immune cells. Greater understanding of cytokine signaling has laid the groundwork for studying the effects of chronic stress.

Acute stress enhances the immune system to fight infections and to promote wound healing (Dhabhar and McEwen 1999; Viswanathan and Dhabhar 2005), but chronic stress dysregulates the immune system. Its dysregulation can have several major outcomes: increased susceptibility to infection (Cohen et al. 1991), delayed wound healing (Kiecolt-Glaser et al. 1993, 1995), an increase in inflammatory molecules in the circulation (Kiecolt-Glaser et al. 2003), and decreased response to immunization (Glaser et al. 1999, 2000).

In chronically stressed humans (Kiecolt-Glaser et al. 2003, 2005), such as those caring for a spouse with Alzheimer's dementia, a dysregulated immune system can lead to delayed early-phase wound healing and a decreased response to influenza vaccinations. In a study that followed such caregivers for 6 years, the rate of increase in one proinflammatory cytokine (IL-6) was 4 times higher than in age-matched noncaregiving control subjects (Kiecolt-Glaser et al. 2003). IL-6, which is increased in most of the diseases of aging, such as coronary heart disease and cancer, has been found to be increased by cigarette smoking, sedentary life style, obesity, and chronic stress. Higher blood concentrations of proinflammatory cytokines were associated with slower healing times in skin wounds in humans (Kiecolt-Glaser et al. 2005). Finally, chronic stress is often associated with fatigue (Teel and Press 1999; Wessely et al. 1998). Although the responsible mechanisms are not known, sleep disorders, depression, and increase in proinflammatory cytokines may all play a role. Studies on cytokines, the inflammatory response, and the immune system provide a framework for understanding how chronic stress might be associated with such a broad array of autoimmune and age-related diseases (Elenkov et al. 2005; Maggio et al. 2006).

Cardiovascular System

In the acute stress response, the sympathetic nervous system stimulates the heart to beat faster, the heart then pumps more glucose to muscles and organs, which provides energy and increased mobility. If glucose stores are insufficient, the body relies on fatty acids from adipose tissue as a backup energy source. With the surge in heart rate comes higher blood pressure against the wall of the artery and an increase in the clotting protein fibrinogen, which protects against blood loss. Chronic stress disturbs those normal cardiovascular functions. Prospective epidemiologic studies that followed people over many years found a relationship between chronic stress and the development of hypertension and other cardiac events (Pickering 2004; Steptoe et al. 2004; Timio et al. 2001).

Alterations in cardiovascular function are integrated with pathologic changes in the immune and endocrine systems. Chronic stress induces cardiovascular abnormalities that appear to be the result of chronic inflammation; chronic inflammation might cause or contribute to early pathologic abnormalities that might progress to disease or disability. The early pathologic changes include abnormalities in heart rate and blood pressure, vascular inflammation, and atherosclerosis.

Acute stress induces immediate rises in heart rate and blood pressure that reverse once the threat disappears. Chronic forms of stress might prolong cardiac reactivity and lead to hypertension and cardiovascular disease. Cardiac reactivity is reflected in blood pressure and heart rate. Several studies have shown that couples that have normal or elevated blood pressure and experience chronic marital distress display greater cardiac reactivity when confronted with a stressful task related to marital conflict, compared to couples without chronic marital distress (Carels et al. 1998; Ewart et al. 1991). Cardiac reactivity is triggered by the sympathetic nervous system's releasing epinephrine to the heart muscle, although other stress hormones (for example, angiotensin II, a vasoconstrictor released by the kidney on stimulation by epinephrine) are also involved (Black and Garbutt 2002).

For decades, chronic stress has been recognized as a risk factor for atherosclerosis[2] and coronary artery disease (Rozanski et al. 1999). The mechanisms underlying the association include long-term immune and endocrine alterations that are associated with chronic stress. The changes include a long-term increase in cortisol, which leads to fat deposition, obesity, increased circulating fatty acids and triglycerides, insulin resistance, activation of the renin-angiotensin system, and a shift towards production of proinflammatory cytokines.

Those endocrine and immune abnormalities are integral to understanding the origins of atherosclerosis as a progressive disease caused by prolonged inflammation of the vascular walls (Greaves and Channon 2002; Libby 2002). The inflammation usually, but not always, occurs in conjunction with higher concentrations of circulating lipids. Indeed, a substantial fraction of people who have cardiovascular disease do not have the traditional risk factor, increased low-density lipoproteins (LDLs) (Libby 2002). Chronic or repeated stress may be the cause of low-

[2]Atherosclerosis can result from fatty deposits on the inner lining of arteries, and calcification of the wall of the arteries. Arteriosclerosis includes a variety of conditions that cause thickening of artery walls and the loss of their elasticity as a result of sustained elevations in blood pressure (hypertension).

grade inflammatory processes that set in motion the pathologic changes that lead to cardiovascular disease (Black and Garbutt 2002; Black et al. 2006). That hypothesis draws from evidence that during the acute stress response, cortisol, catecholamines, angiotensin, and other stress hormones induce the liver and abdominal fat tissue to release proinflammatory cytokines and other inflammatory mediators. Inflammatory molecules, when increased for a long time, lead to a chronic state of inflammation, especially in abdominal fat and vasculature, which contribute to insulin resistance. Inflammation in the vasculature is manifested by recruitment and adherence of white blood cells to the vascular lining and their migration to the inner portions of the lining, binding of receptors to LDL particles, and growth of fibrous tissue. Those processes set the stage for plaque development (Libby 2002). A key marker of the inflammatory process in the circulatory system is C-reactive protein, an independent predictor of cardiovascular risk (Kardys et al. 2006; Libby 2002). In a prospective study, older adults who were current or former caregivers for Alzheimer's disease patients and harbored chronic hostility or pain had more inflammation, as measured by C-reactive protein, when other risk factors were accounted for, than did noncaregiver controls (Graham et al. 2006).

Gastrointestinal System and Brain-Gut Axis

Research is advancing our understanding of the interaction between stress and emotional trauma and the effects on the brain-gut axis, particularly with respect to irritable bowel syndrome (IBS) and other functional gastrointestinal disorders, such as functional dyspepsia (Dilley et al. 2005; Drossman 2005; Longstreth et al. 2006). IBS is the most common gastrointestinal condition seen in primary-care or gastroenterology practice; it is clinically manifested by symptoms of abdominal pain and altered bowel habit (for example, diarrhea, constipation, or both). Those symptoms are produced and amplified by gut-related stressors (such as eating, physical activity, and hormonal changes) or by other stressors, such as abuse, a history of trauma, or psychosocial comorbidities. The stressors appear to disrupt the brain-gut neurophysiologic regulatory pathways that alter intestinal motility and visceral sensation thresholds either centrally or peripherally.

Figure 4-4 shows the relative prevalence of IBS according to severity and shows the relative contributions of peripheral and psychosocial factors to severity. In effect, more severe psychosocial disturbance, including abuse and war trauma, leads to greater symptom reporting, poorer health status, greater psychologic comorbidity, and poorer quality of life.

Several lines of evidence support the concept of dysregulation of stress circuitry in IBS that is linked to and affects gut function (and vice versa). The evidence includes altered CRH and corticotropin reactivity to stress and an increased gut response (motility and pain) to CRH (Dinan et al. 2006; Fukudo et al. 1998; Sagami et al. 2004; Tache et al. 2005) which can be blocked by CRH antagonists (Sagami et al. 2004); increased mucosal inflammatory activity (Chadwick et al. 2002); stress-caused loss of the integrity of the intestinal mucosal barrier to bacterial pathogens and other toxins, which in turn causes entry or release of toxic substances that lead to inflammation and nerve sensitivity (Barbara et al. 2006, 2007; Soderholm et al. 2002; Yang et al. 2006); and altered brain regulation of incoming visceral pain signals leading to an increased pain experience that is enhanced by stress (Chang et al. 2003; Drossman et al. 2003; Naliboff et al. 2001; Ringel et al. 2003a,b). There is also evidence that the mediating mechanisms of reduction in pain can be evaluated with brain imaging (Drossman et al. 2003).

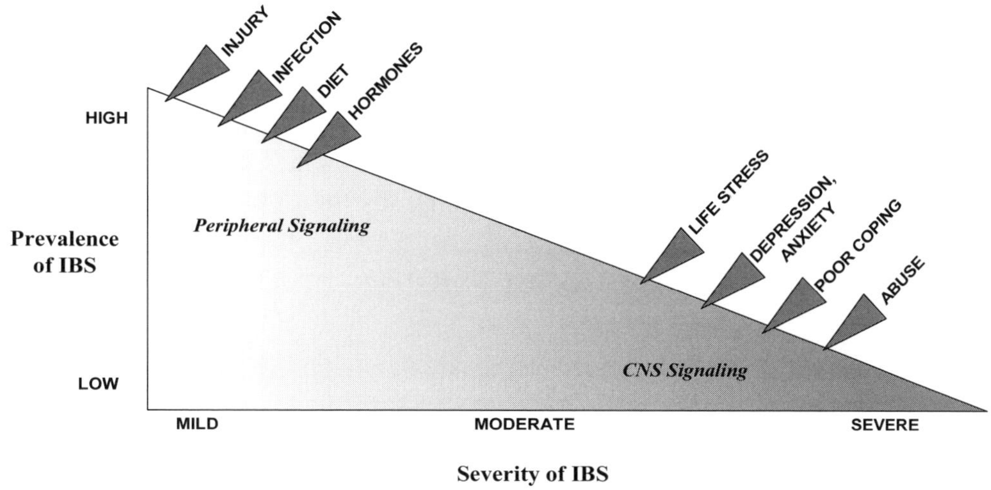

FIGURE 4-4 The brain-gut axis and IBS. Relative prevalence of IBS according to severity, and relative contributions of peripheral (left side of triangle) and psychosocial (right side of triangle) factors to severity. Most patients have mild to moderate IBS symptoms with increased peripheral-nerve signaling. However, a smaller group of patients with moderate to severe symptoms also have impaired modulation of pain at the CNS level, which is enabled by psychosocial factors (such as trauma, abuse, life stress, psychosocial comorbidities, and poor coping). These patients experience increased symptoms at the level of the CNS signaling. Factors that may contribute to CNS signaling include life stress and abuse.

Activation of IBS symptoms results from physiologic dysfunction that occurs peripherally (for example, motility disturbances or intestinal infection with inflammation). The peripheral stimuli send signals from the colon up the spinal cord to the thalamus and then to the brain via two pathways. The brain regions innervated by those pathways, which are activated in response to painful colorectal stimuli, include the somatosensory cortex—the area responsible for localization and intensity of peripheral sensations—and the limbic system, including the thalamus, insula, amygdala, and anterior cingulate cortex, which is linked to emotional stress and cognitive interpretation of pain. The brain has the ability to turn down the incoming signals through descending inhibitory pathways that modulate pain transmission and incoming signals are thus downregulated at the level of the spinal cord. As discussed earlier, CRH secretion and the HPA axis can also regulate inflammation, including that of the bowel mucosa. In IBS, however, the normal regulatory mechanisms of the brain-gut axis are dysfunctional, and there is impaired regulation of visceral pain (Naliboff et al. 2001) and altered HPA reactivity. The latter disrupts normal control of mucosal immune function that results in inflammation via cytokine activation (Dinan et al. 2006). With brain imaging, it can be shown that psychosocial difficulties (such as anxiety and life stress, including abuse or trauma, hypervigilance, and maladaptive coping) can impair those regulatory mechanisms (Drossman 2005). The presence and intensity of symptoms depends on the degree of activity of the peripheral signals and how they are modulated by the CNS in the face of stress or other modifying factors.

That model can be generalized to include other medical conditions. Most people with fibromyalgia, chronic fatigue, or other pain syndromes will have milder symptoms because their dysfunction is mostly peripheral, with little input from the CNS. But patients with more severe symptoms, greater symptom reporting, greater psychosocial disturbance, and poorer health status and quality of life will have greater CNS contributions to their symptoms. With increasing CNS dysregulation, the ability to filter incoming peripheral and visceral signals is impaired, and a person will report more symptoms (Chang et al. 2003; Clauw and Chrousos 1997; Sternberg 1995); this helps to explain the clinical similarity of those conditions when they are severe.

CONCLUSIONS

The stress response, the body's reaction to stress, can be life-saving (and be adaptive) in the short term when a person confronts immediate stressors but can lead to illness or disease (and be maladaptive) in the long term when stressors are severe, recurrent, or persistent. In response to deployment-related stress, physiologic changes occur in the body, may persist for a long time after deployment has ended, and may result in symptoms and disorders that appear soon after exposure to the stressor or become evident only years later.

Some biologic factors and life experiences can modify a person's response to stress, including genes, early-life events, and the degree to which the stressor is perceived to be controllable. Those factors might help to explain the differences in people's reactions to stress and the development of subsequent health effects.

The studies discussed in this chapter provide a context for understanding why people deployed to a war zone may report more symptoms than people who are not deployed—the stress response results in a cascade of physiologic changes that can have profound effects on multiple organ systems. War-zone stressors might produce disruption in brain systems that mediate responses to stress and in central pain regulatory pathways that can result in greater reporting of physical and emotional symptoms. The continuation of altered physiologic states over months and years can contribute to the accumulation of a chronic stress burden that has adverse long-term health consequences. The possible long-term manifestations of those altered states in veterans are discussed in Chapters 5, 6, and 7.

Much progress has been made in understanding the physiologic mechanisms of the stress response, particularly in animal models, but work remains to be done in human studies. Research on the effect of stressors on the endocrine, immune, cardiovascular, and gastrointestinal systems demonstrates the complexity of the interactions between those systems.

REFERENCES

Alheid GF, Heimer L. 1988. New perspectives in basal forebrain organization of special relevance for neuropsychiatric disorders: The striatopallidal, amygdaloid, and corticopetal components of substantia innominata. *Neuroscience* 27(1):1-39.

Amat J, Baratta MV, Paul E, Bland ST, Watkins LR, Maier SF. 2005. Medial prefrontal cortex determined how stressor controllability affects behavior and dorsal raphe nucleus. *Nature Neurosciences* 8:365-371.

Anda RF, Williamson DF, Escobedo LG, Mast EE, Giovino GA, Remington PL. 1990. Depression and the dynamics of smoking. A national perspective. *Journal of the American Medical Association* 264(12):1541-1545.

Barbara G, Stanghellini V, De Giorgio R, Corinaldesi R. 2006. Functional gastrointestinal disorders and mast cells: Implications for therapy. *Neurogastroenterology and Motility* 18(1):6-17.

Barbara G, Wang B, Stanghellini V, de Giorgio R, Cremon C, Di Nardo G, Trevisani M, Campi B, Geppetti P, Tonini M, Bunnett NW, Grundy D, Corinaldesi R. 2007. Mast cell-dependent excitation of visceral-nociceptive sensory neurons in irritable bowel syndrome. *Gastroenterology* 132(1):26-37.

Barr CS, Newman TK, Lindell S, Shannon C, Champoux M, Lesch KP, Suomi SJ, Goldman D, Higley JD. 2004. Interaction between serotonin transporter gene variation and rearing condition in alcohol preference and consumption in female primates. *Archives of General Psychiatry* 61(11):1146-1152.

Black DW, Blum N, Letuchy E, Carney Doebbeling C, Forman-Hoffman VL, Doebbeling BN. 2006. Borderline personality disorder and traits in veterans: Psychiatric comorbidity, healthcare utilization, and quality of life along a continuum of severity. *CNS Spectrums* 11(9):680-689.

Black PH, Garbutt LD. 2002. Stress, inflammation and cardiovascular disease. *Journal of Psychosomatic Research* 52(1):1-23.

Bonne O, Grillon C, Vythilingam M, Neumeister A, Charney DS. 2004. Adaptive and maladaptive psychobiological responses to severe psychological stress: Implications for the discovery of novel pharmacotherapy. *Neuroscience and Biobehavioral Reviews* 28(1):65-94.

Brady KT, Sinha R. 2005. Co-occurring mental and substance use disorders: The neurobiological effects of chronic stress. *American Journal of Psychiatry* 162(8):1483-1493.

Brindley DN. 1995. Role of glucocorticoids and fatty acids in the impairment of lipid metabolism observed in the metabolic syndrome. *International Journal of Obesity and Related Metabolic Disorders* 19(Suppl 1):S69-S75.

Carels RA, Szczepanski R, Blumenthal JA, Sherwood A. 1998. Blood pressure reactivity and marital distress in employed women. *Psychosomatic Medicine* 60(5):639-643.

Caspi A, McClay J, Moffitt TE, Mill J, Martin J, Craig IW, Taylor A, Poulton R. 2002. Role of genotype in the cycle of violence in maltreated children. *Science* 297(5582):851-854.

Chadwick VS, Chen W, Shu D, Paulus B, Bethwaite P, Tie A, Wilson I. 2002. Activation of the mucosal immune system in irritable bowel syndrome. *Gastroenterology* 122(7):1778-1783.

Chang L, Berman S, Mayer EA, Suyenobu B, Derbyshire S, Naliboff B, Vogt B, FitzGerald L, Mandelkern MA. 2003. Brain responses to visceral and somatic stimuli in patients with irritable bowel syndrome with and without fibromyalgia. *American Journal of Gastroenterology* 98(6):1354-1361.

Charney DS. 2004. Psychobiological mechanisms of resilience and vulnerability: Implications for successful adaptation to extreme stress. *American Journal of Psychiatry* 161(2):195-216.

Chourbaji S, Zacher C, Sanchis-Segura C, Dormann C, Vollmayr B, Gass P. 2005. Learned helplessness: Validity and reliability of depressive-like states in mice. *Brain Research. Brain Research Protocols* 16(1-3):70-78.

Chrousos GP, Gold PW. 1992. The concepts of stress and stress system disorders. Overview of physical and behavioral homeostasis. *Journal of the American Medical Association* 267(9):1244-1252.

Clauw DJ, Chrousos GP. 1997. Chronic pain and fatigue syndromes: Overlapping clinical and neuroendocrine features and potential pathogenic mechanisms. *Neuroimmunomodulation* 4(3):134-153.

Cohen S, Tyrrell DA, Smith AP. 1991. Psychological stress and susceptibility to the common cold. *New England Journal of Medicine* 325(9):606-612.

Coplan JD, Andrews MW, Rosenblum LA, Owens MJ, Friedman S, Gorman JM, Nemeroff CB. 1996. Persistent elevations of cerebrospinal fluid concentrations of corticotropin-releasing factor in adult nonhuman primates exposed to early-life stressors: Implications for the pathophysiology of mood and anxiety disorders. *Proceedings of the National Academy of Sciences of the United States of America* 93(4):1619-1623.

Dallman MF, Pecoraro N, Akana SF, La Fleur SE, Gomez F, Houshyar H, Bell ME, Bhatnagar S, Laugero KD, Manalo S. 2003. Chronic stress and obesity: A new view of "comfort food." *Proceedings of the National Academy of Sciences of the United States of America* 100(20):11696-11701.

Danese A, Pariante CM, Caspi A, Taylor A, Poulton R. 2007. Childhood maltreatment predicts adult inflammation in a life-course study. *Proceedings of the National Academy of Sciences of the United States of America* 104(4):1319-1324.

Davis M, Whalen PJ. 2001. The amygdala: Vigilance and emotion. *Molecular Psychiatry* 6(1):13-34.

Dhabhar FS. 2000. Acute stress enhances while chronic stress suppresses skin immunity. The role of stress hormones and leukocyte trafficking. *Annals of the New York Academy of Sciences* 917:876-893.

Dhabhar FS, McEwen BS. 1999. Enhancing versus suppressive effects of stress hormones on skin immune function. *Proceedings of the National Academy of Sciences of the United States of America* 96(3):1059-1064.

Dilley J, Jones M, Drossman D. 2005. Understanding the mind-body connection in the functional GI disorders: Anatomic and physiologic relationships between the central nervous system and digestive tract. In: Jones M, Crowell M, editors. *Contemporary Diagnosis and Management of Functional Digestive Disorders*. 1st Ed. Newton, PA: Handbooks in Health Care.

Dinan TG, Quigley EM, Ahmed SM, Scully P, O'Brien S, O'Mahony L, O'Mahony S, Shanahan F, Keeling PW. 2006. Hypothalamic-pituitary-gut axis dysregulation in irritable bowel syndrome: Plasma cytokines as a potential biomarker? *Gastroenterology* 130(2):304-311.

Drossman DA. 2005. Brain imaging and its implications for studying centrally targeted treatments in irritable bowel syndrome: A primer for gastroenterologists. *Gut* 54(5):569-573.

Drossman DA, Ringel Y, Vogt BA, Leserman J, Lin W, Smith JK, Whitehead W. 2003. Alterations of brain activity associated with resolution of emotional distress and pain in a case of severe irritable bowel syndrome. *Gastroenterology* 124(3):754-761.

Dube SR, Anda RF, Felitti VJ, Edwards VJ, Croft JB. 2002. Adverse childhood experiences and personal alcohol abuse as an adult. *Addictive Behaviors* 27(5):713-725.

Eisch AJ, Harburg GC. 2006. Opiates, psychostimulants, and adult hippocampal neurogenesis: Insights for addiction and stem cell biology. *Hippocampus* 16(3):271-286.

Elenkov IJ, Iezzoni DG, Daly A, Harris AG, Chrousos GP. 2005. Cytokine dysregulation, inflammation and well-being. *Neuroimmunomodulation* 12(5):255-269.

Ewart CK, Taylor CB, Kraemer HC, Agras WS. 1991. High blood pressure and marital discord: Not being nasty matters more than being nice. *Health Psychology* 10(3):155-163.

Fukudo S, Nomura T, Hongo M. 1998. Impact of corticotropin-releasing hormone on gastrointestinal motility and adrenocorticotropic hormone in normal controls and patients with irritable bowel syndrome. *Gut* 42(6):845-849.

Glaser R, Rabin B, Chesney M, Cohen S, Natelson B. 1999. Stress-induced immunomodulation: Implications for infectious diseases? *Journal of the American Medical Association* 281(24):2268-2670.

Glaser R, Sheridan J, Malarkey WB, MacCallum RC, Kiecolt-Glaser JK. 2000. Chronic stress modulates the immune response to a pneumococcal pneumonia vaccine. *Psychosomatic Medicine* 62(6):804-807.

Gold PE, Van Buskirk RB. 1975. Facilitation of time-dependent memory processes with posttrial epinephrine injections. *Behavioral Biology* 13(2):145-153.

Graham JE, Robles TF, Kiecolt-Glaser JK, Malarkey WB, Bissell MG, Glaser R. 2006. Hostility and pain are related to inflammation in older adults. *Brain, Behavior, and Immunity* 20(4):389-400.

Greaves DR, Channon KM. 2002. Inflammation and immune responses in atherosclerosis. *Trends in Immunology* 23(11):535-541.

Hariri AR, Drabant EM, Weinberger DR. 2006. Imaging genetics: Perspectives from studies of genetically driven variation in serotonin function and corticolimbic affective processing. *Biological Psychiatry* 59(10):888-897.

Harlow H. 1974. *Learning to Love*. New York: Jason Aronson.

Herman JP, Schafer MK, Young EA, Thompson R, Douglass J, Akil H, Watson SJ. 1989. Evidence for hippocampal regulation of neuroendocrine neurons of the hypothalamo-pituitary-adrenocortical axis. *Journal of Neuroscience* 9(9):3072-3082.

Ichise M, Vines DC, Gura T, Anderson GM, Suomi SJ, Higley JD, Innis RB. 2006. Effects of early life stress on [11C] DASB positron emission tomography imaging of serotonin transporters in adolescent peer- and mother-reared rhesus monkeys. *Journal of Neuroscience* 26(17):4638-4643.

Judd AM, Call GB, Barney M, McIlmoil CJ, Balls AG, Adams A, Oliveira GK. 2000. Possible function of IL-6 and TNF as intraadrenal factors in the regulation of adrenal steroid secretion. *Annals of the New York Academy of Sciences* 917:628-637.

Kardys I, Knetsch AM, Bleumink GS, Deckers JW, Hofman A, Stricker BH, Witteman JC. 2006. C-reactive protein and risk of heart failure. The Rotterdam Study. *American Heart Journal* 152(3):514-520.

Kempermann G, Neumann H. 2003. Neuroscience. Microglia: The enemy within? *Science* 302(5651):1689-1690.

Kiecolt-Glaser JK, Malarkey WB, Chee M, Newton T, Cacioppo JT, Mao HY, Glaser R. 1993. Negative behavior during marital conflict is associated with immunological down-regulation. *Psychosomatic Medicine* 55(5):395-409.

Kiecolt-Glaser JK, Marucha PT, Malarkey WB, Mercado AM, Glaser R. 1995. Slowing of wound healing by psychological stress. *Lancet* 346(8984):1194-1196.

Kiecolt-Glaser JK, Preacher KJ, MacCallum RC, Atkinson C, Malarkey WB, Glaser R. 2003. Chronic stress and age-related increases in the proinflammatory cytokine IL-6. *Proceedings of the National Academy of Sciences of the United States of America* 100(15):9090-9095.

Kiecolt-Glaser JK, Loving TJ, Stowell JR, Malarkey WB, Lemeshow S, Dickinson SL, Glaser R. 2005. Hostile marital interactions, proinflammatory cytokine production, and wound healing. *Archives of General Psychiatry* 62(12):1377-1384.

Levine S. 1962. Plasma-free corticosteroid response to electric shock in rats stimulated in infancy. *Science* 135:795-796.

Libby P. 2002. Inflammation in atherosclerosis. *Nature* 420(6917):868-874.

Liston C, Miller MM, Goldwater DS, Radley JJ, Rocher AB, Hof PR, Morrison JH, McEwen BS. 2006. Stress-induced alterations in prefrontal cortical dendritic morphology predict selective impairments in perceptual attentional set-shifting. *Journal of Neuroscience* 26(30):7870-7874.

Liu D, Diorio J, Tannenbaum B, Caldji C, Francis D, Freedman A, Sharma S, Pearson D, Plotsky PM, Meaney MJ. 1997. Maternal care, hippocampal glucocorticoid receptors, and hypothalamic-pituitary-adrenal responses to stress. *Science* 277(5332):1659-1662.

Longstreth G, Thompson W, Chey W, Houghton L, Mearin F, Spiller R. 2006. Functional bowel disorders. In: Drossman D, Corazziari E, Delvaux M, Spiller R, Talley N, Thompson W, editors. *Rome III: The Functional Gastrointestinal Disorders*. 3rd Ed. McLean, VA: Degnon Associates, Inc.

MacPherson A, Dinkel K, Sapolsky R. 2005. Glucocorticoids worsen excitotoxin-induced expression of pro-inflammatory cytokines in hippocampal cultures. *Experimental Neurology* 194(2):376-383.

Maggio M, Guralnik JM, Longo DL, Ferrucci L. 2006. Interleukin-6 in aging and chronic disease: a magnificent pathway. *The Journals of Gerontology. Series A, Biological Sciences and Medical Sciences* 61(6):575-584.

Maier SF, Watkins LR. 1998. Stressor controllability, anxiety and serotonin. *Cognitive Therapy and Research* 22(6):595-613.

Maier SF, Watkins LR. 2005. Stressor controllability and learned helplessness: The roles of the dorsal raphe nucleus, serotonin, and corticotropin-releasing factor. *Neuroscience and Biobehavioral Reviews* 29(4-5):829-841.

Maier SF, Seligman MEP, Solomon RL. 1969. Pavlovian fear conditioning and learned helplessness. In: Campbell BA, Church RM, editors. *Punishment*. New York: Appleton-Century-Crofts.

Maier SF, Busch CR, Maswood S, Grahn RE, Watkins LR. 1995. The dorsal raphe nucleus is a site of action mediating the behavioral effects of the benzodiazepine receptor inverse agonist DMCM. *Behavioral Neuroscience* 109(4):759-766.

Malarkey WB, Mills PJ. 2007. Endocrinology: The active partner in PNI research. *Brain, Behavior, and Immunity* 21(2):161-168.

Mathew SJ, Coplan JD, Smith EL, Scharf BA, Owens MJ, Nemeroff CB, Mann JJ, Gorman JM, Rosenblum LA. 2002. Cerebrospinal fluid concentrations of biogenic amines and corticotropin-releasing factor in adolescent non-human primates as a function of the timing of adverse early rearing. *Stress* 5(3):185-193.

McDougall SJ, Widdop RE, Lawrence AJ. 2004. Medial prefrontal cortical integration of psychological stress in rats. *The European Journal of Neuroscience* 20(9):2430-2440.

McEwen B, Lasley E. 2002. *The End of Stress as We Know It.* Washington, DC: Joseph Henry Press.

McEwen BS. 1998. Protective and damaging effects of stress mediators. *New England Journal of Medicine* 338(3):171-179.

McEwen BS. 1999a. Stress and hippocampal plasticity. *Annual Review of Neuroscience* 22:105-122.

McEwen BS. 1999b. Stress and the aging hippocampus. *Frontiers in Neuroendocrinology* 20(1):49-70.

McEwen BS. 2002a. The neurobiology and neuroendocrinology of stress. Implications for post-traumatic stress disorder from a basic science perspective. *The Psychiatric Clinics of North America* 25(2):469-494, ix.

McEwen BS. 2002b. Sex, stress and the hippocampus: Allostasis, allostatic load and the aging process. *Neurobiology of Aging* 23(5):921-939.

McEwen BS. 2005. Stressed or stressed out: What is the difference? *The Journal of Neuropsychiatry and Clinical Neurosciences* 30(5):315-318.

McEwen BS. 2006. Sleep deprivation as a neurobiologic and physiologic stressor: Allostasis and allostatic load. *Metabolism* 55(10 Suppl 2):S20-S23.

McEwen BS. 2007. Physiology and neurobiology of stress and adaptation: Central role of the brain. *Physiological Reviews* 87(3):873-904.

McEwen BS, Wingfield JC. 2003. The concept of allostasis in biology and biomedicine. *Hormones and Behavior* 43(1):2-15.

McEwen BS, Weiss JM, Schwartz LS. 1968. Selective retention of corticosterone by limbic structures in rat brain. *Nature* 220(5170):911-912.

McEwen BS, Gould EA, Sakai RR. 1992. The vulnerability of the hippocampus to protective and destructive effects of glucocorticoids in relation to stress. *The British Journal of Psychiatry.* (Suppl 15):18-23.

McGaugh J, Introini-Collison I, Cahill L, Kim M, Liang K. 1992. Involvement of the amygdala in neuromodulatory influences on memory storage. In: Aggleton J, editor. *The Amygdala: Neurobiological Aspects of Emotion, Memory, and Mental Dysfunction.* New York: Wiley-Liss. Pp. 431-451.

Meaney MJ, Aitken DH, Bodnoff SR, Iny LJ, Tatarewicz JE, Sapolsky RM. 1985. Early postnatal handling alters glucocorticoid receptor concentrations in selected brain regions. *Behavioral Neuroscience* 99(4):765-770.

Meaney MJ, Aitken DH, van Berkel C, Bhatnagar S, Sapolsky RM. 1988. Effect of neonatal handling on age-related impairments associated with the hippocampus. *Science* 239(4841 Pt 1):766-768.

Mineka S, Suomi SJ. 1978. Social separation in monkeys. *Psychological Bulletin* 85(6):1376-1400.

Mirescu C, Gould E. 2006. Stress and adult neurogenesis. *Hippocampus* 16(3):233-238.

Monje ML, Toda H, Palmer TD. 2003. Inflammatory blockade restores adult hippocampal neurogenesis. *Science* 302(5651):1760-1765.

Naliboff BD, Derbyshire SW, Munakata J, Berman S, Mandelkern M, Chang L, Mayer EA. 2001. Cerebral activation in patients with irritable bowel syndrome and control subjects during rectosigmoid stimulation. *Psychosomatic Medicine* 63(3):365-375.

Overmier JB, Seligman ME. 1967. Effects of inescapable shock upon subsequent escape and avoidance responding. *Journal of Comparative and Physiological Psychology* 63(1):28-33.

Pfaff DW. 2005. *Brain Arousal and the Information Theory: Neural and Genetic Mechanisms*. Boston, MA: Harvard University Press.

Pham K, Nacher J, Hof PR, McEwen BS. 2003. Repeated restraint stress suppresses neurogenesis and induces biphasic PSA-NCAM expression in the adult rat dentate gyrus. *The European Journal of Neuroscience* 17(4):879-886.

Pickering TG. 2004. Reflections in hypertension: Work and blood pressure. *Journal of Clinical Hypertension* (Greenwich, Conn) 6(7):403-405.

Radley JJ, Morrison JH. 2005. Repeated stress and structural plasticity in the brain. *Ageing Research Reviews* 4(2):271-287.

Radley JJ, Arias CM, Sawchenko PE. 2006. Regional differentiation of the medial prefrontal cortex in regulating adaptive responses to acute emotional stress. *Journal of Neuroscience* 26(50):12967-12976.

Reaven G, Abbasi F, McLaughlin T. 2004. Obesity, insulin resistance, and cardiovascular disease. *Recent Progress in Hormone Research* 59:207-223.

Reiche EM, Nunes SO, Morimoto HK. 2004. Stress, depression, the immune system, and cancer. *The Lancet Oncology* 5(10):617-625.

Ringel Y, Drossman DA, Turkington TG, Bradshaw B, Hawk TC, Bangdiwala S, Coleman RE, Whitehead WE. 2003a. Regional brain activation in response to rectal distension in patients with irritable bowel syndrome and the effect of a history of abuse. *Digestive Diseases and Sciences* 48(9):1774-1781.

Ringel Y, Drossman D, Leserman J, Lin W, Liu H, Vogt B, Whitehead W. 2003b. Association of anterior cingulate cortex (ACC) activation with psychosocial distress and pain reports. *Gastroenterology* 124(4):A-97.

Roozendaal B, Okuda S, de Quervain DJ, McGaugh JL. 2006. Glucocorticoids interact with emotion-induced noradrenergic activation in influencing different memory functions. *Neuroscience* 138(3):901-910.

Rosmond R, Lapidus L, Marin P, Bjorntorp P. 1996. Mental distress, obesity and body fat distribution in middle-aged men. *Obesity Research* 4(3):245-252.

Rozanski A, Blumenthal JA, Kaplan J. 1999. Impact of psychological factors on the pathogenesis of cardiovascular disease and implications for therapy. *Circulation* 99(16):2192-2217.

Sagami Y, Shimada Y, Tayama J, Nomura T, Satake M, Endo Y, Shoji T, Karahashi K, Hongo M, Fukudo S. 2004. Effect of a corticotropin releasing hormone receptor antagonist on colonic sensory and motor function in patients with irritable bowel syndrome. *Gut* 53(7):958-964.

Sapolsky RM. 2003. Stress and plasticity in the limbic system. *Neurochemical Research* 28(11):1735-1742.

Sapolsky RM, Krey LC, McEwen BS. 1986. The neuroendocrinology of stress and aging: The glucocorticoid cascade hypothesis. *Endocrine Reviews* 7(3):284-301.

Seligman ME, Maier SF. 1967. Failure to escape traumatic shock. *Journal of Experimental Psychology* 74(1):1-9.

Selye H. 1956. *The Stress of Life*. New York: McGraw-Hill.

Shin LM, Orr SP, Carson MA, Rauch SL, Macklin ML, Lasko NB, Peters PM, Metzger LJ, Dougherty DD, Cannistraro PA, Alpert NM, Fischman AJ, Pitman RK. 2004. Regional cerebral blood flow in the amygdala and medial prefrontal cortex during traumatic imagery in male and female Vietnam veterans with PTSD. *Archives of General Psychiatry* 61(2):168-176.

Shumyatsky GP, Malleret G, Shin RM, Takizawa S, Tully K, Tsvetkov E, Zakharenko SS, Joseph J, Vronskaya S, Yin D, Schubart UK, Kandel ER, Bolshakov VY. 2005. Stathmin, a gene enriched in the amygdala, controls both learned and innate fear. *Cell* 123(4):697-709.

Soderholm JD, Yang PC, Ceponis P, Vohra A, Riddell R, Sherman PM, Perdue MH. 2002. Chronic stress induces mast cell-dependent bacterial adherence and initiates mucosal inflammation in rat intestine. *Gastroenterology* 123(4):1099-1108.

Spiegel K, Tasali E, Penev P, Van Cauter E. 2004. Brief communication: Sleep curtailment in healthy young men is associated with decreased leptin levels, elevated ghrelin levels, and increased hunger and appetite. *Annals of Internal Medicine* 141(11):846-850.

Steptoe A, Siegrist J, Kirschbaum C, Marmot M. 2004. Effort-reward imbalance, overcommitment, and measures of cortisol and blood pressure over the working day. *Psychosomatic Medicine* 66(3):323-329.

Sternberg EM. 1995. Neuroendocrine factors in susceptibility to inflammatory disease: Focus on the hypothalamic-pituitary-adrenal axis. *Hormone Research* 43(4):159-161.

Tache Y, Million M, Nelson AG, Lamy C, Wang L. 2005. Role of corticotropin-releasing factor pathways in stress-related alterations of colonic motor function and viscerosensibility in female rodents. *Gender Medicine* 2(3):146-154.

Taheri S, Lin L, Austin D, Young T, Mignot E. 2004. Short sleep duration is associated with reduced leptin, elevated ghrelin, and increased body mass index. *PLoS Medicine* 1(3):e62.

Teel CS, Press AN. 1999. Fatigue among elders in caregiving and noncaregiving roles. *West Journal of Nursing Research* 21(4):498-514; discussion 514-520.

Thayer JF, Brosschot JF. 2005. Psychosomatics and psychopathology: Looking up and down from the brain. *Psychoneuroendocrinology* 30(10):1050-1058.

Timio M, Saronio P, Verdura C, Schiaroli M, Timio F, Monarca C. 2001. A link between psychosocial factors and blood pressure trend in women. *Physiology and Behavior* 73(3):359-363.

Tracey KJ. 2002. The inflammatory reflex. *Nature* 420(6917):853-859.

Vermetten E, Bremner JD. 2002. Circuits and systems in stress. II. Applications to neurobiology and treatment in posttraumatic stress disorder. *Depression and Anxiety* 16(1):14-38.

Viswanathan K, Dhabhar FS. 2005. Stress-induced enhancement of leukocyte trafficking into sites of surgery or immune activation. *Proceedings of the National Academy of Sciences of the United States of America* 102(16):5808-5813.

Vollmayr B, Henn FA. 2001. Learned helplessness in the rat: Improvements in validity and reliability. *Brain Research. Brain Research Protocols* 8(1):1-7.

Vyas A, Mitra R, Shankaranarayana Rao BS, Chattarji S. 2002. Chronic stress induces contrasting patterns of dendritic remodeling in hippocampal and amygdaloid neurons. *Journal of Neuroscience* 22(15):6810-6818.

Weiss JM. 1968. Effects of coping responses on stress. *Journal of Comparative and Physiological Psychology* 65(2):251-260.

Weiss JM, Goodman PA, Losito BG, Corrigan SA, Charry JM, Bailey WH. 1981. Behavioral depression produced by an uncontrollable stressor: Relationship to norepinephrine, dopamine, and serotonin levels in various regions of the rat brain. *Brain Research Reviews* 3:167-205.

Wessely S, Hotopf M, Sharpe M. 1998. *Chronic Fatigue and Its Syndromes*. New York: Oxford University Press.

Will MJ, Watkins LR, Maier SF. 1998. Uncontrollable stress potentiates morphine's rewarding properties. *Pharmacology, Biochemistry, and Behavior* 60(3):655-664.

Wu H, Devi R, Malarkey WB. 1996. Localization of growth hormone messenger ribonucleic acid in the human immune system—a Clinical Research Center study. *The Journal of Clinical Endocrinology and Metabolism* 81(3):1278-1282.

Yang PC, Jury J, Soderholm JD, Sherman PM, McKay DM, Perdue MH. 2006. Chronic psychological stress in rats induces intestinal sensitization to luminal antigens. *American Journal of Pathology* 168(1):104-114.

5

POSTTRAUMATIC STRESS DISORDER

Posttraumatic stress disorder (PTSD) is an anxiety disorder that is defined as resulting from exposure to a traumatic event. War-related traumatic events have been detailed in numerous studies (see Chapter 3). However, not everyone exposed to a war-zone trauma will develop PTSD, nor is the course of the disorder the same for everyone that does develop it. There are many factors that affect a person's response to a traumatic event and there is much research being done to elucidate the biological mechanisms of PTSD.

It is widely recognized that soldiers suffer psychologic consequences of combat (Jones 2006). The constellation of symptoms that has come to be known as PTSD was given other names in earlier wars. During the Civil War, "irritable heart" or "effort syndrome" featured shortness of breath, disturbed sleep, palpitations, and other symptoms. During World War I, effort syndrome was again diagnosed, as was "shell shock," which was first described in British soldiers evacuated from the trenches in France. Marked by blindness, muteness, and amnesia, shell shock was initially thought to be the result of brain concussion from nearby shell explosions, but over time it became clear that effort syndrome and shell shock had psychologic origins (Hyams et al. 1996; Shephard 2001). During World War II, physicians identified an acute psychologic syndrome commonly found in soldiers, which they referred to as battle fatigue or combat exhaustion, so named to avoid stigma and to imply that soldiers would recover naturally with food and rest. Although the sheer number of psychiatric casualties was high, many of the troops were returned to combat after treatment near the front line (Grob 1994; Shephard 2001). Nevertheless, in 1942-1945, 850,000 active-duty U.S. soldiers were admitted to military hospitals for neuropsychiatric care (Starr 1982). A persistent and chronic form of battle fatigue was described among those veterans (Friedman et al. 1994; Grob 1994; Southwick et al. 1994). In World War II, Grinker and Spiegel (1945) described cases of "war neurosis" in members of combat aircrews. The primary symptoms of war neurosis were restlessness, irritability, aggression, fatigue, sleep difficulties, anxiety, startle reaction, tension, depression, personality changes, memory disturbances, tremors, difficulty in concentrating, alcoholism, preoccupation with combat experiences, decrease in appetite, psychosomatic symptoms, irrational fears, and suspiciousness.

The experiences of World War II military psychiatrists were instrumental in spurring the profession into the modern era of psychiatric diagnosis. Military psychiatrists believed that psychiatric disorders among veterans of military combat were more pervasive and serious than had been anticipated before the war. They also believed, contrary to prevailing views, that psychological maladjustment could be triggered by external stress (Grob 1994). Their influence was felt in the first edition of the *Diagnostic and Statistical Manual of Mental Disorders* (*DSM*), published in 1952 by the American Psychiatric Association (APA).

After the Vietnam War, research demonstrated that many veterans, particularly those exposed to severe war-related trauma, and other traumatized populations such as Holocaust survivors, suffered from chronic psychologic problems that often resulted in social and occupational dysfunction. The strength of the evidence led to the formal recognition of PTSD as a psychiatric diagnosis in the third edition of *DSM* (*DSM-III*), published in 1980. Because the *DSM-III* provided a formal operational definition of PTSD, it presented a platform for large-scale studies of PTSD in Vietnam veterans and veterans of later wars.

In the sections below, the committee discusses the diagnosis and clinical features of PTSD; its prevalence in military populations; the course of the disorder; the comorbidity of PTSD with other psychiatric disorders and associated disability of people who have PTSD; risk and protective factors for PTSD; and finally the neurobiology of PTSD.

DIAGNOSIS AND CLINICAL FEATURES

People who are exposed to traumatic events react to them in different ways; some experience temporary distress, and others will go on to develop PTSD or other psychiatric disorders, such as major depression. The criteria for PTSD are listed in the fourth edition of the *DSM* (*DSM-IV-TR*) (Box 5-1) and require that the person have experienced, witnessed, or been confronted with an event that involves actual or threatened death, serious injury, or a threat to the physical integrity of self or others and that the person have responded with intense fear, helplessness, or horror. Symptoms must persist for a month or more and include three symptom clusters:

- Re-experiencing—intrusive recollections of a traumatic event, such as flashbacks or nightmares.
- Avoidance/numbing—efforts to avoid reminders of the event and numbing of emotions.
- Hyperarousal—manifested by, for example, difficulty in sleeping or jumpiness.

Finally, the person must have clinically significant distress or functional impairment resulting from the symptoms (APA 2000).

Two terms are used to describe PTSD in this report: lifetime and current. In lifetime PTSD, the person has met the criteria for a diagnosis of PTSD at some point and may or may not be symptomatic at the time of the assessment. The meaning of current PTSD varies by study; it can mean that the person met the criteria for PTSD at the time of the assessment, within the preceding month, within the preceding 3 months, 6 months, even 12 months. The committee used the terminology and timeframe for PTSD as given in each study. Lifetime and current PTSD may or may not be related to combat or deployment experiences; when PTSD has been related to combat or deployment experiences, the committee has included this information in its discussion.

PTSD should be assessed on the basis of a thorough diagnostic interview; structured or semistructured interviews, such as the Clinician-Administered PTSD Scale, the Structured Clinical Interview for *DSM-IV* (SCID), the Diagnostic Interview Schedule for *DSM-IV* (DIS-IV), and the Composite International Diagnostic Interview (CIDI) are examples of diagnostic interviews. However, many epidemiologic studies use screening instruments to assess the number and frequency of symptoms of PTSD, rather than a full diagnostic interview. Those screening instruments include the Department of Veterans Affairs (VA) Primary Care PTSD Screen, the PTSD Checklist (either military or civilian version), the Mississippi Scale for Combat-Related PTSD, and the Keane Scale of the Minnesota Multiphasic Personality Inventory (MMPI-PK).

BOX 5-1 *DSM-IV* Diagnostic Criteria for Posttraumatic Stress Disorder

A. The person has been exposed to a traumatic event in which both of the following were present:
- (1) The person experienced, witnessed, or was confronted with an event or events that involved actual or threatened death or serious injury, or a threat to the physical integrity of self or others.
- (2) The person's response involved intense fear, helplessness, or horror.

B. The traumatic event is persistently re-experienced in one (or more) of the following ways:
- (1) Recurrent and intrusive distressing recollections of the event, including images, thoughts, and/or perceptions;
- (2) Recurrent distressing dreams of the event;
- (3) Acting or feeling as if the traumatic event were recurring (includes a sense of reliving the experience, illusions, hallucinations, and/or dissociative flashback episodes, including those that occur on awakening or when intoxicated);
- (4) Intense psychological distress at exposure to internal or external cues that symbolize or resemble an aspect of the traumatic event;
- (5) Physiological reactivity on exposure to internal or external cues that symbolize or resemble an aspect of the traumatic event.

C. Persistent avoidance of stimuli associated with the trauma and numbing of general responsiveness (not present before the trauma), as indicated by at least three of the following:
- (1) efforts to avoid thoughts, feelings, and/or conversations associated with the trauma;
- (2) efforts to avoid activities, places, and/or people that arouse recollections of the trauma;
- (3) inability to recall an important aspect of the trauma;
- (4) markedly diminished interest or participation in significant activities;
- (5) feeling of detachment or estrangement from others;
- (6) restricted range of affect (e.g., inability to have loving feelings);
- (7) sense of a foreshortened future (e.g., does not expect to have a career, marriage, children, or a normal life span).

D. Persistent symptoms of increased arousal (not present before the trauma), as indicated by at least two of the following:
- (1) difficulty falling or staying asleep;
- (2) irritability or outbursts of anger;
- (3) difficulty concentrating;
- (4) hypervigilance;
- (5) exaggerated startle response.

E. Duration of the disturbance (symptoms in Criteria B, C, and D) is more than one (1) month.

F. The disturbance causes clinically significant distress and/or impairment in social, occupational, and/or other important areas of functioning.

SOURCE: Reprinted with permission from APA (2000).

PREVALENCE

The National Comorbidity Survey (NCS) conducted in 1990-1992 on a nationally representative sample of 5877 people, found the prevalence of lifetime PTSD to be 7.8% (5% in men and 10% in women) (Kessler et al. 1995). In the NCS replication conducted in 2001-2003 on 9282 people, Kessler et al. (2005b) found the prevalence of PTSD in the previous 12 months to be 3.5%. PTSD was assessed according to the World Health Organization World Mental Health Survey version of the CIDI. In a study of young adults in a health maintenance organization in an urban area, Breslau (2001a) estimated that about 8% of adults may experience lifetime PTSD, or about 15-24% of those who are exposed to traumatic events. Although women's exposure to traumatic events is estimated to be somewhat less than that of men, twice as many women develop PTSD (Breslau 2001a). In a comparison group of 500 civilians in the National Vietnam Veterans Readjustment Study (NVVRS), Kulka et al. (1990) found that 1.2% of men and 0.3% of women had current (6-month) PTSD.

Many people experience traumatic events. Some traumatic events are common and are associated with a relatively low prevalence of PTSD, such as the sudden death of a loved one; other, less common traumatic events, such as rape, are associated with a very high prevalence of PTSD (see Table 5-1). In the case of the 1995 Oklahoma City bombing, it was found that the postdisaster prevalence of PTSD was 34% among all cases identified in 4-8 months after the bombing (North et al. 1999).

TABLE 5-1 Prevalence of Traumatic Events and PTSD in Men and Women

	Prevalence of Event (%)		Prevalence of Lifetime PTSD in Response to Event (%)	
Traumatic Event	**Men**	**Women**	**Men**	**Women**
Rape	0.7	9.2	65.0	45.9
Molestation	2.8	12.3	12.2	26.5
Physical assault	11.1	6.9	1.8	21.3
Accident	25.0	13.8	6.3	8.8
Natural disaster	18.9	15.2	3.7	5.4
Witnessed death or injury	40.1	18.6	9.1	2.8
Learned about a traumatic event	63.1	61.8	1.4	3.2
Sudden death of a loved one	61.1	59.0	12.6	16.2

SOURCE: Adapted with permission from Yehuda (2002).

Combat is one of the most traumatic events a person can experience. Men who named combat as their "worst lifetime traumatic event" were found to be 7 times as likely to have PTSD than men naming other experiences (Prigerson et al. 2001). Nearly 30% of all cases of PTSD in the U.S. population are attributed to combat experience (Prigerson et al. 2002). Numerous studies in military populations have provided estimates of the prevalence of PTSD; some of those are discussed below.

Operation Enduring Freedom and Operation Iraqi Freedom

In U.S. combat troops deployed to Afghanistan and Iraq, the risk of having PTSD 3-4 months after their return was 6.2% for Army troops returning from Afghanistan (odds ratio [OR] 1.26, 95% confidence interval [CI] 0.97-1.64) and 12.9% for Army (OR 2.84, 95% CI 2.17-3.72) and 12.2% for Marines (OR 2.66, 95% CI 2.01-3.51) returning from Iraq. The risk of having PTSD before deployment was 5.0% for all the military personnel screened using the PTSD Checklist (Hoge et al. 2004). A year after their return from Iraq, 16.6% of the U.S. Army combat troops met the screening criteria for PTSD (Hoge et al. 2007). The Department of Defense conducted a mental-health survey of Army soldiers and Marines deployed in Iraq in 2003, 2004, and 2006. In 2003, 16% of the soldiers and Marines met the screening criteria for PTSD while deployed; in 2004, 14% met the criteria; and in 2006, 17% of soldiers and 14% of Marines met the criteria (MHAT 2006).

Gulf War

The effects of the 1991 Gulf War on Army active-duty, and reserve or National Guard units from Pennsylvania and Hawaii were studied about 2 years after the war (Stretch et al. 1996). Of the deployed active-duty and reserve or National Guard soldiers, 8% and 9.2%, respectively, had a symptom complex suggestive of PTSD; of the nondeployed active-duty and reserve or National Guard soldiers, only 1.3% and 2.1%, respectively, had such symptoms. In an earlier study of 11,000 active-duty Gulf War soldiers conducted 6-12 months after the war, current PTSD rates were 12.9-15.5% (Stretch et al. 1996). The lower rates in the Pennsylvania and Hawaiian troops were attributed to their military occupations—support activities—which may have resulted in less exposure to traumatic events than the active-duty Army soldiers who had engaged in combat.

In a 1995-1997 survey of 9476 Gulf War-era veterans and 11,441 Gulf War-deployed veterans in all four services, Kang et al. (2003) found that 12.1% of deployed veterans and 4.3% of nondeployed veterans met the screening criteria for current PTSD using the PTSD Checklist (adjusted OR 3.1, 95% CI 2.7-3.4). The risk of PTSD increased with the severity of the stress, ranging from 3.3% in activated but nondeployed reserve personnel (minimal stress) to 22.6% in Gulf War-deployed veterans who had worn chemical protective gear, heard chemical alarms, been involved in direct combat duty, and witnessed deaths (maximal stress). In a followup to that study, Toomey et al. (2007) found that 6.2% of Gulf War-deployed veterans and 1.1% of nondeployed veterans had a diagnosis of war-related PTSD 10 years after the war (OR 5.78, 95% CI 2.62-12.74; adjusted for age, sex, ethnicity, duty type, service branch, and rank).

Ikin et al. (2004) found that a decade after the Gulf War, 5.1% of Australian Gulf War veterans had PTSD (diagnosed with the CIDI), compared with 1.7% of nondeployed Australian veterans. Few of the Australian veterans experienced direct combat; rather, their stressors were associated with the threat of combat, anticipation of attack with biologic or chemical agents, and the discomfort and isolation of deployment. Similar risks for PTSD were seen in Canadian Gulf War-deployed and nondeployed veterans (Goss Gilroy Inc. 1998). A 1998-2001 mail survey of 23,358 UK Gulf War veterans also found increased self-reports of PTSD and associated symptoms compared with nondeployed military personnel (1.0% vs 0.4%, OR 2.4, 95% CI 1.8-3.1) (Simmons et al. 2004).

Vietnam War

The NVVRS assessed the readjustment to civilian life and the prevalence of PTSD and other psychiatric disorders in 3016 Vietnam veterans 15-20 years after the war (Kulka et al. 1990). It was estimated that 15.2% of all male Vietnam-theater veterans had current (6-month) combat-related PTSD and 30.9% had lifetime combat-related PTSD (the former value is equivalent to about 479,000 of the 3.14 million men who served in the Vietnam theater). Of the 7200 female veterans, it was estimated that 8.5% had current PTSD and 26.9% had lifetime PTSD. The prevalence of current PTSD (35.8%) was 4 times as high in men (7 times as high as in women) exposed to high levels of war-zone stress as in men exposed to low or moderate war-zone stress (8.5%); 2-3 times as high as in those with service-connected physical disabilities (wounded in combat), and twice as high as in men (5 times as high in women) with lifetime substance-abuse disorders (Schlenger et al. 1992). Exposure to war-zone stress was more predictive of PTSD in the NVVRS study than were predisposing factors (Keane 1998).

Dohrenwend et al. (2006) reanalyzed the military records of 1200 male Vietnam-theater veterans from the NVVRS with a records-based military-history measure of exposure to war-zone stressors. Over 86% of the veterans with war-related PTSD described events that were personally life-threatening or involved witnessing death of or physical harm to others. A diagnosis of PTSD was based on the SCID. A dose-response relationship was established: fewer than 1% of low-exposed veterans had a diagnosis of current (as of 1988) war-related PTSD vs 28.1% of those in the high-exposure category. When adjusted for impairment of functioning and documentation of exposure to war-related traumatic events, the prevalence of lifetime and current war-related PTSD was 18.7% and 9.1%, respectively.

The Vietnam Experience Study (VES) was conducted by the Centers for Disease Control and Prevention in 1984 on a random sample of 2490 Vietnam theater and 1972 era Army veterans via telephone interview. A subsample of the respondents received a physical examination by a clinician and were interviewed with the DIS for assessment of psychiatric disorders (CDC 1988). Lifetime and current (1-month) PTSD rates were 14.7% and 2.2%, respectively, in the theater veterans 13 years after the end of the war. PTSD prevalence in the era veterans was not given. Using the same dataset, but including noncombat PTSD with combat-related PTSD, Boscarino (1995) found the prevalence of current PTSD in theater and era veterans to be 12% and 2%, respectively. PTSD was positively associated with reported combat exposure (OR 2.42, $p < 0.001$).

In an effort to reconcile the different prevalences of combat-related PTSD in Vietnam veterans reported in the NVVRS and the VES, Thompson et al. (2006) noted that the discrepancies could be minimized if the same definition of PTSD were applied to both studies. Rates determined with particularly broad and sensitive criteria were about 5 times those determined with more restrictive criteria. The authors concluded that consistent methods of diagnosis are needed to compare rates of PTSD in different studies of veteran populations.

O'Toole et al. (1996) found the prevalence of lifetime PTSD to be 21% in Australian Vietnam veterans (diagnosed with the SCID) and 12% for current PTSD, 20-25 years after the war.

World War II and Korean War

Veterans of World War II and the Korean War who are participating in the Normative Aging Study, a long-term study established by the VA in Boston that has screened and tracked over 6000 men for a variety of health conditions since its inception in 1961, were screened for PTSD in 1990 (Spiro et al. 1994). The Mississippi Scale for Combat-Related PTSD was used to assess 809 World War II veterans (54% of whom experienced combat) and 401 Korean War veterans (19% of whom experienced combat); the Combat Exposure Scale and two additional questions on length of time in combat and exposure to combat outcomes were used to assess combat-exposure severity. The estimated prevalence of PTSD was 0.74% in World War II veterans (whether combat-exposed or not) and 0.25% in Korean War veterans (whether combat-exposed or not). On the basis of combat exposure of the World War II veterans, the estimated prevalence of PTSD increased from 0.94% in those with light to moderate exposure to 3.45% in those with moderate to heavy exposure. None of the 76 combat-exposed Korean War veterans screened positively for PTSD, although 0.31% of the Korean War veterans who were not exposed to combat did.

Kang et al. (2006) compared the health status of 19,442 U.S. World War II prisoners of war with a randomly selected control group of 9728 veterans who had served in the military during World War II but had not been prisoners of war. On the basis of computerized VA inpatient medical records for 1990-2000 and outpatient medical records for 1997-2000 or computerized medical records from the Health Care Financing Administration, they found that 113 of the control group (1.16%) had a diagnosis of PTSD. PTSD had been diagnosed in 3254 (16.7%) of the POWs, 71% of whom had been interned in Europe. The study did not indicate whether the control group had been engaged in combat or where they had served during the war.

Table 5-2 summarizes the prevalence or risk of PTSD in numerous studies of U.S. military personnel. Some of the difference in rates might be attributed to the definition of PTSD being used (*DSM-III-R* or *DSM-IV-TR*) and the instruments used to screen for or diagnose it.

COURSE

DSM-IV recognizes that the onset of PTSD may be acute, beginning within 6 months of exposure to the traumatic event, or delayed, beginning more than 6 months after the traumatic event. Symptoms typically begin shortly after exposure—even on the first day (North et al. 1999). The lag time between exposure and development of enough symptoms to meet the diagnostic criteria is variable and may be years (Bremner et al. 1996; Bryant and Harvey 2002; Carty et al. 2006; Gray et al. 2004; Green et al. 1990a; Op den Velde et al. 1996; Port et al. 2001; Ruzich et al. 2005). It is considered to be chronic by *DSM-IV-TR* criteria if symptoms persist for 3 months or longer. PTSD can be chronic with no remission, or it can be recurrent with periods of remission and recurrence (Friedman 2003).

Of the veterans with PTSD in the NVVRS, Schnurr et al. (2003) found that PTSD resulted from traumatic experiences before their Vietnam deployment in 8%; for those with PTSD related to Vietnam, it began in 31% in the same year that they went to Vietnam; it began in 31% in the following year, it began in 32% within 2-5 years of entry into Vietnam, and it began in 6% even later. More than 40% of the veterans had symptoms that had persisted for more than 2 decades. Symptoms began earlier in men than in women. Among men, members of ethnic minority groups were slower to develop symptoms.

TABLE 5-2 Estimated Prevalence of PTSD in U.S. Military Populations

Population	PTSD Prevalence	How Measured	When Assessed	Reference
OEF combat troops	Current: predeployment 5%; 6% postdeployment (n = 1962)	PTSD Checklist	Army: 3-4 months after return from combat duty	Hoge et al. 2004
OIF combat troops	Current: 5% predeployment; 12-13% postdeployment Iraq (n = 1709)	PTSD Checklist	Army: 1 week before deployment and 3-4 months after return from combat duty Marines: 3-4 months after return from combat duty	Hoge et al. 2004
	Current: 14-17% (n = 1767)	PTSD Checklist	9 months into deployment	MHAT 2006
Gulf War veterans	Current: 3.4% (n = 967)	CIDI	February 2000-October 2001	Fiedler et al. 2006
	Current: Ft. Devens 5%, 8% (n = 148) New Orleans 7%, 8% (n = 58) (according to CAPS and Mississippi Scale, respectively)	CAPS for 75% of subjects Mississippi Scale for Desert Storm War Personnel for 99% of subjects	Ft. Devens cohort: initial survey within 5 days of return (spring 1991) and winter 1992/spring 1993 New Orleans cohort: initial survey within 9 months of return in 1991 and summer 1994/fall 1995	Proctor et al. 1998
	Current: 12% (n = 11441)	PTSD Checklist	November 1995-1997	Kang et al. 2003
	Lifetime: 6.2% (n = 1061)	CAPS	10 years after war	Toomey et al. 2007
	Current: 8-9.2% (n = 1524)	17-item questionnaire based on *DSM-III-R* criteria Impact of Event Scale Brief Symptom Inventory	1.5-2 years after war	Stretch et al. 1996
Vietnam veterans	Current: 15% men (n = 1200), 8.5% women (n = 432) Lifetime: 30.6% men, 26.9% women	Mississippi Scale for Combat-Related PTSD DIS MMPI PTSD Scale SCID	15 or more years after service	Kulka et al. 1990
	Current: 9.1% Lifetime: 18.7% (n = 1200)	Military records Historical accounts Diagnostic histories of PTSD MMPI SCID	1988 for NVVRS	Dohrenwend et al. 2006
	Current: 2.2% Lifetime: 14.7% post deployment (n = 2490)	DIS MMPI	11-12 years after Vietnam War; 15-20 years after Army service	CDC 1988

TABLE 5-2 Continued

Population	PTSD Prevalence	How Measured	When Assessed	Reference
Korean War veterans	Current: 0.25% (n = 401)	Mississippi Scale for Combat-Related PTSD Combat Exposure Scale	Normative Aging Study cohort; questionnaires sent in 1990	Spiro et al. 1994
World War II veterans	Current: 0.74% (n = 809)	Mississippi Scale for Combat-Related PTSD Combat Exposure Scale	Normative Aging Study cohort; questionnaires sent in 1990	Spiro et al. 1994

NOTE: CAPS = Clinician-Administered PTSD Scale, CIDI = Composite International Diagnostic Interview, DIS = Diagnostic Interview Schedule, MMPI = Minnesota Multiphasic Personality Inventory, OEF = Operation Enduring Freedom, OIF = Operation Iraqi Freedom, SCID = Structured Clinical Interview for *DSM-IV*.

In a small study, Bremner et al. (1996) found that of 61 Vietnam veterans with combat-related PTSD, 0 (15%) developed PTSD during their combat tour and 38 (62%) met the criteria for PTSD within 2 years of the end of their combat tour, and 8 patients (13%) did not meet the full criteria for PTSD until 10 or more years after their tours ended. The first symptoms reported were typically in the hyperarousal cluster. Symptoms typically increased during the first few years and then leveled off.

Increasing PTSD symptoms and symptom severity were observed Wolfe et al. (1999) in a larger cohort of 2119 male and 194 female Gulf War veterans screened for PTSD. Five days after their return from the gulf, 3% of the veterans (8% of women and 3% of men) exceeded the PTSD screening cutoff; at 18-24 months, the percentage of veterans exceeding the cutoff had more than doubled to 8% (16% of women and 7% of men).

Similar results were seen in 84 National Guard troops (medical and military police units) returning from the Gulf War (Southwick et al. 1993b, 1995). Most of the PTSD symptoms reported at 2 years after deployment were present by 6 months, but symptom severity continued to increase. The hyperarousal symptom cluster was more prevalent than the intrusive-memories cluster, which was more prevalent than the avoidance-numbing cluster. PTSD symptom severity did not differ between the units or between the sexes. Those who were highly symptomatic at 6 months continued to be symptomatic at 2 years.

In many cases, PTSD will remit naturally (McFarlane 1997). Most (60%) PTSD remissions in the general population occur within 1 year. More than one-third of cases do not remit, however, regardless of whether the person receives treatment (Connor and Butterfield 2003; Kessler et al. 1995). In the NCS, the median time to remission among people who ever sought professional treatment was 36 months, but it was 64 months for those who did not (Kessler et al. 1995). Factors associated with PTSD chronicity in the general population are a greater number of symptoms (especially numbing and arousal symptoms), comorbid alcohol abuse or other psychiatric or medical illness, being female, having a family history of antisocial behavior, and having a history of childhood trauma (Breslau 2001b).

Marshall et al. (2006) found that NVVRS veterans with chronic war-related PTSD had more numbing symptoms and, to a lesser extent, more hyperarousal symptoms than veterans with PTSD in remission; re-experiencing symptoms did not appear to be related to PTSD chronicity.

The above studies indicate that the development and course of PTSD are variable. Some people may have no or few symptoms of PTSD initially but develop more symptoms over time and others may rapidly develop symptoms that meet the full diagnostic criteria for PTSD. Some recover or experience a reduction in symptoms, others suffer longstanding PTSD symptoms (Friedman et al. 1994; Kulka et al. 1990; Schnurr et al. 2003), and still others will follow an episodic course. Even those who appear to have recovered entirely from PTSD may experience a recurrence of symptoms years later, especially if exposed to additional trauma or other important life events, such as the death of a spouse (Friedman et al. 1994).

COMORBIDITY AND DISABILITY

People with PTSD tend to report poor health and impaired function in many life activities. Several studies indicate that veterans with PTSD report more symptoms of adverse health and disability than do veterans without PTSD (see Chapter 6 for more information on symptom reporting). On examination, many people with PTSD are found to have other psychiatric disorders that increase the complexity of diagnosing PTSD. The presence of those additional psychiatric disorders may also play a role in the adverse health effects seen with PTSD.

In Chapter 6, studies are assessed for the strength of the association between deployment to a war zone and PTSD; those studies are found in the section on psychiatric disorders. The body of evidence that addresses specific health effects that may occur in veterans with PTSD is also reviewed in Chapter 6 for each relevant health effect. The psychosocial effects seen in veterans with PTSD, including effects on family and employment, are considered in Chapter 7.

Comorbidity

In veteran and general population samples, PTSD frequently co-occurs with other psychiatric or substance-use disorders. In the NVVRS, male and female theater veterans with PTSD were 10-15 times more likely to have depression and dysthymia and 20 times more likely to have an anxiety disorder than their counterparts without PTSD (Kulka et al. 1990). Zatzick et al. (1997a) found that the risk of having PTSD was significantly greater in male NVVRS veterans with major depression (OR 17.6, 95% CI 6.5-47.4), alcohol abuse or dependence (OR 3.2, 95% CI 1.9-5.4), drug abuse or dependence (OR 7.4, 95% CI 2.2-24.5), or panic disorder (OR 22.6, 95% CI 3.1-163.5) that in those with the disorders. Among female veterans, PTSD was seen in 51% of those with major depression, 40.7% of those with alcohol abuse or dependence, and 70.1% of those with panic disorder (Zatzick et al. 1997b).

High rates of comorbidity are also seen in the general population. In the NCS, 88.3% of men and 79.0% of women with PTSD had a life history of mood, anxiety, or substance-use disorders (Kessler et al. 1995). The temporal relationship between PTSD and other psychiatric and substance-use disorders is complex. Psychiatric comorbidity increases the likelihood of PTSD, as found in the NCS. However, PTSD also increases the likelihood of developing the other disorders (Schnurr et al. 2000a, 2002; Shalev et al. 1998). Trauma can also lead to the simultaneous development of PTSD and other psychiatric disorders, such as major depression (Shalev et al. 1998). For example, in a study of 262 World War II and Korean War prisoners of war (Engdahl et al. 1998), half of whom developed war-related PTSD, 66% of those with PTSD but only 34% of those without PTSD had another anxiety, mood, or substance-use disorder. The majority of the other disorders began in the same year as PTSD. Although the high rate of psychiatric and substance-use comorbidity can be partly explained by symptom overlap in *DSM-IV*, it does not diminish the diagnostic integrity of PTSD; rather, it suggests the importance of complete clinical evaluations to elucidate the full clinical picture of each patient.

Disability

PTSD can result in profound and long-term impairment of functioning and quality of life. This section considers the functional outcomes and disability that may occur in veterans with PTSD. Psychosocial effects and the impact of PTSD on family, friends, and others are discussed in Chapter 7. *DSM-IV* requires that a diagnosis of PTSD include "clinically significant distress and/or impairment in social, occupational, and/or other important areas of functioning" (APA 2000). Therefore, it is important to understand the distress and disability that may be associated with it.

Zatzick et al. evaluated 1190 male and 432 female Vietnam veterans by using data from the NVVRS (1997a,b). Of the men, 242 (15.3%) were diagnosed with PTSD and more than 90% of those men reported having one or more of 30 chronic nonpsychiatric medical conditions within the preceding 12 months. Of the veterans with no nonpsychiatric medical disorders, less than 10% had PTSD, whereas of the 141 veterans reporting four or more medical disorders, 31.9% had PTSD. Among the women, 8.9% had PTSD diagnosed, of whom 70% reported having one or more of 37 chronic medical conditions within the preceding 12 months. PTSD was present in only 4.2% of the female veterans with no chronic medical conditions but in 19.1% of those reporting four or more medical conditions. Veterans with PTSD reported significantly ($p < 0.05$) more functional impairment than veterans without PTSD, including inability to work, fair or poor health, diminished well-being, current limitation in physical functioning, and more days in bed in the preceding 3 months.

Dohrenwend et al. (2006) also reanalyzed the NVVRS data, including the Global Assessment of Functioning (GAF) scale that is traditionally used by VA to assess a veteran's functional impairment. Of the sample of 260 veterans who had no diagnosis of PTSD or a diagnosis of past PTSD, 47% and 44%, respectively, were rated as having good functioning, although none of the veterans who had a diagnosis of current PTSD had good functioning in all GAF areas. Of those with current PTSD, 15% had only slight impairment, 41% had some difficulty, and 37% had moderate or serious impairment. The GAF scores were related to the severity of the PTSD.

A study of 70 UK active-duty military personnel referred to a PTSD clinic found that a diagnosis of PTSD, major depression, or alcohol dependence did not predict disability in work, relationships, or social activities, although symptoms of depression accounted for much of any total functional impairment, particularly in family life (Neal et al. 2004). Bleich and Solomon (2004) found that in Israeli veterans, PTSD symptoms resulted in more impairment in occupational functioning than in interpersonal functioning or activities of daily living.

World War II veterans 70-74 years old, who had PTSD as a result of their participation in secret military tests of mustard gas during the war were assessed for health-related disability (Schnurr et al. 2000b). As of 1996, compared with similarly exposed veterans without PTSD, veterans with PTSD had decreased functioning and increased impairment on all measures: physical function, social function, physical role impairment, emotional role impairment, lifetime disability, and current unemployment.

Men and women appear to suffer equal degrees of impairment from PTSD, although women are more likely to seek medical help and take medication. In a study of PTSD in the general population, Breslau (2001b) found that when symptoms were most severe, about 25% of both men and women in a population of young adults felt that they were unable to work during the entire 30-day period during which they experienced the symptoms. When inability to work was added to reports of reduced activity, almost 39% of the 20 men and 44% of 44 women reported that they were unable to do their jobs or had to reduce their activities. When young people with a diagnosis of PTSD, other psychiatric diagnoses, or no psychiatric diagnosis were compared, the limitation of activities from PTSD was twice that from the other diagnoses and 4 times that associated with no diagnosis.

RISK AND PROTECTIVE FACTORS

Risk and protective factors influence responses to stressors or traumatic events. In the case of veterans, those factors might determine the extent of the response to a deployment-related stressor and whether PTSD will develop. The following discussion is not exhaustive and is meant to provide the reader with an overview of the types of risk and protective factors that may influence each veteran. Some of the risk and protective factors that have been noted in the development of PTSD are: sex; age; race and ethnicity; developmental history and early-life stressors; personal psychiatric history; hardiness, a sense of control, and coping strategies; socioeconomic status and military status; social support; exposure to combat; and physical injury. None of those factors occurs in isolation; they may interact with one another before, during, and after deployment (Benotsch et al. 2000; Stein et al. 2005). Although many of the studies discussed below focus on PTSD, other health effects, primarily other psychiatric disorders, are also discussed when the results are applicable to them.

Sex

As in the general population (Kessler et al. 1995), female veterans of both the Vietnam War and the Gulf War are more likely than their male counterparts to suffer from PTSD (Fiedler et al. 2006; Kang et al. 2003; Kulka et al. 1990; Wolfe 1996; Wolfe et al. 1993b, 1999; Zatzick et al. 1997b). After the Gulf War, Fiedler et al. (2006) found that deployed women were more likely than deployed men to experience PTSD (4.0% of women and 3.4% of men), other anxiety disorders (25.3% of women and 15.3% of men), and major depression (25.3% of women and 14.2% of men), but they were less likely than men to have drug or alcohol disorders; these findings are mirrored in the general population (Kessler et al. 1995, 2005a). In a study assessing the prevalence of PTSD and chronic fatigue syndrome (CFS) in Gulf War veterans, women made up 18.6% of the 11,441 veterans in the study; 24.3% of the women met the screening criteria for PTSD, and 16.7% had CFS symptoms (Kang et al. 2003). Female Gulf War veterans were more likely than men to have PTSD symptoms when assessed 5 days after their return from the gulf (8% vs 3%, respectively, OR 3.2, 95% CI 1.9-5.5) and after controlling for the effects of combat and other risk factors; 18-24 months later, the prevalence was still higher for women than men (16% vs 7%, respectively, OR 2.3, 95% CI 1.5-3.5) (Wolfe et al. 1999). However, Sutker et al. (1995a) found that female Gulf War veterans (14% of sample) reported similar levels of psychologic distress and had no more PTSD symptoms than their male counterparts.

As discussed in Chapter 3, sexual assault is one of the two leading risk factors (combat is the other) for PTSD (Breslau et al. 2002; Kessler et al. 1995). Sexual victimization in military women was found to have a dose-response relationship with PTSD, according to two studies (Murdoch et al. 2006; Wolfe et al. 1993a), and sexual assault is associated with poorer health outcomes in female veterans (Goldzweig et al. 2006). Kang et al. (2005) found that among 2131 female and 9310 male Gulf War veterans, PTSD was associated with in-theater sexual harassment and assault in women (OR 5.41, 95% CI 3.19-9.17) and men (OR 6.21, 95% CI 2.26-17.04). The risk of having PTSD associated with combat was almost identical in men (OR 4.45, 95% CI 3.54-5.60) and women (OR 4.03, 95% CI 1.97-8.23) and showed a dose-response relationship with increasing combat. Sexual assault, however, was a greater risk factor for PTSD than was combat exposure in both men and women.

Race and Ethnicity

Research results on the role of race and ethnicity as risk factors for stress-related illness are mixed but in general support the conclusion that blacks and Hispanics are at greater risk for developing psychiatric disorders, particularly PTSD, as a result of deployment. In the VES, nonwhite veterans had a poorer psychologic status 15-20 years after the war than did white veterans (CDC 1988). Findings from the NVVRS indicate that black and Hispanic veterans had a higher prevalence of PTSD than whites (Kulka et al. 1990). Among theater veterans, the prevalence of current PTSD in the NVVRS was 27.9% in Hispanics, 20.6% in blacks, and 13.7% in whites and others (Kulka et al. 1990). Those proportions held even when racial differences in combat exposure were controlled for as minority groups had a greater number of war-zone exposures.

The Hawaii Vietnam Veterans Project (HVVP), modeled on the NVVRS, determined that veterans of Japanese ancestry had a lower prevalence of PTSD than whites (Friedman et al. 2004). Schnurr et al. (2003) studied 530 veterans drawn from the NVVRS and the HVVP, and found that black, Hispanic, and native Hawaiian men were more likely and Americans of Japanese descent were less likely than white men to have a lifetime diagnosis of PTSD and that Hispanic male veterans were more likely to have current PTSD than males in other ethnic groups (Schnurr et al. 2004). In a study of 1377 American Legionnaires who had served in Vietnam and were followed for 14 years, minority race contributed to a more chronic course of PTSD; however, the minority sample was too small for further investigation (Koenen et al. 2003). It has been suggested that the racial gap in prevalence or course of PTSD in Vietnam veterans might stem from racism in the military, overidentification with a nonwhite enemy, exacerbation of existing stress by institutional racism, and lower financial or emotional resources after the war (Marsella et al. 1993).

Several studies of Gulf War veterans have also found that minority-group veterans had a greater prevalence of PTSD. In a study by Kang et al. (2003), nonwhite veterans had a greater prevalence of PTSD than white veterans, but the category "nonwhites" was not divided into minority subgroups, and there was no adjustment for socioeconomic factors other than age and marital status. There was no difference between whites and nonwhites in prevalence of CFS. A study of 653 Gulf War veterans from Louisiana with relatively high minority-group participation (35%) found that minority-group troops, particularly men, tended to report greater psychologic distress and more PTSD symptoms than white men (Sutker et al. 1995a); however, as in the Kang study, there was no stratification beyond "nonwhite status" and no adjustment for other factors that may have contributed to the reporting differences. Adjusted for age, sex, race, rank, branch, and military status, Black et al. (2004) found that nonwhite Gulf War veterans were at almost twice the risk of an anxiety disorder as white veterans (OR 1.9, 95% CI 0.7-5.3).

Hoge et al. (2002) assessed the incidence of first hospitalization for a mental disorder in active-duty military personnel in 1990-1999. The rates of hospitalization per 1000 person-years were 9.34 for whites, 9.25 for Hispanics, 8.30 for blacks, 5.97 for Asians and Pacific Islanders, and 18.27 for American Indians and Alaskan Natives. Fontana et al. (2000) found that among U.S. peacekeepers in Somalia, PTSD symptoms were more severe in blacks, although there was no adjustment for socioeconomic factors in the model.

Age

Research results on age as a risk factor for PTSD and other psychiatric disorders are mixed. Studies of Vietnam veterans (Bremner et al. 1993; CDC 1988; Green et al. 1990b; Kulka et al. 1990) and Gulf War veterans (Wolfe et al. 1999) generally found lower age to be a risk factor for PTSD. Kulka et al. (1990) in the NVVRS found that older men (born before 1945) had a lower prevalence of PTSD (4-10%) than those born later (18-19%).

Ikin et al. (2004) found that although Australian Gulf War-deployed veterans were at increased risk for any postwar anxiety disorder compared with nondeployed veterans, the risk did not vary significantly among four age groups (less than 20 years old, 20-24, 25-34, and 35 and higher). Black et al. (2004) also found that being 25 years old or younger did not significantly increase the risk of having a current anxiety condition among Gulf War veterans (OR 1.3; 95% CI 0.8-2.0). During the 1990s, however, active-duty military personnel aged 18-24 were at greater risk for hospitalization for a mental disorder than older veterans (Hoge et al. 2002).

Seal et al. (2007) found that active-duty Operation Enduring Freedom (OEF) and Operation Iraqi Freedom (OIF) male veterans 18-24 years old were more likely to have a diagnosis of PTSD or any other mental health disorder than were older veterans. The risk of having a diagnosis of PTSD or any mental health diagnosis decreased with increasing age. Compared with veterans 40 years and older, the relative risk for PTSD was 8.88 (95% CI 7.49-10.54) for the youngest veterans, 6.91 (95% CI 5.82-8.21) for those 25-29 years old, and 6.07 (95% CI 5.05-7.28) for those 30-39 years old.

Developmental History and Early-Life Stress

Numerous epidemiologic studies of Vietnam and Gulf War veterans and of civilians have found that childhood trauma from physical or sexual abuse is a risk factor for PTSD, regardless of later combat exposure. The strongest evidence of the impact of early-life stress comes from large studies of Vietnam veterans (Fontana and Rosenheck 1994a; Kulka et al. 1990) and Gulf War veterans (Sutker et al. 1995b).

Fontana et al. (1994a) analyzed data from the NVVRS, assigning weights to the major contributors to PTSD in female veterans. A history of child abuse contributed nearly as much to the risk of having PTSD as did military sexual trauma although combat exposure was twice as likely to contribute to the risk of PTSD (Fontana and Rosenheck 1994a). King et al. (1999) also found that a history of early-life trauma was linked to the development of PTSD in male and female Vietnam veterans; it also predicted the likelihood of stressful life events after the war. Childhood sexual and physical abuse is common in Gulf War and Vietnam veterans seeking treatment for psychiatric disorders including PTSD, with studies that assessed this endpoint finding that 25-60% of veterans with a psychiatric disorder had been abused (Bremner et al. 1993; Engel et al. 1993; Lapp et al. 2005).

Psychiatric History

Having been diagnosed previously with a psychiatric disorder increases the likelihood of PTSD after exposure to a traumatic event. People with a history of a psychiatric disorder may have an increased likelihood of engaging in risky behavior which increases the likelihood of their exposure to traumatic events and their potential for PTSD or other stress-related disorders. Someone with a pre-existing psychiatric disorder who is exposed to wartime trauma may respond ineffectively to the traumatic event because of pre-existing symptoms, inadequate coping styles, low social support, and poor self-esteem, all of which increase the likelihood of PTSD or related disorders.

A study of Gulf War veterans by Black et al. (2004) found that the greatest risk of postwar anxiety disorder resulted from the presence of pre-existing anxiety disorders of any kind (OR 10.4, 95% CI 2.9-37.0), and pre-existing depressive disorders (OR 4.1, 95% CI 1.9-8.9). The overall likelihood of postwar anxiety disorders was increased by a factor of 4 (range, 2.2-8.9) by a previous history of any psychiatric disorder. A study of Australian Gulf War veterans by Ikin et al. (2004) found that similar percentages of Gulf War-deployed veterans (31%) and a comparison group of era veterans (33.7%) reported having had a psychiatric disorder before deployment. Most frequently, the pre-existing disorders were substance-use disorders (25-28%) and anxiety disorders (6-8%).

Hoge et al. (2004) screened 2530 U.S. infantry soldiers for mental health disorders before their deployment to Iraq in 2003. They found that 14.3% reported a moderate or severe mental health problem, 5.3% met the patient health questionnaire definition of depression, 6.4% met the definition of anxiety, 5.0% met the definition for PTSD, 17.3% reported using more alcohol than they meant to, and 12.5% had felt they wanted to cut down on their drinking. Those findings highlights that a substantial portion of military personnel may enter combat at increased risk for a psychiatric disorder on the basis of psychiatric history alone.

Hardiness, Coping Strategies, and Sense of Control

The occurrence and severity of stress-related health effects are not solely the result of interaction of physiologic processes with a threatening environment. Studies of Vietnam and Gulf War veterans indicate that particular personality or psychologic characteristics can affect a person's reactions to deployment-related stress. Personality includes inherent tendencies toward optimism or pessimism, coping styles, resilience, and hardiness that would be expected to affect one's ability to manage stressful events. Those characteristics are determined or modulated by the action of life experiences on genetic makeup.

One personality trait, hardiness, has been defined as a combination of commitment (feeling deeply involved in life activities), feeling in control of one's experiences, and maintaining a sense of challenge (a positive anticipation of change). Dolan and Adler (2006) adapted the definition of hardiness in a military population to mean the degree to which military personnel are committed to and feel a sense of control over their work experiences. They surveyed U.S. Army soldiers during and after a 6-month peacekeeping mission in Kosovo. Military hardiness was correlated with psychologic but not physical health during and after deployment. Among soldiers who experienced high levels of deployment stressors, those with greater levels of hardiness had less postdeployment depression. Studies of deployed Gulf War veterans have found that hardiness was protective against the adverse effects of combat stress and stressful life events and that the level of hardiness was a significant predictor of health outcomes (Bartone 1999). Those with greater hardiness reported fewer physical symptoms than those with lower hardiness regardless of the intensity of the combat exposure or the reported level of stressful life events. For military personnel with long exposure to war-zone stressors, hardiness and perceived social support may gradually diminish, and the diminution can result in deterioration of physical health (Taft et al. 1999).

The types of physiologic changes seen in animals after exposure to uncontrollable stressors have also been observed in humans (see Chapter 4 for a discussion of the animal studies). In a prospective study of 348 Gulf War veterans (all military reservists), Benotsch et al. (2000) measured sense of control with the 45-item Dispositional Resilience Scale 14 months after the conflict (time 1) and 13 months after that (time 2). Veterans' perceptions of their personal resources, particularly the hardiness components of control and (to a lesser degree) commitment, and problem-focused coping decreased significantly between time 1 and time 2. Conversely, coping with stress through avoidance increased significantly between the two times. Storzbach et al. (2000) found that veterans with unexplained illness reported feeling less control over stressful events that they had recently experienced than did veterans without such illness.

Coping strategies are also associated with ability to respond to stressors. In a study of Vietnam combat veterans, positive coping strategies were found to protect against the development of PTSD symptoms (Wolfe et al. 1993c). When assessed 15 years after their deployment, veterans who used negative coping strategies—such as mental escapism, externalization, and behavioral avoidance—had poorer psychological functioning and more PTSD symptoms than veterans who used nonavoidant coping styles, regardless of the level of combat exposure in each group. Vaillant (1977) found that avoidant behavior was also a major predictor of a downward trajectory in life in a civilian population. It has been shown in other stressful circumstances that ineffective coping strategies, especially avoidant or passive coping as opposed to active problem-solving strategies, predict adverse mental-health outcomes (Arata et al. 2000; Gibbs 1989; North 1995; North et al. 1994, 2001).

In addition to a positive coping style, a perception that some benefit derives from military experience is associated with reduced potential for adverse health effects after combat exposure. Lee et al. (1995), in a 50-year prospective study of World War II combat veterans, found premorbid characteristics to be significantly associated with postcombat psychopathology. Aldwin et al. (1994) conducted a study of 1287 male veterans 44-91 years old, 40% of whom had been engaged in combat. The majority of veterans responded with positive comments about their military service (for example, a sense of mastery, enhanced self-esteem, and effective coping), and there was a linear relationship between perceived benefits and combat exposure. Similar results were seen by Jennings et al. (2006), who found that veterans in the Normative Aging Study (mean age, 74 years) with moderate combat exposure had higher levels of wisdom later in life than veterans with no or high combat exposure; wisdom was assessed with the Adult Self-Transcendence Inventory. Wisdom also correlated positively with perception of benefits of military experience and with positive coping strategies. The studies suggest that a favorable appraisal of one's combat experience or personal attributes associated with it may mitigate long-term adverse health consequences, such as PTSD.

Socioeconomic Status and Military Status

In civilian studies, socioeconomically disadvantaged populations are at greater risk for psychiatric and somatic disorders (Neeleman et al. 2001); those in the lowest social and economic strata have 2-3 times the risk of psychiatric disorders, especially depression and anxiety disorders, of those in the highest strata (U.S. Department of Health and Human Services 1999). Not surprisingly, similar relationships are apparent in veteran populations. Low income and lack of education are associated with chronic stress-related disorders—for example, anxiety disorders, major depression, and substance-use disorders—in Gulf War and Vietnam veterans (Black et al. 2004; Boscarino 1995; Brewin et al. 2000; Fiedler et al. 2006).

Low military rank (enlisted personnel vs officers) is also associated with greater risk of a stress-related disorder (Black et al. 2004; Fiedler et al. 2006; Kang et al. 2003; Kulka et al. 1990). Two studies found that being an officer or being college-educated reduced the risk of developing anxiety or depressive disorders after deployment by at least half (Black et al. 2004; Fiedler et al. 2006). Slusarcick et al. (2001) found that aboard a U.S. Navy hospital ship during the Gulf War, junior enlisted health-care providers had the highest levels of depression followed by junior officers, senior enlisted, and senior officers, in that order. By occupation, corpsmen were the most depressed, and physicians the least. However, Ikin et al. (2004) found that although Australian Gulf War-deployed veterans were at higher risk for any postwar anxiety disorder than were nondeployed veterans, the risk did not vary significantly by rank, whether officer or enlisted.

Social Support

Social support has been linked to favorable mental-health outcomes (Bland et al. 1997; Regehr et al. 2001) especially among men (Solomon et al. 1987). Studies have shown that good social support is a protective factor against the onset of PTSD (Benotsch et al. 2000; Fontana and Rosenheck 1994b; Fontana et al. 1997).

Two meta-analyses found that lack of social support was the factor most strongly associated with the development of PTSD after a traumatic event for veterans of the Vietnam War and the Gulf War (Benotsch et al. 2000; Brewin et al. 2000; Fontana et al. 1997; Koenen et al. 2003; Ozer et al. 2003). Vietnam veterans with low levels of social support 10 years after the war had more symptoms of PTSD than those with high levels of social support; and when combined with high levels of combat exposure, those with low social support had far more symptoms of PTSD (Barrett and Mizes 1988). The role of social-support networks in the Vietnam-Era Adjustment Survey was explored in nursing and combat personnel (Stretch 1985, 1986; Stretch et al. 1985). The rates of PTSD were highest in men and women who had lacked positive social supports from family, friends, and society in general. Hispanic Vietnam veterans who were highly symptomatic for PTSD expressed fewer social contacts, more adverse social encounters, and smaller family and social networks (Escobar et al. 1983).

One study, conducted in 1978, explored the burden of war and social bonding in 149 veterans of World War II and the Korean War. Painful memories of war and symptoms of stress in later life were diminished through involvement with a supportive community of service mates and partners (Elder and Clipp 1988). Prospective studies reveal a downward spiral: as PTSD symptoms worsen, veterans lose more social support, the lack of which in turn exacerbates their PTSD symptoms (Benotsch et al. 2000).

Although most studies of social support deal with PTSD, particularly in Vietnam veterans, the same findings are applicable to major depression and other stress-related illnesses (Boscarino 1995; Fontana et al. 1997; Green et al. 1990b). Those studies all showed that low social support increased the risk of depression and other psychiatric disorders, such as generalized anxiety disorder.

Most findings regarding social support come from studies of homecoming support, whether given by family, friends, or community. A perceived lack of family cohesion has also been associated with PTSD in Gulf War veterans (Sutker et al. 1995b). Few studies have specifically investigated social support during the period of deployment to a war zone. In one such study of Vietnam-theater and Vietnam-era veterans (Stretch 1985), social support during and after deployment was found to be a major factor in development of PTSD symptoms (social support accounted for 12% of explained variance).

The lack of studies of the role of social support during deployment is an important gap because U.S. military personnel consistently report "being away from family" as a leading deployment stressor, according to several periodic DoD surveys of more than 12,000 active-duty military personnel serving in Iraq (MHAT 2006). The committee notes that it is difficult to determine whether low social support leads to mental-health sequelae, psychiatric problems reduce social support, or the relationship is indirect with other variables, such as the association of personality with both social support and other psychopathology.

Combat Exposure

One of the major risk factors for PTSD is exposure to combat. Combat as a deployment-related stressor was discussed in Chapter 3.

PTSD appears to be associated with intensity and length of combat exposure. Studies of veterans from the Vietnam War and the Gulf War have confirmed a dose-response relationship between level of combat exposure and likelihood of PTSD. A study of 641 Australian Vietnam veterans conducted 20-25 years after the war found a dose-response relationship between exposure to combat and PTSD (O'Toole et al. 1996). The prevalence of lifetime combat-related PTSD was 20.9% with the Australian version of the SCID and 11.7% with the DIS; the prevalence of current (1-month) PTSD was 11.6% with the SCID. When the prevalence of lifetime or current PTSD (based on the SCID) was compared with responses to a 21-item combat index, there was a linear dose-response relationship with increasing combat exposure. The OR for each combat-score quartile for lifetime PTSD was 1.00, 3.03, 5.36, and 9.18; for current PTSD, the OR was 1.00, 2.11, 6.97, and 10.33 for each quartile increase in combat exposure.

Dohrenwend et al. (2006) used NVVRS data on 1200 Vietnam-theater veterans to assess exposure to war-zone stressors. A diagnosis of PTSD was based on the SCID. A dose-response relationship between PTSD and exposure to war-zone stressors was established. Current (as of 1988) war-related PTSD was diagnosed in 0.3% of low-exposure veterans, 14.4% of moderate-exposure, 27.0% of high-exposure, and 28.1% of very-high-exposure.

Longer and more intense combat exposure is associated with a greater prevalence of current PTSD. One study of male twins discordant for serving in Vietnam found more PTSD symptoms in the Vietnam veterans than in their twins who did not serve in Vietnam, even 15 years after the war (Goldberg et al. 1990). Roy-Byrne et al. (2004) also compared PTSD in twins, of whom one had substantial combat exposure in Vietnam and the other had low or no combat exposure or did not serve in Vietnam. Over the 10-year followup, the number of PTSD symptoms in veterans with greater combat exposure gradually decreased, but it was never reduced to the number seen in veterans with low or no combat exposure.

One study of 1709 Marines and soldiers deployed to OIF found that the number of veterans who screened positively for PTSD 3-4 months after their return increased linearly with the number of reported firefights with the enemy: 4.5% for no firefights, 9.3% for 1-2 firefights, 12.7% for 3-5 firefights, and 19.3% for more than 5 firefights. PTSD rates for 1962 Army soldiers deployed to Afghanistan were 4.5%, 8.2%, 8.3%, and 18.9%, respectively (Hoge et al. 2004).

Other combat-related factors influence the risk of PTSD and its course. Vietnam veterans (n = 1377) were questioned about possible PTSD symptoms in 1984 and again in 1998 (Koenen et al. 2003). The estimated prevalence of current (1 month) PTSD decreased from 11.8% in 1984 to 10.5% in 1998; 5.3% of those surveyed had symptoms of PTSD at both times, 6.5% met the criteria only in 1984, and 5.2% met the criteria only in 1998. Veterans who experienced high or medium combat exposure, perceived adverse community attitudes, or had discomfort in disclosing their war experience were more likely to have PTSD at either time. Discomfort in disclosing their Vietnam experience was associated with increased risk for developing PTSD but not with its course. For veterans with PTSD in 1984, high combat exposure increased the likelihood of having PTSD in 1998 and was the most important predictor of the course of PTSD. A veteran was also more likely to have PTSD in 1998 if he had symptoms of depression or anger in 1984, regardless of whether he had PTSD (Koenen et al. 2003). Combat-related lifetime PTSD is associated with increased current PTSD symptoms and a lower rate of remission among a group of 255 Hispanic and American Indian Vietnam veterans with PTSD. PTSD severity was greater in the 106 veterans who reported having had a traumatic experience associated with combat, 90% of whom were in combat units and the remaining veteran had served in roles related to combat such as medic or helicopter crews. The other 149 veterans had PTSD that was not related to combat experiences (Brinker et al. 2007).

In 1996, Schnurr et al. (2000b) assessed 363 World War II veterans for PTSD. The veterans had participated in secret military tests during the war that exposed them to mustard gas (and lewisite). Even 50 years after the war, 32% of the veterans had mustard-gas-related PTSD. Risk factors that had the greatest impact on the development of PTSD were having physical symptoms during the test, seeing others in distress during the test, and being prohibited from disclosing participation in the test; having volunteered for the test lowered the risk of PTSD.

Different combat-related traumas may result in different prominence of particular PTSD symptoms as manifestations of the disorder. For example, participation in atrocities might result in more avoidant symptoms, whereas heavy combat might result in more intrusive rather than avoidant symptoms (Yehuda et al. 1992b).

Physical Injury

Being wounded in combat significantly increases the risk of having current PTSD, regardless of the severity of the injury or the severity of the traumatic event that caused the injury (Koren et al. 2005). Veterans with injuries are at far greater the risk of PTSD than their noninjured counterparts (Gill et al. 2005; Koren et al. 2005; Kulka et al. 1990; Pitman et al. 1989). In a study of 13 Vietnam combat veterans who had been wounded and 21 who had not, of those who were wounded, only 1 had never had PTSD, 2 had PTSD that was in remission, and 10 (77%) had current PTSD, compared with 8, 7, and 6, respectively, of the nonwounded. Although the sample was small, the study suggests a strong association between being wounded and developing PTSD (Buydens-Branchey et al. 1990). Hoge et al. (2007) found that of 2863 OIF combat veterans surveyed a year after their return from Iraq, those who had been wounded or injured at least once were more than twice as likely to have PTSD as veterans who had never been wounded (31.8% vs 13.6%). Being wounded is also associated with increased risk of suicide in veterans. Bullman and Kang (1996) found a dose-response relationship between the number of times a Vietnam veteran was wounded in combat and the likelihood of suicide (see the Chapter 6 section on suicide for more details).

Grieger et al. (2006) found that the prevalence of PTSD in combat-wounded soldiers increased with time. A month after their injury, 4.2% of the OEF and OIF soldiers screened positive for likelihood of PTSD, but PTSD likelihood increased to 12% at 7 months after injury. Lee et al. (1995) found that all the World War II men who were wounded in the war reported later symptoms of PTSD regardless of the level of combat to which they were exposed. It has been suggested that veterans with chronic physical disabilities as a result of war-related injuries have higher rates of PTSD, particularly chronic PTSD. The disability may serve as a constant reminder of the traumatic incident, possibly contributing to the likelihood of PTSD and its persistence (Friedman et al. 1994).

NEUROBIOLOGY

Most neurobiologic research in PTSD has concentrated on two systems critical for survival: the sympathetic nervous system and the hypothalamus-pituitary-adrenal (HPA) axis (as discussed in Chapter 4). This discussion of PTSD focuses on the noradrenergic system and the HPA axis, but it is important to emphasize that numerous neurobiologic systems—such as the serotonin system, the opiate system, and sex steroidal systems—are also involved in pathologic and protective responses to stress, although less is known about their involvement in the genesis of PTSD.

Sympathetic Nervous System Alterations

Findings from clinical physiologic, receptor-binding, and pharmacologic-challenge studies have provided evidence of noradrenergic hyperreactivity in traumatized people who have PTSD (Bremner et al. 1999; Pitman and Orr 1990; Southwick and Friedman 2001). The exaggerated activity is generally not present under baseline or resting conditions but is evident during stress, especially stress associated with traumatic reminders. Numerous psychophysiologic studies have documented heightened sympathetic nervous system arousal in combat veterans who suffer from PTSD (Orr et al. 1990; Prins et al. 1995). Trauma victims with PTSD respond with greater psychophysiologic reactivity (particularly heart rate) to trauma-relevant stimuli than do comparison groups, such as trauma victims without PTSD and nontraumatized controls. Some studies have reported a higher baseline resting heart rate in those with PTSD than in control groups, but most studies have found no differences (Pitman and Orr 1990; Prins et al. 1995). In addition, response to generic stressors has typically been the same in groups with and without PTSD (Pitman and Orr 1990). Thus, trauma survivors with PTSD appear to have normal resting sympathetic nervous system activity as reflected in heart rate and blood pressure that become abnormally reactive in response to specific reminders of a personally experienced trauma but not in response to generic stressors (Murburg et al. 1994; Prins et al. 1995).

Biochemical correlates of the heightened sympathetic nervous system activation in veterans and civilians with PTSD include increased excretion of epinephrine and norepinephrine (Davidson and Baum 1986; Kosten et al. 1987; Yehuda et al. 1992a) and decreased numbers of alpha-2 adrenergic receptors on the surface of platelets (Perry 1994; Perry et al. 1987). As noted in Chapter 4, chronic increases in circulating epinephrine and norepinephrine may lead to a decrease in the number of adrenergic receptors.

These increases in epinephrine and norepinephrine may not be present during resting states. However, it appears that PTSD subjects respond to a variety of stressors with greater increases in catecholamines than do healthy controls (McFall et al. 1990; Murburg et al. 1994; Southwick et al. 1995). Greater increases in epinephrine have been observed in veterans with war-related PTSD than in controls during and after viewing of a combat film but not in response to a film of an automobile accident (McFall et al. 1990). Auditory reminders of trauma have also been used as in vivo probes of noradrenergic responsivity in combat veterans with PTSD. In a study of 15 combat veterans with PTSD and 6 combat veterans without a mental disorder, Blanchard et al. (1991) sampled plasma norepinephrine before and after exposure to combat-related auditory stimuli. The PTSD group showed a 30% increase in plasma norepinephrine and heart rate in contrast with no change in the combat control group.

Pharmacologic provocation studies have also revealed exaggerated catecholamine responses in patients with PTSD. To assess adrenergic responsivity of the peripheral and central nervous system more directly, yohimbine was administered to 20 Vietnam combat veterans with PTSD and 18 healthy controls (Southwick et al. 1993a). Yohimbine is an alpha-2 adrenergic receptor antagonist that activates noradrenergic neurons by blocking the alpha-2 adrenergic auto receptor, thereby increasing the release of endogenous norepinephrine. Yohimbine caused a marked increase in anxiety and PTSD-specific symptoms: 70% of combat veterans with PTSD experienced yohimbine-induced panic attacks, and 40% had flashbacks, but there were no panic attacks and only one flashback in the placebo group. Subjects with PTSD also had significantly greater increases in heart rate and more than twice the plasma 3-methoxy-4-hydroxy phenylglycol, which is a breakdown product of norepinephrine. In the Southwick et al. (1993a) study, the yohimbine-induced increase in catecholamine activity may have produced a biologic response that resembled the biologic state at the time when the traumatic memory was encoded, which then facilitated the retrieval of traumatic memories, a phenomenon known as "state-dependent recall." Those findings suggest a dysfunction of the locus coeruleus-norepinephrine function in patients with PTSD.

Interventions designed to suppress noradrenergic hyperreactivity directly in trauma survivors with PTSD have been limited to trials with the antiadrenergic agents clonidine (Kinzie and Leung 1989), guanfacine (Horrigan 1996), prazosin (Raskind et al. 2002), and propranolol (Pitman et al. 2002). Pitman et al. (2002), in a pilot study, administered propranolol to survivors of car accidents within 6 hours of the accidents. Although PTSD symptom scores 1 and 3 months after the trauma did not differ significantly between the two groups, the propranolol group at 3 months demonstrated significantly less psychophysiologic reactivity (in heart rate, skin conductance, and corrugator electromyography) to mental imagery that symbolized or resembled the index trauma. Positive results with propanolol have also been reported in accident victims who presented at an emergency room with tachycardia (Vaiva et al. 2003). Those preliminary studies with propranolol need replication, however, to determine whether it will be an effective treatment after trauma exposure to prevent PTSD. The propranolol results are consistent with data on healthy people. Southwick et al. (1993a) found a positive association between enhanced noradrenergic activity and enhanced long-term memory, and Cahill et al. (1994) reported that propranolol blocked enhanced memory of an arousing story. However, it is important to note that evidence has shown that propranolol can block extinction of fear-related memories (Cain et al. 2004). Taken together, the above evidence suggests that at least a subgroup of people with PTSD has increased responsivity of the sympathetic nervous system that is most clearly evident when people are restressed (Southwick et al. 1995).

HPA-Axis Alterations

That cortisol concentrations are increased during stress and that the magnitude of stress response is associated with the magnitude of increases in cortisol led to the hypothesis that cortisol would be increased in PTSD. However, the first report, 20 years ago, of cortisol in PTSD yielded counterintuitive results: the mean 24-hour urinary excretion of cortisol was lower in patients with PTSD than in other psychiatric patients (Mason et al. 1986).

Ambiguity has persisted in the literature regarding the direction of any PTSD, associated change in cortisol concentrations as some investigators have reported increased urinary cortisol excretion in PTSD. Yehuda et al. (2002) noted that PTSD is associated with a dysregulation of the cortisol response rather than with a clear-cut directional response (cortisol that is "too low" or "too high"). Present evidence supports the hypothesis that pre-existing low cortisol is associated with increased risk of PTSD. Several recent studies have found that trauma victims who develop PTSD have lower initial cortisol responses to a traumatic event than do trauma victims who do not develop PTSD (McFarlane 1997; Resnick et al. 1997). In combat veterans with chronic PTSD, low plasma cortisol has been recorded throughout the day and night, especially in the early morning and late evening (Yehuda et al. 2002). Finally, in a randomized double-blind placebo-controlled study, Schelling et al. (2001, 2006) assessed the effect of hydrocortisone administered during septic shock. Physiologically stressful doses of hydrocortisone did have a moderately protective effect against PTSD.

Receptor-binding studies have found higher numbers of glucocorticoid receptors in subjects with PTSD than in controls without PTSD (Yehuda 1997; Yehuda et al. 1995). As discussed in Chapter 4, an increased number of receptors would enhance sensitivity by providing more binding sites for cortisol. It is consistent with increased receptor number and sensitivity that subjects with PTSD hyperrrespond to administration of dexamethasone, a synthetic glucocorticoid that acts like cortisol (Yehuda 1997; Yehuda et al. 2004). Usually, when dexamethasone is administered to healthy people, it engages glucocorticoid receptors that serve as part of a negative feedback mechanism. When engaged, the receptors signal the hypothalamus and pituitary to decrease the release of corticotropin-releasing hormone (CRH) and corticotropin; this results in decreased stimulation of the adrenal gland and diminished release of endogenous cortisol. In several different populations of trauma survivors with PTSD, dexamethasone has had an exaggerated effect and endogenous cortisol release has been reduced to a greater degree than in healthy controls. The HPA-axis findings in PTSD differ markedly from findings in studies of major depressive disorder, in which cortisol tends to be increased, and the cortisol response to dexamethasone reduced.

Additional findings in subjects with PTSD include increased CRH in cerebrospinal fluid (Baker et al. 1997; Bremner et al. 1997), blunted corticotropin response to CRH infusion (Smith et al. 1989), and increased corticotropin response to metyrapone (Yehuda et al. 2004). Those findings are consistent with studies in primates that have experienced early-life stress (Coplan et al. 1996). Animal data on the effects of a nonpeptide CRH receptor-1 antagonist (antalarmin) that penetrates the blood-brain barrier have shown that it blocks the development, consolidation, and expression of conditioned fear (Deak et al. 1999). Recent studies in rhesus monkeys showed that oral administration of antalarmin significantly inhibited stress-induced increases in plasma norepinephrine, cortisol, and anxiety-related behaviors (Habib et al. 2000). If applicable to humans, those data suggest that a CRH antagonist could be helpful after an acute traumatic event or in preventing harmful central nervous system changes that occur during chronic stress (Gold et al. 2005).

In summary, most PTSD studies demonstrate alterations consistent with increased feedback inhibition of the HPA axis and increased CRH activity. The degree to which those abnormalities represent predisposing neurobiologic risk factors for PTSD rather than consequences of trauma or of living with PTSD is not clear (Yehuda et al. 2002).

Fear Conditioning

Several investigators have noted that the behavioral and physiologic responses of veterans with PTSD are similar to the effects of fear conditioning in animals (Kardiner and Spiegel 1947; Kolb 1987). Fear conditioning can be adaptive. A person who can anticipate a threat by responding to conditioned contextual cues can rapidly engage in appropriate defensive behaviors. Clinically, specific environmental stimuli may be linked to a traumatic event, a spontaneous panic attack, or an embarrassing social situation in such a way that exposure to a similar cue produces a recurrence of symptoms of anxiety and fear. For example, a Vietnam veteran may associate the smell of stir-fried pork with unpleasant memories of Vietnam or the sound of thunder with being in combat. Fear conditioning occurs outside conscious awareness (LeDoux 1996). For the Vietnam veteran, a formerly neutral stimulus has become frightening because it has been transformed into a fear-conditioned stimulus. Clinically, that means that a traumatized person, when exposed to a fear-conditioned cue, may become frightened, anxious, or irritable for reasons that he or she does not understand. Fear-conditioned responses, once they are established, can persist for long periods. Theoretically, once a conditioned fear stimulus is no longer associated with an aversive outcome, the conditioned fear response should extinguish. However, evidence in animals suggests that extinction is an active process that may involve new learning and that the old fear-conditioned association may persist indefinitely and under the right circumstances become reactivated (Bouton and Nelson 1994).

In addition to the formation of vivid memories, patients with PTSD may fail to recover because fear is not extinguished after trauma. Most trauma survivors appear to respond with the re-experiencing, avoidance, and arousal symptoms of PTSD in the immediate aftermath of trauma. However, most of those fear reactions extinguish over time, and people do not develop chronic PTSD. Prospective studies indicate that those who recover from PTSD show a decrease in PTSD symptoms beginning soon after the trauma, but those who do not recover show a different pattern: their PTSD symptoms decrease in the first month after trauma but then remain fairly steady (Rothbaum et al. 1992); they do not worsen, but their original fear reactions are not extinguished to the extent found in non-PTSD people.

People with PTSD do not seem to benefit from safety signals, such as the presence of a spouse, that potentially could help them to cope with painful fear memories (Herman 1992). An example might be a female rape victim who, before the rape, had a close, intimate relationship with her husband (a safety signal) but now feels unsafe with him and with other men. Similarly, despite the passage of many years and being in an environment very different from Vietnam, a war veteran's fear can persist despite the presence of many potential safety signals, such as being in the United States instead of Vietnam, being in regular clothes instead of battle fatigues, and being back with loved ones.

Thus, although a great deal is known about brain systems involved in fear generation, much less is known about brain systems involved in fear inhibition (extinction and safety signals). The need to understand the biologic mechanisms of fear inhibition is just beginning to be appreciated (Myers and Davis 2007).

Startle Reflex

Exaggerated startle reflex is commonly associated with PTSD. Metzger et al. (1999) in a meta-analysis of the eye-blink component of the startle reflex in PTSD, concluded that the weighted effect sizes across all 11 studies provide support for exaggerated startle as a symptom of PTSD. Eight of 11 of the studies found medium to large-sized effects for eye-blink electromyogram startle-response magnitude to acoustic stimuli. Studies included Vietnam and Gulf War combat veterans and victims of sexual assault and mixed trauma.

In a comprehensive review of the startle reflex in PTSD, Grillon and Baas (2003) concluded that abnormalities of both a tonic and a phasic nature may exist in PTSD. They suggest that exposure to a traumatic event probably prompts a sensitization process that leads to an initial exaggerated startle. As the trauma becomes more distant in time, the enhanced startle response may gradually subside. The exaggerated startle response in patients with chronic PTSD may be a phasic symptom that is elicited by later trauma-related stimuli or by stressful environments and may involve different brain circuits over time. The amygdala may be involved in the early sensitization and in conditioned emotional responses (Hitchcock and Davis 1986; Hitchcock et al. 1989), whereas in chronic PTSD sufferers the exaggeration of startle in stressful contexts suggests that excessive release of CRH leads to involvement of the bed nucleus of the stria terminal (see Chapter 4). The most robust findings of exaggerated startle in PTSD are seen in patients with recent onset (within the preceding 5 years). The results in patients with chronic PTSD (onset more than 10 years earlier) are less clear. Vietnam veterans with chronic PTSD showed exaggerated startle response when assessed under stressful experimental conditions, but only one of the five studies that assessed the veterans with PTSD under nonstressful conditions found exaggerated startle response (Grillon and Baas 2003).

Sleep Disturbances

PTSD is characterized by trauma-related nightmares and sleep disturbance, which are often refractory to treatment (Friedman 2002; Ross et al. 1989; Taylor et al. 2007; Van Liempt et al. 2006). It has been hypothesized that increased noradrenergic function in the brain might contribute to PTSD-associated sleep symptoms (Mellman et al. 1995a). For example, increased noradrenergic activity could account for the abnormalities in rapid-eye-movement (REM) sleep in people with PTSD. The abnormalities include increased phasic motor activity, stage shifts, and arousal (Ross et al. 1994; Breslau et al. 2004), and REM fragmentation during early PTSD development (Mellman et al. 1995b). Furthermore, disruption in REM sleep could be related to nightmares (Mellman et al. 1995b, 2002) and the cognitive processing of traumatic events (Stickgold 2007). It is consistent with those findings that prazosin, an alpha-1 adrenergic antagonist, has been demonstrated to be an effective treatment for trauma nightmares and sleep disturbance in PTSD (Raskind et al. 2003, 2007; Taylor and Raskind 2002) by increasing total sleep time, REM sleep time, and REM-period duration (Taylor et al. 2007). See Chapter 6 for more discussion of PTSD and sleep disturbance.

Neuroimaging Studies

Neuroimaging studies have been used to identify the neural circuits that may be involved in the development of PTSD. Neuroimaging studies, using magnetic resonance imaging (MRI), of people with PTSD have focused primarily on the amygdala, the hippocampus, the medial prefrontal cortex, and the anterior cingulate cortex. Reduced hippocampal volume has been reported in a diverse population of adults with PTSD, both those with a history of childhood trauma and those who suffered trauma as adults. A recent neuroimaging study of identical twin children of veterans who had PTSD and reduced hippocampal volume found that the twin children also had reduced hippocampal volume despite having had no exposure to combat and no history of PTSD (Gilbertson et al. 2002). In some people, smaller hippocampal volumes may predate their trauma exposure and PTSD and be a risk factor for PTSD rather than a consequence of it.

However, not all studies report smaller hippocampal findings in subjects with PTSD (Bonne et al. 2001), and the literature is ambiguous about whether PTSD is associated with reduced hippocampal volume in children (De Bellis et al. 2001). Recent studies suggest that traumatic stress in early development may have diffuse effects on total brain volume rather than only effects on hippocampal volume (De Bellis et al. 2002a,b). Possible explanations for discrepant findings on hippocampal volume in PTSD include variability in intensity and duration of trauma exposure, the presence of comorbid psychiatric disorders, differences in imaging methods (Vythilingam et al. 2005), and the lack of an effect of PTSD on hippocampal volume.

Functional MRI studies that measure regional cerebral blood flow (rCBF) using cognitive activation models, script-driven imagery, or other methods that provoke PTSD re-experiencing symptoms have generally found exaggerated activation of the amygdala or reduced activation of the prefrontal cortex. The overactive amygdala may be receiving insufficient negative feedback from the anterior cingulate gyrus and the medial prefrontal cortex.

Although most functional imaging studies have examined responses to threat- or trauma-relevant stimuli, it is also important to sort out how neural networks function in PTSD in the absence of threat-related stimuli. One study explored PTSD responses to a selective attention task that engages anterior cingulate cortex networks but in response to a nonthreatening stimulus. Bryant and Guthrie (2005) investigated whether anterior cingulate-amygdala dysregulation in PTSD was specific to processing threat-related stimuli or generalized to more generic, nonthreatening stimuli. They believe that their findings of enhanced anterior cingulate responses, and activation in the left amygdala and posterior parietal networks in response to nonthreatening stimuli, may reflect generalized hypervigilance. The nature and anatomic bases of attention and working-memory deficits in PTSD are also being studied with functional neuroimaging. With proton-emission tomography, working-memory deficits in PTSD have been found to be associated with reduced left dorsolateral prefrontal cortical activity (Clark et al. 2003).

In summary, many structural MRI studies have found that decreased hippocampal volume is associated with PTSD in adults. In general, functional neuroimaging studies in trauma survivors with PTSD have reported exaggerated rCBF in the amygdala and other paralimbic regions and relative decreases in prefrontal cortical rCBF. Increased stress-induced activation of the amygdala in combination with reduced inhibition by the prefrontal cortex might leave a trauma survivor with an exaggerated and relatively unchecked amygdala-driven fight-or-flight stress response.

CONCLUSIONS

Characterized by symptoms of hyperarousal, numbing or avoidance, and re-experiencing of a traumatic event, PTSD may be evident shortly after exposure to the traumatic event or take years to produce symptoms sufficient to meet the diagnostic criteria; once developed, the symptoms may persist for many years. PTSD (or symptoms associated with it) has been reported in veterans from World War II, the Korean War, the Vietnam War, the Gulf War, and OEF and OIF. The prevalence of PTSD in the Vietnam War, Gulf War, and OEF and OIF have been estimated to be 14-19% (lifetime), 5-9% (lifetime), and 12-16% (current), respectively. Across a variety of precipitating events, women have twice the PTSD prevalence as men both in veteran populations and in the general population. In the general population, the prevalence of lifetime PTSD is estimated to be about 5% for men and 10% for women. The prevalence of PTSD in veterans increases as combat exposure increases, in some cases showing a linear dose-response relationship. PTSD is also highly comorbid with other psychiatric disorders, particularly major depression, general anxiety disorder, and substance-use disorders. PTSD is also associated with more disability and impaired functioning in veterans.

Although military personnel may be exposed to identical stressors during their deployment to a war zone, their short-term and long-term responses to those stressors vary. The variation is due to a host of individual risk and protective factors that influence the likelihood of long-term health effects after exposure. The committee found that among the most significant risk factors for PTSD or other psychiatric disorders are being in combat and being physically wounded. Other important risk factors include childhood maltreatment, the presence of a pre-existing psychiatric disorder, poor social support on homecoming, negative coping styles, being a minority, and a lack of hardiness. Protective factors include better education, higher military rank, having a stable family life, and having a sense of control.

Research has shown heightened sympathetic nervous system activation in people with PTSD, which includes increased excretion of epinephrine and norepinephrine. PTSD subjects respond to a variety of stressors with greater increases in catecholamines than do healthy controls. Pre-existing low cortisol is associated with increased risk of PTSD, and most PTSD studies demonstrate physiologic alterations consistent with enhanced feedback inhibition of the HPA axis and increased HPA reactivity. PTSD has also been associated with a lack of fear extinction after trauma.

REFERENCES

Aldwin CM, Levenson MR, Spiro A 3rd. 1994. Vulnerability and resilience to combat exposure: Can stress have lifelong effects? *Psychology and Aging* 9(1):34-44.

APA (American Psychiatric Association). 2000. *Diagnostic and Statistical Manual of Mental Disorders, Fourth Edition, Text Revision (DSM-IV-TR)*. Washington, DC: American Psychiatric Publishing Association.

Arata CM, Picou JS, Johnson GD, McNally TS. 2000. Coping with technological disaster: An application of the conservation of resources model to the Exxon Valdez oil spill. *Journal of Traumatic Stress* 13(1):23-39.

Baker DG, West SA, Orth DN, Hill KK, Nicholson WE, Ekhator NN, Bruce AB, Wortman MD, Keck PE Jr., Geracioti TD Jr. 1997. Cerebrospinal fluid and plasma beta-endorphin in combat veterans with post-traumatic stress disorder. *Psychoneuroendocrinology* 22(7):517-529.

Barrett TW, Mizes JS. 1988. Combat level and social support in the development of posttraumatic stress disorder in Vietnam veterans. *Behavior Modification* 12(1):100-115.

Bartone PT. 1999. Hardiness protects against war-related stress in Army Reserve forces. *Consulting Psychology Journal: Practice and Research* 51(2):72-82.

Benotsch EG, Brailey K, Vasterling JJ, Uddo M, Constans JI, Sutker PB. 2000. War zone stress, personal and environmental resources, and PTSD symptoms in Gulf War veterans: A longitudinal perspective. *Journal of Abnormal Psychology* 109(2):205-213.

Black DW, Carney CP, Peloso PM, Woolson RF, Schwartz DA, Voelker MD, Barrett DH, Doebbeling BN. 2004. Gulf War veterans with anxiety: Prevalence, comorbidity, and risk factors. *Epidemiology* 15(2):135-142.

Blanchard EB, Kolb LC, Prins A, Gates S, McCoy GC. 1991. Changes in plasma norepinephrine to combat-related stimuli among Vietnam veterans with posttraumatic stress disorder. *Journal of Nervous and Mental Disease* 179(6):371-373.

Bland SH, O'Leary ES, Farinaro E, Jossa F, Krogh V, Violanti JM, Trevisan M. 1997. Social network disturbances and psychological distress following earthquake evacuation. *Journal of Nervous and Mental Disease* 185(3):188-194.

Bleich A, Solomon Z. 2004. Evaluation of psychiatric disability in PTSD of military origin. *Israel Journal of Psychiatry and Related Sciences* 41(4):268-276.

Bonne O, Brandes D, Gilboa A, Gomori JM, Shenton ME, Pitman RK, Shalev AY. 2001. Longitudinal MRI study of hippocampal volume in trauma survivors with PTSD. *American Journal of Psychiatry* 158(8):1248-1251.

Boscarino JA. 1995. Post-traumatic stress and associated disorders among Vietnam veterans: The significance of combat exposure and social support. *Journal of Traumatic Stress* 8(2):317-336.

Bouton ME, Nelson JB. 1994. Context-specificity of target versus feature inhibition in a feature-negative discrimination. *Journal of Experimental Psycholology: Animal Behavior Processes* 20(1):51-65.

Bremner J, Southwick SM, Darnell A, Charney DS. 1996. Chronic PTSD in Vietnam combat veterans: Course of illness and substance abuse. *American Journal of Psychiatry* 153(3):369-375.

Bremner JD, Southwick SM, Johnson DR, Yehuda R, Charney DS. 1993. Childhood physical abuse and combat-related posttraumatic stress disorder in Vietnam veterans. *American Journal of Psychiatry* 150(2):235-239.

Bremner JD, Licinio J, Darnell A, Krystal JH, Owens MJ, Southwick SM, Nemeroff CB, Charney DS. 1997. Elevated CSF corticotropin-releasing factor concentrations in posttraumatic stress disorder. *American Journal of Psychiatry* 154(5):624-629.

Bremner JD, Staib LH, Kaloupek D, Southwick SM, Soufer R, Charney DS. 1999. Neural correlates of exposure to traumatic pictures and sound in Vietnam combat veterans with and without posttraumatic stress disorder: A positron emission tomography study. *Biological Psychiatry* 45(7):806-816.

Breslau N. 2001a. The epidemiology of posttraumatic stress disorder: What is the extent of the problem? *Journal of Clinical Psychiatry* 62(Suppl 17):16-22.

Breslau N. 2001b. Outcomes of posttraumatic stress disorder. *Journal of Clinical Psychiatry* 62(Suppl 17):55-59.

Breslau N, Chase GA, Anthony JC. 2002. The uniqueness of the DSM definition of post-traumatic stress disorder: Implications for research. *Psychological Medicine* 32(4):573-576.

Breslau N, Roth T, Burduvali E, Kapke A, Schultz L, Roehrs T. 2004. Sleep in lifetime posttraumatic stress disorder: A community-based polysomnographic study. *Archives of General Psychiatry* 61:508-516.

Brewin CR, Andrews B, Valentine JD. 2000. Meta-analysis of risk factors for posttraumatic stress disorder in trauma-exposed adults. *Journal of Consulting and Clinical Psychology* 68(5):748-766.

Brinker M, Westermeyer J, Thuras P, Canive J. 2007. Severity of combat-related posttraumatic stress disorder versus noncombat-related posttraumatic stress disorder: A community-based study in American Indian and Hispanic veterans. *Journal of Nervous and Mental Disease* 19598):655-661.

Bryant RA, Guthrie RM. 2005. Maladaptive appraisals as a risk factor for posttraumatic stress: A study of trainee firefighters. *Psychological Science* 16(10):749-752.

Bryant RA, Harvey AG. 2002. Delayed-onset posttraumatic stress disorder: A prospective evaluation. *Australian and New Zealand Journal of Psychiatry* 36(2):205-209.

Bullman TA, Kang HK. 1996. The risk of suicide among wounded Vietnam veterans. *American Journal of Public Health* 86(5):662-667.

Buydens-Branchey L, Noumair D, Branchey M. 1990. Duration and intensity of combat exposure and posttraumatic stress disorder in Vietnam veterans. *Journal of Nervous and Mental Disease* 178(9):582-587.

Cahill L, Prins B, Weber M, McGaugh JL. 1994. Beta-adrenergic activation and memory for emotional events. *Nature* 371(6499):702-704.

Cain CK, Blouin AM, Barad M. 2004. Adrenergic transmission facilitates extinction of conditional fear in mice. *Learning and Memory* 11(2):179-187.

Carty J, O'Donnell ML, Creamer M. 2006. Delayed-onset PTSD: A prospective study of injury survivors. *Journal of Affective Disorders* 90(2-3):257-261.

CDC (Centers for Disease Control). 1988. Health status of Vietnam veterans. I. Psychosocial characteristics. The Centers for Disease Control Vietnam Experience Study. *Journal of the American Medical Association* 259(18):2701-2707.

Clark CR, McFarlane AC, Morris P, Weber DL, Sonkkilla C, Shaw M, Marcina J, Tochon-Danguy HJ, Egan GF. 2003. Cerebral function in posttraumatic stress disorder during verbal working memory updating: A positron emission tomography study. *Biological Psychiatry* 53(6):474-481.

Connor KM, Butterfield MI. 2003. Posttraumatic stress disorder. *Focus* 1(3):247-262.

Coplan JD, Andrews MW, Rosenblum LA, Owens MJ, Friedman S, Gorman JM, Nemeroff CB. 1996. Persistent elevations of cerebrospinal fluid concentrations of corticotropin-releasing factor in adult nonhuman primates exposed to early-life stressors: Implications for the pathophysiology of mood and anxiety disorders. *Proceedings of the National Academy of Sciences of the United States of America* 93(4):1619-1623.

Davidson LM, Baum A. 1986. Chronic stress and posttraumatic stress disorders. *Journal of Consulting and Clinical Psychology* 54(3):303-308.

De Bellis MD, Hall J, Boring AM, Frustaci K, Moritz G. 2001. A pilot longitudinal study of hippocampal volumes in pediatric maltreatment-related posttraumatic stress disorder. *Biological Psychiatry* 50(4):305-309.

De Bellis MD, Keshavan MS, Frustaci K, Shifflett H, Iyengar S, Beers SR, Hall J. 2002a. Superior temporal gyrus volumes in maltreated children and adolescents with PTSD. *Biological Psychiatry* 51(7):544-552.

De Bellis MD, Keshavan MS, Shifflett H, Iyengar S, Beers SR, Hall J, Moritz G. 2002b. Brain structures in pediatric maltreatment-related posttraumatic stress disorder: A sociodemographically matched study. *Biological Psychiatry* 52(11):1066-1078.

Deak T, Nguyen KT, Ehrlich AL, Watkins LR, Spencer RL, Maier SF, Licinio J, Wong ML, Chrousos GP, Webster E, Gold PW. 1999. The impact of the nonpeptide corticotropin-releasing hormone antagonist antalarmin on behavioral and endocrine responses to stress. *Endocrinology* 140(1):79-86.

Dohrenwend B, Turner J, Turse N, Adams B, Koenen K, Marshal R. 2006. The psychological risks of Vietnam for U.S. veterans: A revisit with new data and methods. *Science* 313(5789):979-982.

Dolan CA, Adler AB. 2006. Military hardiness as a buffer of psychological health on return from deployment. *Military Medicine* 171(2):93-98.

Elder GH Jr., Clipp EC. 1988. Wartime losses and social bonding: Influences across 40 years in men's lives. *Psychiatry* 51(2):177-198.

Engdahl B, Dikel TN, Eberly R, Blank A Jr. 1998. Comorbidity and course of psychiatric disorders in a community sample of former prisoners of war. *American Journal of Psychiatry* 155(12):1740-1745.

Engel CC Jr., Engel AL, Campbell SJ, McFall ME, Russo J, Katon W. 1993. Posttraumatic stress disorder symptoms and precombat sexual and physical abuse in Desert Storm veterans. *Journal of Nervous and Mental Disease* 181(11):683-688.

Escobar JI, Randolph ET, Puente G, Spiwak F, Asamen JK, Hill M, Hough RL. 1983. Post-traumatic stress disorder in Hispanic Vietnam veterans. Clinical phenomenology and sociocultural characteristics. *Journal of Nervous and Mental Disease* 171(10):585-596.

Fiedler N, Ozakinci G, Hallman W, Wartenberg D, Brewer NT, Barrett DH, Kipen HM. 2006. Military deployment to the Gulf War as a risk factor for psychiatric illness among U.S. troops. *British Journal of Psychiatry* 188:453-459.

Fontana A, Rosenheck R. 1994a. Posttraumatic stress disorder among Vietnam theater veterans. A causal model of etiology in a community sample. *Journal of Nervous and Mental Disease* 182(12):677-684.

Fontana A, Rosenheck R. 1994b. Traumatic war stressors and psychiatric symptoms among World War II, Korean, and Vietnam War veterans. *Psychology and Aging* 9(1):27-33.

Fontana A, Rosenheck R, Horvath T. 1997. Social support and psychopathology in the war zone. *Journal of Nervous and Mental Disease* 185(11):675-681.

Fontana A, Litz B, Rosenheck R. 2000. Impact of combat and sexual harassment on the severity of posttraumatic stress disorder among men and women peacekeepers in Somalia. *Journal of Nervous and Mental Disease* 188(3):163-169.

Friedman M. 2003. *Post Traumatic Stress Disorder*. Kansas City, MO: Compact Clinicals.

Friedman MJ. 2002. Future pharmacotherapy for post-traumatic stress disorder: Prevention and treatment. *Psychiatry Clinics of North America* 25:427-441.

Friedman MJ, Schnurr PP, McDonagh-Coyle A. 1994. Post-traumatic stress disorder in the military veteran. *Psychiatry Clinics of North America* 17(2):265-277.

Friedman MJ, Schnurr PP, Sengupta A, Holmes T, Ashcraft M. 2004. The Hawaii Vietnam Veterans Project: Is minority status a risk factor for posttraumatic stress disorder? *Journal of Nervous and Mental Disease* 192(1):42-50.

Gibbs MS. 1989. Factors in the victim that mediate between disaster and psychopathology: A review. *Journal of Traumatic Stress* 2(4):489-514.

Gilbertson MW, Shenton ME, Ciszewski A, Kasai K, Lasko NB, Orr SP, Pitman RK. 2002. Smaller hippocampal volume predicts pathologic vulnerability to psychological trauma. *Nature Neuroscience* 5(11):1242-1247.

Gill JM, Szanton SL, Page GG. 2005. Biological underpinnings of health alterations in women with PTSD: A sex disparity. *Biological Research for Nursing* 7(1):44-54.

Gold SD, Marx BP, Soler-Baillo JM, Sloan DM. 2005. Is life stress more traumatic than traumatic stress? *Journal of Anxiety Disorders* 19(6):687-698.

Goldberg J, True WR, Eisen SA, Henderson WG. 1990. A twin study of the effects of the Vietnam War on posttraumatic stress disorder. *Journal of the American Medical Association* 263(9):1227-1232.

Goldzweig CL, Balekian TM, Rolon C, Yano EM, Shekelle PG. 2006. The state of women veterans' health research: Results of a systematic literature review. *Journal of General Internal Medicine* 21(Suppl 3):S82-S92.

Goss Gilroy Inc. 1998. *Health Study of Canadian Forces Personnel Involved in the 1991 Conflict in the Persian Gulf*. Ottawa, Canada: Goss Gilroy Inc. Department of National Defence.

Gray MJ, Bolton EE, Litz BT. 2004. A longitudinal analysis of PTSD symptom course: Delayed-onset PTSD in Somalia peacekeepers. *Journal of Consulting and Clinical Psychology* 72(5):909-913.

Green BL, Grace MC, Lindy JD, Gleser GC. 1990a. War stressors and symptom persistence in posttraumatic stress disorder. *Journal of Anxiety Disorders* 4(1):31-39.

Green BL, Grace MC, Lindy JD, Gleser GC, Leonard A. 1990b. Risk factors for PTSD and other diagnoses in a general sample of Vietnam veterans. *American Journal of Psychiatry* 147(6):729-733.

Grieger TA, Cozza SJ, Ursano RJ, Hoge C, Martinez PE, Engel CC, Wain HJ. 2006. Posttraumatic stress disorder and depression in battle-injured soldiers. *American Journal of Psychiatry* 163(10):1777-1783.

Grillon C, Baas J. 2003. A review of the modulation of the startle reflex by affective states and its application in psychiatry. *Clinical Neurophysiology* 114:1557-1579.

Grinker RR, Spiegel JP. 1945. *Men Under Stress.* Philadelphia, PA: Blakiston.

Grob GN. 1994. *The Mad Among Us: A History of the Care of America's Mentally Ill.* New York: Free Press.

Habib KE, Weld KP, Rice KC, Pushkas J, Champoux M, Listwak S, Webster EL, Atkinson AJ, Schulkin J, Contoreggi C, Chrousos GP, McCann SM, Suomi SJ, Higley JD, Gold PW. 2000. Oral administration of a corticotropin-releasing hormone receptor antagonist significantly attenuates behavioral, neuroendocrine, and autonomic responses to stress in primates. *Proceedings of the National Academy of Sciences of the United States of America* 97(11):6079-6084.

Herman J. 1992. *Trauma and Recovery*. New York: Basic Books.

Hitchcock JM, Davis M. 1986. Lesions of the amygdala, but not of the cerebellum or red nucleus, block conditioned fear as measured with the potentiated startle paradigm. *Behavioral Neuroscience* 100:11-22.

Hitchcock JM, Sananes CB, Davis M. 1989. Sensitization of the startle reflex by footshock: Blockade by lesions of the central nucleus of the amygdala or its efferent pathway to the brainstem. *Behavioral Neuroscience* 103:509-518.

Hoge CW, Lesikar SE, Guevara R, Lange J, Brundage JF, Engel CC Jr., Messer SC, Orman DT. 2002. Mental disorders among U.S. military personnel in the 1990s: Association with high levels of health care utilization and early military attrition. *American Journal of Psychiatry* 159(9):1576-1583.

Hoge CW, Castro CA, Messer SC, McGurk D, Cotting DI, Koffman RL. 2004. Combat duty in Iraq and Afghanistan, mental health problems, and barriers to care. *New England Journal of Medicine* 351(1):13-22.

Hoge CW, Terhakopian A, Castro CA, Messer SC, Engel CC. 2007. Association of posttraumatic stress disorder with somatic symptoms, health care visits, and absenteeism among Iraq War veterans. *American Journal of Psychiatry* 164(1):150-153.

Horrigan JP. 1996. Guanfacine for PTSD nightmares. *Journal of the American Academy of Child Adolescent Psychiatry* 35(8):975-976.

Hyams KC, Wignall FS, Roswell R. 1996. War syndromes and their evaluation: From the U.S. Civil War to the Persian Gulf War. *Annals of Internal Medicine* 125(5):398-405.

Ikin JF, Sim MR, Creamer MC, Forbes AB, McKenzie DP, Kelsall HL, Glass DC, McFarlane AC, Abramson MJ, Ittak P, Dwyer T, Blizzard L, Delaney KR, Horsley KW, Harrex WK, Schwarz H. 2004. War-related psychological stressors and risk of psychological disorders in Australian veterans of the 1991 Gulf War. *British Journal of Psychiatry* 185:116-126.

Jennings PA, Aldwin CM, Levenson MR, Spiro A 3rd, Mroczek DK. 2006. Combat exposure, perceived benefits of military service, and wisdom in later life: Findings from the Normative Aging Study. *Research on Aging* 28(1):115-134.

Jones E. 2006. Historical approaches to post-combat disorders. *Philosophical Transactions of the Royal Society of London—Series B: Biological Sciences* 361(1468):533-542.

Kang H, Dalager N, Mahan C, Ishii E. 2005. The role of sexual assault on the risk of PTSD among Gulf War veterans. *Annals of Epidemiology* 15(3):191-195.

Kang HK, Natelson BH, Mahan CM, Lee KY, Murphy FM. 2003. Post-traumatic stress disorder and chronic fatigue syndrome-like illness among Gulf War veterans: A population-based survey of 30,000 veterans. *American Journal of Epidemiology* 157(2):141-148.

Kang HK, Bullman TA, Taylor JW. 2006. Risk of selected cardiovascular diseases and posttraumatic stress disorder among former World War II prisoners of war. *Annals of Epidemiology* 16(5):381-386.

Kardiner A, Spiegel H. 1947. *War Stress and Neurotic Illness*. New York: Paul B. Hoeber.

Keane TM. 1998. Psychological effects of military combat. In: Dohrenwend BP, editor. *Adversity, Stress, and Psychopathology*. Oxford, UK: Oxford University Press. Pp. 52-65.

Kessler RC, Sonnega A, Bromet E, Hughes M, Nelson CB. 1995. Posttraumatic stress disorder in the National Comorbidity Survey. *Archives of General Psychiatry* 52(12):1048-1060.

Kessler RC, Berglund P, Demler O, Jin R, Merikangas KR, Walters EE. 2005a. Lifetime prevalence and age-of-onset distributions of DSM-IV disorders in the National Comorbidity Survey Replication. *Archives of General Psychiatry* 62(6):593-602.

Kessler RC, Chiu WT, Demler O, Merikangas KR, Walters EE. 2005b. Prevalence, severity, and comorbidity of 12-month DSM-IV disorders in the National Comorbidity Survey Replication. *Archives of General Psychiatry* 62(6):617-627.

King DW, King LA, Foy DW, Keane TM, Fairbank JA. 1999. Posttraumatic stress disorder in a national sample of female and male Vietnam veterans: Risk factors, war-zone stressors, and resilience-recovery variables. *Journal of Abnormal Psychology* 108(1):164-170.

Kinzie JD, Leung P. 1989. Clonidine in Cambodian patients with posttraumatic stress disorder. *Journal of Nervous and Mental Disease* 177(9):546-550.

Koenen KC, Stellman JM, Stellman SD, Sommer JF Jr. 2003. Risk factors for course of posttraumatic stress disorder among Vietnam veterans: A 14-year follow-up of American Legionnaires. *Journal of Consulting and Clinical Psychology* 71(6):980-986.

Kolb LC. 1987. A neuropsychological hypothesis explaining posttraumatic stress disorders. *American Journal of Psychiatry* 144(8):989-995.

Koren D, Norman D, Cohen A, Berman J, Klein EM. 2005. Increased PTSD risk with combat-related injury: A matched comparison study of injured and uninjured soldiers experiencing the same combat events. *American Journal of Psychiatry* 162(2):276-282.

Kosten TR, Mason JW, Giller EL, Ostroff RB, Harkness L. 1987. Sustained urinary norepinephrine and epinephrine elevation in post-traumatic stress disorder. *Psychoneuroendocrinology* 12(1):13-20.

Kulka RA, Schlenger WE, Fairbank JA, Hough RL, Jordan BK, Marmar CR, Weiss DS. 1990. *Trauma and the Vietnam War Generation: Report of Findings from the National Vietnam Veterans Readjustment Study*. New York: Brunner/Mazel Publishers.

Lapp KG, Bosworth HB, Strauss JL, Stechuchak KM, Horner RD, Calhoun PS, Meador KG, Lipper S, Butterfield MI. 2005. Lifetime sexual and physical victimization among male veterans with combat-related post-traumatic stress disorder. *Military Medicine* 170(9):787-790.

LeDoux J. 1996. Emotional networks and motor control: A fearful view. *Progress in Brain Research* 107:437-446.

Lee KA, Vaillant GE, Torrey WC, Elder GH. 1995. A 50-year prospective study of the psychological sequelae of World War II combat. *American Journal of Psychiatry* 152(4):516-522.

Marsella AJ, Friedman MJ, Spain EH. 1993. Ethnocultural aspects of posttraumatic stress disorder. In: Oldham JM, Riba MB, Tasman A, editors. *Review of Psychiatry*. Washington, DC: American Psychiatric Press.

Marshall RD, Turner JB, Lewis-Fernandez R, Koenan K, Neria Y, Dohrenwend BP. 2006. Symptom patterns associated with chronic PTSD in male veterans: New findings from the National Vietnam Veterans Readjustment Study. *Journal of Nervous and Mental Disease* 194(4):275-278.

Mason JW, Giller EL, Kosten TR, Ostroff RB, Podd L. 1986. Urinary free-cortisol levels in posttraumatic stress disorder patients. *Journal of Nervous and Mental Disease* 174(3):145-149.

McFall ME, Murburg MM, Ko GN, Veith RC. 1990. Autonomic responses to stress in Vietnam combat veterans with posttraumatic stress disorder. *Biological Psychiatry* 27(10):1165-1175.

McFarlane AC. 1997. The prevalence and longitudinal course of PTSD. Implications for the neurobiological models of PTSD. *Annals of the New York Academy of Sciences* 821:10-23.

Mellman TA, Kumar A, Kulick-Bell R, Kumar M, Nolan B. 1995a. Nocturnal/daytime urine noradrenergic measures and sleep in combat-related PTSD. *Biological Psychiatry* 38:174-179.

Mellman TA, Kulick-Bell R, Ashlock L, Nolan B. 1995b. Sleep events among veterans with combat-related posttraumatic stress disorder. *American Journal of Psychiatry* 152:110-115.

Mellman TA, Bustamante V, Fins AL, Pigeon WR, Nolan B. 2002. REM sleep and the early development of posttraumatic stress disorder. *American Journal of Psychiatry* 159:1696-1701.

Metzger LJ, Orr SP, Berry NJ, Ahern CE, Lasko NB, Pitman RK. 1999. Physiologic reactivity to startling tones in women with posttraumatic stress disorder. *Journal of Abnormal Psychology* 108:347-352.

MHAT (Mental Health Advisory Team). 2006. *Mental Health Advisory Team (MHAT) IV Operation Iraqi Freedom 05-07: Final Report.* [Washington, DC]: Office of the Surgeon Multinational Force-Iraq and Office of the Surgeon General United States Army Medical Command. [Online]. Available: http://www.armymedicine.army.mil/news/mhat/mhat_iv/MHAT_IV_Report_17NOV06.pdf.

Murburg MM, McFall ME, Ko GN, Veith RC. 1994. Stress-induced alterations in plasma catecholamines and sympathetic nervous system funuction in PTSD. In: Murburg MM, editor. *Catecholamine Function in Post-Traumatic Stress Disorder: Emerging Concepts*. 1st Ed. Washington, DC: American Psychiatric Press. Pp. 189-202.

Murdoch M, Polusny MA, Hodges J, Cowper D. 2006. The association between in-service sexual harassment and post-traumatic stress disorder among Department of Veterans Affairs disability applicants. *Military Medicine* 171(2):166-173.

Myers KM, Davis M. 2007. Mechanisms of fear extinction. *Molecular Psychiatry* 12(2):120-150.

Neal LA, Green G, Turner MA. 2004. Post-traumatic stress and disability. *British Journal of Psychiatry* 184:247-250.

Neeleman J, Ormel J, Bijl RV. 2001. The distribution of psychiatric and somatic ill health: Associations with personality and socioeconomic status. *Psychosomatic Medicine* 63(2):239-247.

North CS. 1995. Human response to violent trauma. *Balliere's Clinical Psychiatry* 1:225-245.

North CS, Smith EM, Spitznagel EL. 1994. Posttraumatic stress disorder in survivors of a mass shooting. *American Journal of Psychiatry* 151(1):82-88.

North CS, Nixon SJ, Shariat S, Mallonee S, McMillen C, Spitznagel EL, Smith EM. 1999. Psychiatric disorders among survivors of the Oklahoma City bombing. *Journal of the American Medical Association* 282(8):755-762.

North CS, Spitznagel EL, Smith EM. 2001. A prospective study of coping after exposure to a mass murder episode. *Annals of Clinical Psychiatry* 13(2):81-87.

Op den Velde W, Hovens JE, Aarts PG, Frey-Wouters E, Falger PR, Van Duijn H, De Groen JH. 1996. Prevalence and course of posttraumatic stress disorder in Dutch veterans of the civilian resistance during World War II: An overview. *Psychological Reports* 78(2):519-529.

Orr SP, Claiborn JM, Altman B, Forgue DF, de Jong JB, Pitman RK, Herz LR. 1990. Psychometric profile of posttraumatic stress disorder, anxious, and healthy Vietnam veterans: Correlations with psychophysiologic responses. *Journal of Consulting Clinical Psychology* 58(3):329-335.

O'Toole BI, Marshall RP, Grayson DA, Schureck RJ, Dobson M, French M, Pulvertaft B, Meldrum L, Bolton J, Vennard J. 1996. The Australian Vietnam Veterans Health Study: III. Psychological health of Australian Vietnam veterans and its relationship to combat. *International Journal of Epidemiology* 25(2):331-340.

Ozer EJ, Best SR, Lipsey TL, Weiss DS. 2003. Predictors of posttraumatic stress disorder and symptoms in adults: A meta-analysis. *Psychological Bulletin* 129(1):52-73.

Perry BD. 1994. Neurobiological squeal of childhood trauma: Post-traumatic stress disorder in children. In: Murburg M, editor. *Catecholamine Function in Post Traumatic Stress Disorder: Emerging Concepts*. Washington, DC: American Psychiatric Press. Pp. 253-276.

Perry BD, Giller EL Jr., Southwick SM. 1987. Altered platelet alpha 2-adrenergic binding sites in posttraumatic stress disorder. *American Journal of Psychiatry* 144(11):1511-1512.

Pitman RK, Orr SP. 1990. Twenty-four hour urinary cortisol and catecholamine excretion in combat-related posttraumatic stress disorder. *Biological Psychiatry* 27(2):245-247.

Pitman RK, Altman B, Macklin ML. 1989. Prevalence of posttraumatic stress disorder in wounded Vietnam veterans. *American Journal of Psychiatry* 46(5):667-669.

Pitman RK, Sanders KM, Zusman RM, Healy AR, Cheema F, Lasko NB, Cahill L, Orr SP. 2002. Pilot study of secondary prevention of posttraumatic stress disorder with propranolol. *Biological Psychiatry* 51(2):189-192.

Port CL, Engdahl B, Frazier P. 2001. A longitudinal and retrospective study of PTSD among older prisoners of war. *American Journal of Psychiatry* 158(9):1474-1479.

Prigerson HG, Maciejewski PK, Rosenheck RA. 2001. Combat trauma: Trauma with highest risk of delayed onset and unresolved posttraumatic stress disorder symptoms, unemployment, and abuse among men. *Journal of Nervous and Mental Disease* 189(2):99-108.

Prigerson HG, Maciejewski PK, Rosenheck RA. 2002. Population attributable fractions of psychiatric disorders and behavioral outcomes associated with combat exposure among U.S. men. *American Journal of Public Health* 92(1):59-63.

Prins A, Kaloupek DG, Keane TM. 1995. Psychophysiological evidence for autonomic arousal and startle in traumatized adult populations. In: Friedman MJ, Charney DS, Deutch AY, editors. *Neurobiological and Clinical Consequences of Stress: From Normal Adaptation to PTSD*. Philadelphia, PA: Lippincott-Raven. Pp. 291-314.

Proctor SP, Heeren T, White RF, Wolfe J, Borgos MS, Davis JD, Pepper L, Clapp R, Sutker PB, Vasterling JJ, Ozonoff D. 1998. Health status of Persian Gulf War veterans: Self-reported symptoms, environmental exposures and the effect of stress. *International Journal of Epidemiology* 27(6):1000-1010.

Raskind MA, Thompson C, Petrie EC, Dobie DJ, Rein RJ, Hoff DJ, McFall ME, Peskind ER. 2002. Prazosin reduces nightmares in combat veterans with posttraumatic stress disorder. *Journal of Clinical Psychiatry* 63(7):565-568.

Raskind MA, Peskind ER, Kanter ED, Petrie EC, Radant A, Thompson CE, Dobie DJ, Hoff D, Rein RJ, Straits-Troster K, Thomas RJ, McFall MM. 2003. Reduction of nightmares and other PTSD symptoms in combat veterans by prazosin: A placebo-controlled study. *American Journal of Psychiatry* 160:371-373.

Raskind MA, Peskind ER, Hof DJ, Hart KL, Homes HA, Warren D, Schofer J, O'Connell J, Taylor F, Gross C, Rohde K, McFall ME. 2007. A parallel group placebo controlled study of prazosin for trauma nightmares and sleep disturbances in combat veterans with posttraumatic stress disorder. *Biological Psychiatry* 61:928-934.

Regehr C, Hemsworth D, Hill J. 2001. Individual predictors of posttraumatic distress: A structural equation model. *Canadian Journal of Psychiatry* 46(2):156-161.

Resnick HS, Yehuda R, Acierno R. 1997. Acute post-rape plasma cortisol, alcohol use, and PTSD symptom profile among recent rape victims. *Annals of the New York Academy of Sciences* 821:433-436.

Ross RJ, Ball WA, Sullivan KA, Caroff SN. 1989. Sleep disturbance as the hallmark of posttraumatic stress disorder. *American Journal of Psychiatry* 146:697-707.

Ross RJ, Ball WA, Dinges DF, Kribbs NB, Morrison AR, Silver SM, Mulvaney FD. 1994. Motor dysfunction during sleep in posttraumatic stress disorder. *Sleep* 17:723-732.

Rothbaum B, Foa E, Riggs D, Murdock T, Walsh W. 1992. A prospective examination of post-traumatic stress disorder in rape. *Journal of Traumatic Stress* 5:455-475.

Roy-Byrne P, Arguelles L, Vitek ME, Goldberg J, Keane TM, True WR, Pitman RK. 2004. Persistence and change of PTSD symptomatology—a longitudinal co-twin control analysis of the Vietnam Era Twin Registry. *Social Psychiatry and Psychiatric Epidemiology* 39(9):681-685.

Ruzich MJ, Looi JC, Robertson MD. 2005. Delayed onset of posttraumatic stress disorder among male combat veterans: A case series. *American Journal of Geriatric Psychiatry* 13(5):424-427.

Seal KH, Bertenthal D, Miner CR, Sen S, Marmar C. 2007. Bringing the war back home: Mental health disorders among 103,788 U.S. veterans returning from Iraq and Afghanistan seen at Department of Veterans Affairs facilities. *Archives of Internal Medicine* 167:476-482.

Schelling G, Briegel J, Roozendaal B, Stoll C, Rothenhausler HB, Kapfhammer HP. 2001. The effect of stress doses of hydrocortisone during septic shock on posttraumatic stress disorder in survivors. *Biological Psychiatry* 50(12):978-985.

Schelling G, Roozendaal B, Krauseneck T, Schmoelz M, DE Quervain D, Briegel J. 2006. Efficacy of hydrocortisone in preventing posttraumatic stress disorder following critical illness and major surgery. *Annals of the New York Academy of Sciences* 1071:46-53.

Schlenger WE, Kulka RA, Fairbank JA, Hough RL. 1992. The prevalence of post-traumatic stress disorder in the Vietnam generation: A multimethod, multisource assessment of psychiatric disorder. *Journal of Traumatic Stress* 5(3):333-363.

Schnurr PP, Spiro A, Paris AH. 2000a. Physician-diagnosed medical disorders in relation to PTSD symptoms in older male military veterans. *Health Psychology* 19(1):91-97.

Schnurr PP, Ford JD, Friedman MJ, Green BL, Dain BJ, Sengupta A. 2000b. Predictors and outcomes of posttraumatic stress disorder in World War II veterans exposed to mustard gas. *Journal of Consulting and Clinical Psychology* 68(2):258-268.

Schnurr PP, Friedman MJ, Bernardy NC. 2002. Research on posttraumatic stress disorder: Epidemiology, pathophysiology, and assessment. *Journal of Clinical Psychology* 58(8):877-889.

Schnurr PP, Lunney CA, Sengupta A, Waelde LC. 2003. A descriptive analysis of PTSD chronicity in Vietnam veterans. *Journal of Traumatic Stress* 16(6):545-553.

Schnurr PP, Lunney CA, Sengupta A. 2004. Risk factors for the development versus maintenance of posttraumatic stress disorder. *Journal of Traumatic Stress* 17(2):85-95.

Shalev AY, Freedman S, Peri T, Brandes D, Sahar T, Orr SP, Pitman RK. 1998. Prospective study of posttraumatic stress disorder and depression following trauma. *American Journal of Psychiatry* 155(5):630-637.

Shephard B. 2001. *A War of Nerves: Soldiers and Psychiatrists in the Twentieth Century*. Cambridge, MA: Harvard University Press.

Simmons R, Maconochie N, Doyle P. 2004. Self-reported ill health in male UK Gulf War veterans: A retrospective cohort study. *BMC Public Health* 4(1):27.

Slusarcick AL, Ursano RJ, Dinneen MP, Fullerton CS. 2001. Factors associated with depression on a hospital ship deployed during the Persian Gulf War. *Military Medicine* 166(3):248-252.

Smith MA, Davidson J, Ritchie JC, Kudler H. 1989. The corticotropin-releasing hormone test in patients with posttraumatic stress disorder. *Biological Psychiatry* 26(4):349-355.

Solomon SD, Smith EM, Robins N, Fischbach RL. 1987. Social involvement as a mediator of disaster-induced stress. *Journal of Applied Social Psychology* 17(12):1092-1112.

Southwick S, Friedman MJ. 2001. Neurolobiological models of posttraumatic stress disorder. In: Gerrity E, Keane TM, Tuma F, editors. *The Mental Health Consequences of Torture*. New York: Kluwer. Pp. 73-87.

Southwick SM, Krystal JH, Morgan CA, Johnson D, Nagy LM, Nicolaou A, Heninger GR, Charney DS. 1993a. Abnormal noradrenergic function in posttraumatic stress disorder. *Archives of General Psychiatry* 50(4):266-274.

Southwick SM, Morgan A, Nagy LM, Bremner D, Nicolaou AL, Johnson DR, Rosenheck R, Charney DS. 1993b. Trauma-related symptoms in veterans of Operation Desert Storm: A preliminary report. *American Journal of Psychiatry* 150(10):1524-1528.

Southwick SM, Bremner D, Krystal JH, Charney DS. 1994. Psychobiologic research in post-traumatic stress disorder. *Psychiatric Clinics of North America* 17(2):251-264.

Southwick SM, Morgan CA 3rd, Darnell A, Bremner D, Nicolaou AL, Nagy LM, Charney DS. 1995. Trauma-related symptoms in veterans of Operation Desert Storm: A 2-year follow-up. *American Journal of Psychiatry* 152(8):1150-1155.

Spiro A 3rd, Schnurr PP, Aldwin CM. 1994. Combat-related posttraumatic stress disorder in older men. *Psychology and Aging* 9(1):17-26.

Starr P. 1982. *The Social Transformation of American Medicine*. New York: Basic Books.

Stein AL, Tran GQ, Lund LM, Haji U, Dashevsky BA, Baker DG. 2005. Correlates for posttraumatic stress disorder in Gulf War veterans: A retrospective study of main and moderating effects. *Journal of Anxiety Disorders* 19(8):861-876.

Stickgold R. 2007. Of sleep, memories, and trauma. *Nature Neurosciences* 10:540-542.

Storzbach D, Campbell KA, Binder LM, McCauley L, Anger WK, Rohlman DS, Kovera CA. 2000. Psychological differences between veterans with and without Gulf War unexplained symptoms. Portland Environmental Hazards Research Center. *Psychosomatic Medicine* 62(5):726-735.

Stretch RH. 1985. Posttraumatic stress disorder among U.S. Army Reserve Vietnam and Vietnam-era veterans. *Journal of Consulting and Clinical Psychology* 53(6):935-936.

Stretch R. 1986. PTSD among Vietnam and Vietnam-era veterans. In: Figley CR, editor. *Trauma and Its Wake: The Study and Treatment of Post-Traumatic Stress Disorder*. New York: Brunner/Mazel. Pp. 156-192.

Stretch RH, Marlowe DH, Wright KM, Bliese PD, Knudson KH, Hoover CH. 1996. Post-traumatic stress disorder symptoms among Gulf War veterans. *Military Medicine* 161(7):407-410.

Stretch RH, Vail JD, Maloney JP. 1985. Posttraumatic stress disorder among Army Nurse Corps Vietnam veterans. *Journal of Consulting and Clinical Psychology* 53(5):704-708.

Sutker PB, Davis JM, Uddo M, Ditta SR. 1995a. Assessment of psychological distress in Persian Gulf troops: Ethnicity and gender comparisons. *Journal of Personality Assessment* 64(3):415-427.

Sutker PB, Davis JM, Uddo M, Ditta SR. 1995b. War zone stress, personal resources, and PTSD in Persian Gulf War returnees. *Journal of Abnormal Psychology* 104(3):444-452.

Taft CT, Stern AS, King LA, King DW. 1999. Modeling physical health and functional health status: The role of combat exposure, posttraumatic stress disorder, and personal resource attributes. *Journal of Traumatic Stress* 12(1):3-23.

Taylor F, Raskind MA. 2002. The α_1-adrenergic antagonist prazosin improves sleep and nightmares in civilian trauma posttraumatic stress disorder. *Journal of Clinical Psychopharmacology* 22:82-85.

Taylor FB, Martin P, Thompson C, Williams J, Mellman TA, Gross C, Peskind ER, Raskind MA. 2007. Prazosin effects on objective sleep measures and clinical symptoms in civilian trauma posttraumatic stress disorder: A placebo-controlled study. *Biological Psychiatry* (Sep 12). Available: http://www.sciencedirect.com.

Thompson WW, Gottesman II, Zalewski C. 2006. Reconciling disparate prevalence rates of PTSD in large samples of U.S. male Vietnam veterans and their controls. *BMC Psychiatry* 6:19.

Toomey R, Kang HK, Karlinsky J, Baker DG, Vasterling JJ, Alpern R, Reda DJ, Henderson WG, Murphy FM, Eisen SA. 2007. Mental health of U.S. Gulf War veterans 10 years after the war. *British Journal of Psychiatry* 190:385-393.

U.S. Department of Health and Human Services. 1999. *Mental Health: A Report of the Surgeon General*. Rockville, MD: U.S. Department of Health and Human Services, Substance Abuse and Mental Services Administration, Center for Mental Health Services, National Institutes of Health, and National Institute of Mental Health.

Vaillant GE. 1977. *Adaptation to Life*. Boston, MA: Little Brown.

Vaiva G, Ducrocq F, Jezequel K, Averland B, Lestavel P, Brunet A, Marmar CR. 2003. Immediate treatment with propranolol decreases posttraumatic stress disorder two months after trauma. *Biological Psychiatry* 54(9):947-949.

Van Liempt S, Vermetten E, Geuze E, Westenberg HGM. 2006. Pharmacotherapy for disordered sleep in posttraumatic stress disorder: A systematic review. *International Clinical Psychopharmacology* 21:193-202.

Vythilingam M, Luckenbaugh DA, Lam T, Morgan CA 3rd, Lipschitz D, Charney DS, Bremner JD, Southwick SM. 2005. Smaller head of the hippocampus in Gulf War-related posttraumatic stress disorder. *Psychiatry Research* 139(2)89-99.

Wolfe J. 1996. *Female Gender and Other Potential Predictors of Functional Health Status Among Persian Gulf War Veterans*. Boston, MA: Tufts University.

Wolfe J, Brown PJ, Furey J, Levin KB. 1993a. Development of a wartime stressor scale for women. *Psychological Assessment* 5(3):330-335.

Wolfe J, Brown PJ, Kelley JM. 1993b. Reassessing war stress: Exposure and the Persian Gulf War. *Journal of Social Issues* 49(4):15-31.

Wolfe J, Keane T, Kaloupek D. 1993c. Patterns of positive readjustment in Vietnam combat veterans. *Journal of Traumatic Stress* 6(2):179-193.

Wolfe J, Erickson DJ, Sharkansky EJ, King DW, King LA. 1999. Course and predictors of posttraumatic stress disorder among Gulf War veterans: A prospective analysis. *Journal of Consulting and Clinical Psychology* 67(4):520-528.

Yehuda R. 1997. Stress and glucocorticoid. *Science* 275(5306):1662-1663.

Yehuda R. 2002. Post-traumatic stress disorder. *New England Journal of Medicine* 346(2):108-114.

Yehuda R, Southwick S, Giller EL, Ma X, Mason JW. 1992a. Urinary catecholamine excretion and severity of PTSD symptoms in Vietnam combat veterans. *Journal of Nervous and Mental Disease* 180(5):321-325.

Yehuda R, Southwick SM, Giller EL Jr. 1992b. Exposure to atrocities and severity of chronic posttraumatic stress disorder in Vietnam combat veterans. *American Journal of Psychiatry* 149(3):333-336.

Yehuda R, Teicher MH, Giller EL. 1995. Lack of significant cortisol and growth hormone changes in Israeli civilians during the Gulf War. *American Journal of Psychiatry* 152(4):652-653.

Yehuda R, Halligan SL, Grossman R, Golier JA, Wong C. 2002. The cortisol and glucocorticoid receptor response to low dose dexamethasone administration in aging combat veterans and Holocaust survivors with and without posttraumatic stress disorder. *Biological Psychiatry* 52(5):393-403.

Yehuda R, Golier JA, Yang RK, Tischler L. 2004. Enhanced sensitivity to glucocorticoids in peripheral mononuclear leukocytes in posttraumatic stress disorder. *Biological Psychiatry* 55(11):1110-1116.

Zatzick DF, Marmar CR, Weiss DS, Browner WS, Metzler TJ, Golding JM, Stewart A, Schlenger WE, Wells KB. 1997a. Posttraumatic stress disorder and functioning and quality of life outcomes in a nationally representative sample of male Vietnam veterans. *American Journal of Psychiatry* 154(12):1690-1695.

Zatzick DF, Weiss DS, Marmar CR, Metzler TJ, Wells K, Golding JM, Stewart A, Schlenger WE, Browner WS. 1997b. Post-traumatic stress disorder and functioning and quality of life outcomes in female Vietnam veterans. *Military Medicine* 162(10):661-665.

6

HEALTH EFFECTS

The studies discussed in this chapter demonstrate that veterans' reactions to deployment to a war zone and its inherent stressors are varied. Some veterans suffer no ill consequences and may even benefit from deployment, and some experience initial distress but become acclimated to some of the stressors; but the body of evidence suggests that most veterans perceive deployment to a war zone as stressful (Gifford et al. 2006; MHAT 2006b). Given that few studies provide a good indication of the deployment-related stressors to which veterans were exposed and the amount of stress experienced during those exposures, the committee decided that deployment to a war zone itself was sufficient to elicit a stress response and that deployment would serve as a surrogate for deployment-related stress (the stress response is discussed in detail in Chapter 4). Therefore, military personnel deployed to a war zone would constitute the study group of interest and military personnel serving at the same time but not deployed to a war zone would be the appropriate comparison group. The studies reviewed in this chapter generally compared Gulf War veterans or veterans of other deployments, such as to Vietnam, with veterans who were deployed during the same period to noncombat areas within the United States or elsewhere (for example, Germany). In some cases, the committee included studies of other military personnel, such as peacekeepers, or civilians that had similar exposures if the studies appeared to be relevant to the discussion.

ORGANIZATION OF THIS CHAPTER

The committee discusses health effects in the order they occur in the *International Statistical Classification of Diseases and Related Health Problems, 10th Edition (ICD-10,)*[1] except for the last section, which examines the many reports of increased health symptoms in deployed veterans. The committee did not examine health effects related to or resulting from infectious and parasitic diseases as the Institute of Medicine (IOM) Committee on Gulf War and Health: Infectious Diseases has examined those outcomes and released its report (IOM 2007). The committee also did not consider health effects that are most likely to be associated with exposures to environmental agents—such as sarin nerve gas, the defoliant Agent Orange, or combustion products from oil-well fires—or with the use of various vaccines and other

[1]The *International Statistical Classification of Diseases and Related Health Problems (ICD)* provides a detailed description of known diseases and injuries. Every disease (or group of related diseases) is given a unique code. *ICD* is periodically revised and is currently in its 10th edition (*ICD-10*) and available at http://www.who.int/classifications/apps/icd/icd10online/.

prophylactic measures, although anticipation of exposure to such agents may be a deployment-related stressor, as indicated in Chapter 3. Those stressors have already been thoroughly evaluated by other IOM committees.

In general, for each health effect presented in this chapter, the committee identifies first the primary studies and then the secondary or supporting studies, as defined by the criteria in Chapter 2. A primary study had to include information about the putative exposure (deployment) and specific health effects, demonstrate rigorous methods, include details of its methods, include an appropriate control or reference group, have adequate statistical power to detect effects, and provide appropriate adjustment for confounders. Many of the large cohort studies examined multiple effects and so might be referred to in more than one place. A given study might be deemed a primary study for one or more health effects and be a secondary study for another effect, as determined by how the particular health effects were defined and measured. For example, a study that was well designed for assessing a neurobehavioral effect might not be well designed for assessing a psychiatric disorder. In general, only primary studies appear in the evidence tables that accompany the discussions of health effects.

A secondary study was typically a study that had methodologic limitations, such as not including a rigorous or well-defined measure of exposure, that is, deployment to a war zone or posttraumatic stress disorder (PTSD) as a marker of trauma (see Chapter 1). Some studies assessed past trauma that was not necessarily peculiar to war-zone deployment, so they were included as secondary studies. The secondary studies were reviewed and included in the discussion because they evaluated the same health effects and in some cases provided useful information on veteran populations from the same conflicts as the primary studies; they add information that might increase or decrease confidence in the conclusions based on the primary studies. Confidence in a secondary study is substantially reduced if the statistical analysis did not adjust for confounders, if the data were obtained from self-reported cross-sectional surveys or from screening instruments that relied solely on self-reported answers, or if response rates were unacceptably low. Without evidence from primary studies, the potential for unreliable findings due to bias, chance, or multiple comparisons may outweigh the extent to which secondary studies may contribute, even collectively, to the overall conclusion of the committee about an association between deployment-related stress and any specific health effect. Understanding the relationship between a health effect and deployment-related stress may be hampered by the exposure not being explicitly defined as deployment or, more commonly, by many potentially harmful exposures being compared with multiple effects.

With rare exceptions, the chapter excludes studies of participants in Gulf War registries established by the Department of Veterans Affairs (VA) or the Department of Defense (DoD), which were not intended to be representative of the entire group of Gulf War veterans. Registry participants can not be considered representative of all Gulf War veterans in that they are self-selected subjects, many of whom have joined the registries because they believe that they have symptoms of a new medical syndrome; they were not randomly selected from all Gulf War military personnel, and there is no nondeployed control group. One main exception to the use of registries occurs for studies in which the groups of interest are veterans with and without PTSD. As discussed in Chapter 5, PTSD can be diagnosed only after exposure to a traumatic event, thus, the committee agreed that studies of veterans with deployment-related PTSD compared with deployed veterans who had not developed PTSD were appropriate comparison populations when determining whether health effects were associated with deployment-related PTSD.

Many of the studies had other limitations. Few studies measured the stress that troops experienced during deployment; rather, most asked veterans about exposure to possible stressors after their return from deployment. Some studies—such as the congressionally mandated National Vietnam Veterans Readjustment Study (NVVRS), the Vietnam Experience Study (VES), and some Gulf War studies—assessed veterans' war-zone exposures many years after they had returned home. Furthermore, many studies did not verify veterans' reported exposures against military records. Finally, although many studies used various scales, such as the Combat Exposure Scale, to determine possible exposures during deployment, the scales did not ascertain the emotional response of the veterans to the exposures; that is, the studies asked only whether exposure to a stressor occurred and not about the degree to which the veterans found the experience to be stressful. Studies that did ascertain veterans' reactions to stressors, such as seeing a comrade wounded or firing a gun at the enemy, and that asked veterans to rate their responses on a scale, such as "never" to "always," are rare.

The committee acknowledges that many of the health effects associated with deployment were discussed in a previous volume of the *Gulf War and Health* series, *Volume 4: Health Effects of Serving in the Gulf War*. In that volume, the health effects that had been found in deployed Gulf War veterans were identified, and their prevalence compared with the prevalence of the same effects in nondeployed Gulf War veterans. However, that review was restricted to Gulf War veterans; veterans of other conflicts—such as the Vietnam War, World War II, the Korean War, and Operation Enduring Freedom (OEF) and Operation Iraqi Freedom (OIF)—were not considered. Furthermore, that report did not seek to establish whether there was any association between being deployed and specific health effects. As a consequence, although the present committee reviewed many of the same studies as the committee that prepared *Volume 4*, the assessment process used here is different, as are some of the conclusions because a broader array of studies were considered using defined categories of association.

CANCER

Each year over a million people receive a diagnosis of cancer in the United States. About one of two American men and one of three American women will have cancer at some point in their lives. Cancer can develop at any age, but about 77% of all cancers are diagnosed in people 55 years old or older. Military personnel during the Gulf War had a mean age of 28 years and therefore are now in their mid-40s. Insufficient time had elapsed for most forms of cancer to be detected among Gulf War veterans by surveys conducted in the 1990s and early 2000s. That is not the case, however, for veterans of the Vietnam War, many of whom are now at an age when most cancers are likely to be diagnosed. Therefore, given the substantial differences in ages between veterans of the Vietnam War and the Gulf War, the studies are discussed separately.

Primary studies for this health effect were those that compared deployed vs nondeployed veteran populations from either the Vietnam War or the Gulf War. A primary study must have indicated that the presence of cancer or death from cancer was confirmed, as by physical examination, medical record review, or death certificates. Of particular concern in studies of Vietnam veterans is possible confounding from exposure to Agent Orange, a toxic herbicide sprayed on foliage in Vietnam.

Most of the studies reviewed in this section did not distinguish between the type of cancers that were seen in or reported by veterans, so the occurrence of cancer is addressed as a specific endpoint. The few studies reporting specific results on testicular cancer, which occurs predominantly in younger men, and on skin cancer, which is relatively common, are discussed in separate sections. The occurrence of cancer in veterans with PTSD is discussed at the end of the section. The primary studies for cancer are summarized in Table 6-1 at the end of the section.

All Cancers

Vietnam War

The committee identified three primary studies that examined the effect of deployment to Vietnam on the development of cancer in veterans of the Vietnam War (CDC 1988b; Selected Cancers Cooperative Study Group 1990a,b,c; Watanabe and Kang 1995). Two other primary studies (Dalager et al. 1995; Kang et al. 2000c) focused exclusively on cancers in female Vietnam veterans.

In response to a congressional mandate, Centers for Disease Control and Prevention (CDC) undertook the VES to assess the health status of the 5 million Vietnam-theater and Vietnam-era veterans who served in the U.S. Army during 1965-1971; the study was completed in 1988, about 15-20 years after the war (CDC 1988b). It consisted of a nationally representative random sample of 7924 theater veterans and 7364 era veterans who completed a phase 1 telephone interview. In phase 2, a random subsample of 2490 theater veterans and 1972 era veterans also completed physical- and psychologic-health screening examinations in 1985-1986 at a medical facility. On examination, 1.9% of theater veterans and 1.3% of era veterans had cancers (unspecified); the study findings were not significant (odds ratio [OR] 1.4, 95% confidence interval [CI] includes 1.0, $p > 0.05$). The OR was adjusted for age at enlistment, race, year of enlistment, enlistment status, score on a general technical test, and primary military occupational specialty. The study had the advantage of including a physical examination and a large study population, but it is limited in that information on exposure to herbicides, particularly Agent Orange, was not provided, the types of cancer that were screened for were not indicated, the study was not designed to assess the presence of relatively rare cancers, and the participation rate of 75% and 63% for the theater and era veterans, respectively.

As a followup to the VES, CDC conducted a further population-based case-control assessment for six cancers in Vietnam-theater and Vietnam-era veterans: non-Hodgkin's lymphoma (NHL), Hodgkin's lymphoma, soft-tissue and other sarcomas, nasal cancer, nasopharyngeal cancer, and primary liver cancer. Those cancers were chosen because cancers of the liver, nasal cavity, and nasopharnyx, and Hodgkin's disease have been associated with exposure to phenoxy herbicides, such as Agent Orange, in some animal studies and a few human studies. Study participants were all men born in 1929-1953 who were first diagnosed as having cancer in 1984-1988 and were listed in any of eight city or state cancer registries—those in Atlanta, Detroit, San Francisco, Seattle, Miami, Connecticut, Iowa, and Kansas. Controls were selected by random-digit telephone dialing in the relevant locations and frequency-matched by age to the men with cancer. All cancers were confirmed pathologically. An analysis of 1157 men with NHL and 1776 controls found that the risk of NHL in men who served in Vietnam compared with those who served in the military in 1964-1972 but not in Vietnam was 1.52 (95% CI 1.00-2.32, $p = 0.01$) when adjusted for registry, age group in 1968, ethnicity, education, and other covariates, including reported exposures to pesticides, reported medical history and medication use, smoking, marital status, and being raised as Jewish (Selected Cancers Cooperative Study Group 1990a). There was no suggestion of an increasing trend in risk of NHL corresponding to service in support units (OR 1.50, 95% CI 1.02-2.21), combat-support units (OR 1.18, 95% CI 0.65-2.15), or combat units (OR 1.25, 95% CI 0.63-2.45).

With respect to soft-tissue and other sarcomas, the same eight cancer registries showed that 342 men had confirmed cancers compared with the 1776 controls. The OR for soft-tissue and other sarcomas in Vietnam-theater veterans compared with Vietnam-era veterans is a nonsignificant 0.74 (95% CI 0.39-1.41) with the same adjustment factors as for NHL (Selected Cancers Cooperative Study Group 1990b). Again, there was no trend in cancer risk in men who served in support units (OR 0.76, 95% CI 0.37-1.53), combat-support units (OR 1.03, 95% CI 0.44-2.41), or combat units (OR 0.76, 95% CI 0.25-2.28).

Combining data from the eight cancer registries shows that 28 of the 310 men with Hodgkin's disease had served in Vietnam, two of the 48 with nasal carcinoma, three of the 80 with nasopharyngeal carcinoma, and eight of the 130 with primary liver cancer (Selected Cancers Cooperative Study Group 1990c). Although the power of the study was good for Hodgkin's disease (96%), it was less robust for the other cancers. In comparisons of Vietnam-theater veterans with Vietnam-era veterans with the same adjustments as for NHL, the OR was 1.23 for Hodgkin's disease (95% CI 0.65-2.32), 0.31 for nasal carcinoma (95% CI 0.04-2.20, additionally adjusted for occupational exposures), and 0.53 for primary liver cancer (95% CI 0.14-1.94, additionally adjusted for occupational exposures); the OR for nasopharyngeal carcinoma could not be calculated with conditional logistic regression. There was no trend ($p = 0.17$) in risk of Hodgkin's disease related to serving in Vietnam in a support unit (OR 1.58, 95% CI 0.90-2.77), a combat-support unit (OR 0.50, 95% CI 0.14-1.76), or a combat unit (OR 0.94, 95% CI 0.34-2.59). The relationship of combat to the other three cancers was not assessed.

Although the authors did not sample blood for possibly elevated dioxin levels, they asserted that, based on their locations and occupations during the war, the Vietnam-veteran study participants were not at greater risk of exposure to Agent Orange than the nondeployed veterans. Those studies are limited by the small sample sizes for some cancers.

Postservice mortality was assessed in 10,716 Marines who served in Vietnam and 9346 Marines who were not deployed to Vietnam (Watanabe and Kang 1995). An analysis of death certificates showed that as of 1991, for Marines who had served in Vietnam, there were no statistically significant increases in all-cancer mortality (rate ratio 1.08, 95% CI 0.84-1.39), cancer of the larynx (rate ratio 2.60, 95% CI 0.27-25.0), lung cancer (rate ratio 1.12, 95% CI 0.71-1.76), or lymphosarcoma and reticulosarcoma (rate ratio 1.21, 95% CI 0.27-5.41). No statistically significant increase was seen for all cancers or for lung cancer. The relative-risk (RR) estimates based on the Cox proportional-hazards model were 1.20 (95% CI 0.93-1.55) for all cancers and 1.33 (95% CI 0.84-2.10) for lung cancer, adjusted for year of birth and military rank. Death certificates were obtained from VA regional offices, federal records centers, and state vital-statistics offices. Comparisons with the U.S. male population showed slightly increased standardized mortality ratios for laryngeal cancer and for lymphosarcoma and reticulosarcoma, but the increases were not statistically significant. The authors considered the latent period for many cancers to be 15-20 years but found no difference in RRs in cancer deaths whether veterans were followed for less than or more than 16 years. The authors suggested that there may have been insufficient observation time since the war to detect excess deaths from cancer and that there was insufficient statistical power to detect rare causes of death. They also noted that many of the Marines were posted to areas in Vietnam where Agent Orange was used.

A similar study of cancer mortality was conducted in female Vietnam veterans (Dalager et al. 1995). The vital status of 4586 female Vietnam veterans and 5325 female Vietnam-era veterans was compared more than 20 years after the war. Vital status as of 1991 was determined from VA beneficiary records, information from the Social Security Administration and the Internal Revenue Service, the National Death Index, and military personnel records; copies of official death certificates were used to determine cause of death. The Cox proportional-hazard multivariate regression model was used to derive cause-specific mortality risks for female Vietnam theater veterans vs female Vietnam-era veterans adjusted for rank, nursing status, duration of military service, and age at entry into followup. The RR for all cancer mortality was 1.00 (95% CI 0.75-1.34). The authors noted that there were increased risks of cancer of the pancreas, uterine corpus, brain, and other parts of the central nervous system in female Vietnam veterans, but the number of deaths was small and did not reach statistical significance, and adjustment for confounders was not possible. Female theater veterans had a lower mortality than female era veterans from lymphopoietic cancer and lung cancer. This study and that by Watanabe and Kang (1995) discussed above had the advantage of being conducted after a sufficient latent period for many cancers to be evident, however the number of cancer cases was small in each study, and their study populations were to small to have much potential to identify changes in the incidence of relatively rare cancers.

Not all cancers result in death, so a second study of the prevalence of gynecologic cancers among female Vietnam veterans was undertaken (Kang et al. 2000c). The prevalence of malignant tumors was ascertained in 4140 female Vietnam-theater veterans and 4140 female Vietnam-era veterans. Participants were given a structured health questionnaire via telephone interview, and self-reported gynecologic (breast, ovarian, uterine, or cervical) cancer was confirmed by review of medical or hospital records. The response rate of the 6430 women interviewed was 83-87%. A multivariate logistic model was used to calculate the ORs and 95% CIs. The adjusted OR was 1.14 (95% CI 0.94-1.40) for any gynecologic cancer; 1.18 (95% CI 0.91-1.51) for breast cancer, 1.83 (95% CI 0.72-4.61) for ovarian cancer, 1.00 (95% CI 0.61-1.61) for uterine cancer, and 1.11 (95% CI 0.74-1.66) for cervical cancer. Adjustments included age, race, branch of service, pay grade, marital status, nursing occupation, smoking, drinking, family history of cancer, use of birth-control pills, and postmenopausal estrogen and progestin use. Medical records were used to confirm self-reported cancer; 222 records were reviewed, and 99% of self-reported breast cancers, 76% of cervical cancers, 78% of ovarian cancers, and 61% of uterine cancers were confirmed. However, 10% of the self-reported cancers were not confirmed, and 5% of the medical records had no information on cancer. This study indicates that service in Vietnam did not increase the risk of gynecologic cancer in female Vietnam veterans. The study had a high response rate and relatively high validation rate for the diagnosis of gynecologic cancers that had a sufficient latent period for detection. It is limited by lack of information on possible exposures during service in Vietnam, including exposure to Agent Orange.

Gulf War

There was only one primary study in Gulf War-deployed veterans compared with their nondeployed counterparts, which indicated an increased risk of cancer. McCauley et al. (2002b) looked at cancer rates in Gulf War veterans residing in Oregon, Washington, California, Georgia, and North Carolina in 1999 as part of a larger study to assess neurologic and neurophysiologic signs and symptoms in veterans who may have been exposed to chemical-warfare agents as a result of the destruction of munitions at Khamisiyah, Iraq. Names of possible participants were obtained from the Defense Manpower Data Center (DMDC) maintained by the DoD. Gulf War-deployed veterans were categorized as those who were within a 50-km radius of Khamisiyah between March 4 and March 13, 1991, and were therefore potentially exposed to chemical agents (n = 653), and Gulf War veterans who were deployed to Southwest Asia but outside of the 50-km radius (n = 610). A control group consisted of nondeployed veterans in the military at that time but not deployed to Southwest Asia (n = 516). A structured telephone interview asked veterans about physician-diagnosed medical conditions, hospitalizations, and disability during and after return from the Gulf War. The frequency of any cancer was 1.2% for veterans deployed in the Khamisiyah region, and 2.1% for those deployed outside the Khamisiyah region, for an OR of 0.4 (95% CI 0.1-1.4); the frequency of any cancer for nondeployed veterans was 0.6%. When the 21 cases of cancer among all deployed veterans (Khamisiyah region or elsewhere in the gulf combined) were compared with the 3 among nondeployed veterans, there was a nonsignificant increase in cancer frequency among the deployed troops (OR 3.0, 95% CI 1.0-13.1). All statistics were adjusted for age, gender, race, and region of residence. Twenty of the 24 deployed and nondeployed veterans reporting a diagnosis of cancer were asked for details on year of diagnosis and cancer type. When the 7 cases of skin cancer and the 4 cases of cancer for which details were not obtained were removed from the analysis, the resulting OR for non-skin cancers in deployed vs nondeployed was 4.94 (95% CI 0.6-38.1); there was no apparent trend for any specific type of cancer among the remaining 9 cancer cases. This study is limited by the small sample size and few reports of cancer and by the incomplete verification of the diagnosis with medical records or examination. A potential confounder of stress as a risk factor, exposure to chemical-warfare agents, was the target of the researchers' investigation: although this exposure is subject to great uncertainty, the primary result for proximity to Khamisiyah (OR = 0.4) argues against its importance in the development of cancer.

Macfarlane et al. (2003) assessed all first diagnoses of malignant cancer in a cohort of UK military personnel. The deployed group consisted of all military personnel who served in the Persian Gulf during September 1990-June 1991 (n = 51,721). The comparison group was randomly selected from members of the armed services who were in service on January 1, 1991, but not deployed in the Persian Gulf and was stratified to match the Gulf War cohort on age, sex, service branch, rank, and level of fitness for active service (n = 50,755). Followup was from April 1, 1991, until diagnosis of cancer, emigration, death, or July 31, 2002, whichever was earlier. Cancers were identified through the National Health Service Central Register. During followup, 270 incident cases of cancer were identified among the Gulf War veterans and 269 cases among the nondeployed group; the RR—after adjustment for sex, age group, service branch, and rank—was 0.99 (95% CI 0.83-1.17). Thus, there was no evidence of an association of Gulf War service with site-specific cancers. In subgroups of cohort members who participated in morbidity surveys that yielded more information on potential risk factors (28,518 deployed veterans and 20,829 nondeployed veterans), the RR was 1.11 (95% CI 0.86-1.44). That result did not change after adjustment for smoking or alcohol use, and there was no evidence of associations with exposure to pesticides; multiple vaccinations against anthrax, plague, and pertussis; or reported exposure to depleted uranium.

Two studies by Gray et al. (1996, 2000) attempted to determine whether Gulf War veterans were at increased risk for hospitalization after the war compared with nondeployed veterans. DoD hospital records on 547,076 active-duty Gulf War veterans and 618,335 nondeployed active-duty veterans in all service branches were examined with demographic information from military records. The multiple logistic-regression models were adjusted for sex, age, race or ethnic group, marital status, branch of service, rank, salary, occupation, and prewar hospitalizations. Using August 1991 as the end of the war, Gray et al. (1996) found a slightly increased risk of hospitalization for any neoplasm in the last 5 months of 1991 in deployed vs nondeployed veterans (standardized rate ratio about 1.10, 95% CI 1.0-1.2), but this dropped to about 0.92 (95% CI about 0.87-1.0) in 1992 and about 0.94 (95% CI about 0.87-1.1) in 1993. Most of the neoplasms diagnosed in 1991 were benign (for example, benign neoplasms of bone, articular cartilage, connective tissue and other soft tissue, skin, breast, and digestive system). In 1991, hospitalizations for malignant neoplasm of the testis were slightly higher in deployed men (rate ratio 2.12, 95% CI 1.11-4.02), but no difference was seen in 1992 or 1993. Expanding this study to include National Guard and reserve veterans, Gray et al. (2000) examined hospital records from the DoD, VA, and California Office of Statewide Health Planning and Development hospital systems for 1991-1994. The authors could not directly compare rates of hospitalization in the three hospital systems, so they compared proportional morbidity ratios (PMRs) of hospital-discharge diagnoses (14 diagnostic categories from *ICD-9*) in Gulf War-deployed and nondeployed veterans. PMRs for neoplasms were not higher in deployed veterans in any of the hospital systems.

Several other large secondary studies looked at cancer in large populations of Gulf War veterans and found that there was no significant increase in any cancer in deployed veterans compared with nondeployed veterans. Although the studies below used self-reports of medical conditions, they used structured telephone interviews by trained interviewers or in-person interviews of the veterans. The Iowa Persian Gulf Study Group (1997) used a cross-sectional telephone-interview survey of Gulf War-deployed and nondeployed veterans who claimed Iowa as their place of residence in their military records. Randomly selected subjects were stratified on age, sex, rank, race, and branch of military service. Of the 4886 eligible subjects, 3695 (76%) completed the interview (1896 deployed and 1799 nondeployed). Deployed and nondeployed veterans had a similar prevalence of any cancer (prevalence 1.0% and 1.9% in deployed regular military and reserves, respectively, vs 1.0% and 0.6% in nondeployed regular military and reserves; Cochran-Mantel-Haenszel rate difference 0.8, 95% CI 0.2-1.4, $p \leq 0.05$) and aplastic anemia (prevalence 0.1% and 0.0%, respectively, vs 0.0% for all nondeployed veterans; rate difference 0.1, 95% CI -0.1-0.2). Although deployed veterans were asked about exposure to unspecified psychologic stressors, similar data on nondeployed veterans are not provided. This study was limited by restriction of participants to Iowans, a sample size that may not be sufficient to detect cancers, lack of specificity as to reported cancers, and the use of self-reports of health effects.

Kang et al. (2000b) used a nationally representative stratified random sample of Gulf War veterans and nondeployed veterans to assess the health of veterans with telephone interviews. On the basis of responses from 11,441 deployed veterans and 9476 nondeployed veterans, the authors estimated the population prevalence of self-reported cancers other than skin cancer during the preceding 12 months to be 0.7% in deployed and 0.6% in nondeployed for a statistically significant increased rate difference of 0.18 (95% CI 0.15-0.21, $p \leq 0.05$). Prevalence was controlled for sex, age, race, marital status, rank, branch, unit component, active-duty status, and exposures. This study was limited by the use of self-reports and the lack of information on the number of cancer cases reported in the surveyed veterans.

In 1998, Steele (2000) assessed the prevalence of cancer and other medical conditions in a stratified random sample of Kansas Gulf War veterans (n = 1545) and veterans who were not deployed to the gulf (n = 435), using names supplied by the DMDC. The study was conducted to identify cases of Gulf War illness. In telephone interviews, participants were asked whether they had ever had a diagnosis or treatment by a physician for any of 16 specific medical conditions or for any medical conditions in five general categories and, if so, when the conditions had developed. Deployed veterans were also asked whether they had been notified by DoD about being in the area of the Khamisiyah munitions demolition. Cancers, other than skin cancer, were diagnosed after 1990 in 1% each of deployed and nondeployed veterans for a nonsignificant risk of 1.21 (95% CI 0.40-3.69), adjusted for sex, age, income, and education level.

Kang and Bullman (2001) studied causes of postwar mortality in Gulf War veterans through 1997. They ascertained vital status of a stratified random sample of Gulf War-deployed veterans and nondeployed veterans from VA and Social Security Administration databases, and death certificates were obtained from VA and the National Death Index database. From 1990 to 1997, there were 4506 deaths among 621,902 Gulf War veterans, and causes of death were obtained for 94.7% of them. The OR for mortality from any cancer during this period was 0.90 (95% CI 0.81-1.01) in men and 1.11 (95% CI 0.78-1.57) in women adjusted for age, race, branch of service, unit component, and marital status. The main strength of this study was the large sample. As in previous studies of Gulf War veterans, the latent period for most cancers is too long for their manifestation during the study period, and there was also a lack of information on risk factors.

Several secondary studies also looked at the prevalence of any cancer in Gulf War veterans. Eisen et al. (1991) and Proctor et al. (2001) examined U.S. veterans, Simmons et al. (2004) surveyed a large cohort of UK veterans, Goss Gilroy Inc. (1998) surveyed all Canadian Gulf War veterans, and O'Toole et al. (1996b) surveyed the entire Australian cohort of Gulf War veterans. Each of those studies found no significant increases in any cancer, on the basis of self-reports, in veterans deployed to the gulf compared with nondeployed veterans.

Testicular Cancer

Two studies have focused specifically on testicular cancer. Testicular cancer is relatively uncommon in the United States. The annual age-adjusted incidence is 5.3 cases per 100,000 men. However, it is one of the few cancers whose usual age of onset is in the same range as the age of the Gulf War veterans, about 20-44 (Ries et al. 2005).

Knoke et al. (1998) examined testicular cancer in 517,223 deployed and 1,291,323 nondeployed male veterans on active duty during the time of the Gulf War. The authors identified cases of all first hospital admissions, in U.S. military hospitals worldwide, for a principal diagnosis of testicular cancer. Cases were identified by examining the DoD hospitalization database through April 1, 1997. A total of 505 cases were ascertained: 134 in the deployed and 371 in the nondeployed. In Cox proportional-hazards models adjusted for race and ethnicity, age, and occupation, no association with deployment status was observed (RR 1.05, 95% CI 0.86-1.29). The deployed did have an increased risk in the early months after the end of the deployment period. The initial increase in risk was originally reported in a study of all hospitalizations in the cohort by Gray et al. (1996) discussed above. However, by the end of 1996, the cumulative probability of hospitalization of the two groups was the same (0.034% for deployed and 0.035% for nondeployed). There was no interaction between covariates and deployment status. The authors also assessed the association of testicular cancer with specific occupations for both deployed and nondeployed veterans. The highest RRs were observed for men engaged in electronic-equipment repair (RR 1.56, 95% CI 1.23-2.00), construction-related trades (RR 1.42, 95% CI 0.93-2.17), and electric or mechanical repair (RR 1.26, 95% CI 1.01-1.58). The followup period was short for a cancer assessment, but it did include the age range

(22-31 years) when the disease might appear. No specific Gulf War exposures were assessed, although risk by occupational group was calculated.

There was some evidence of an association of testicular cancer with Gulf War deployment in a pilot cancer-registry-based study. Levine et al. (2005) matched a stratified random sample of 621,902 Gulf War deployed active-duty, reserve, and National Guard veterans and 746,248 nondeployed veterans with the central cancer registries of New Jersey and the District of Columbia. From 1991 to 1999, 17 deployed and 11 nondeployed veterans were identified with testicular cancer for a proportional incidence rate of 2.33 (95% CI 0.95-5.70) adjusted for state of residence, deployment status, race, and age. The greatest proportions of testicular cancer were in deployed men in the age groups of 25-29 and 30-34 years (standardized incidence ratio 1.42) and in nondeployed men in age groups of 30-34 and 35-39 years (standardized incidence ratio 0.94). The number of excess cases peaked 4-5 years after deployment, as opposed to the findings in the Knoke et al. study, which found the excess in the first few months after the soldiers returned home.

Gray et al. (1996) analyzed hospital records from DoD facilities for the last 5 months of 1991 and all of 1992 and 1993. In 1991, hospitalizations for malignant neoplasm of the testis were slightly higher in deployed men (rate ratio 2.12, 95% CI 1.11-4.02), but no difference was seen in 1992 or 1993.

Skin Cancer

There are two types of skin cancer: melanoma, which forms in the skin cells that make pigment and is less common, and the more common nonmelanoma skin cancer, which typically begins in cells that do not make pigments—basal cells (small round cells in the base of the outer layer of skin) or squamous cells (flat cells that form the surface of the skin). The annual age-adjusted incidence of melanoma of the skin is about 18.5 per 100,000 people. Skin cancer was assessed separately by the committee because of the potential for military personnel to be exposed to ultraviolet radiation and environmental toxicants and because several of the studies considered by the committee provided an analysis of skin cancer as distinct from other cancers.

The committee identified only one primary study that assessed the prevalence of skin cancer in Vietnam veterans: CDC (1988b) looked for skin cancer as part of the VES. The prevalence of skin cancer on dermatologic examination was 0.6% in Vietnam-theater veterans and 0.7% in Vietnam-era veterans for a nonsignificant OR of 0.8 (95% CI 0.4-1.7) adjusted for age at enlistment, race, year of enlistment, enlistment status, score on general technical test, and primary military occupation.

One primary study that assessed the risk of skin cancer in Gulf War veterans was identified. As of 2002, when Australian Gulf War veterans were compared with their nondeployed counterparts, they had no increase in prevalence of probable or possible skin cancers diagnosed after 1991 (Kelsall et al. 2004a). The entire Australian cohort of 1871 veterans who were deployed to Southeast Asia was compared with nondeployed veterans frequency matched for service type, sex, and age. Participants completed a self-report questionnaire about medical conditions that had been diagnosed or treated by a medical doctor and about when the conditions had been diagnosed. Participants also underwent a comprehensive health assessment by specially trained health professionals who were blinded to the deployment status of the participants and asked further questions about the diagnoses and determined whether the self-reports were unlikely, possible, or probable according to pre-established criteria. The participation rate was 80.5% for Gulf War veterans and 50.5% for the control group. This study has the advantage of a good participation rate for the deployed veterans and use of criteria for assessing self-reports of health but is limited in that self-reports were not verified by a physical examination and the participation rate for the control group was poor. Although the veterans were asked about psychologic stressors experienced during their deployment, the results of this questionnaire were not correlated with specific health outcomes.

Three secondary studies also estimated the risk of skin cancer in Gulf War veterans on the basis of self-reports. As discussed above, the Iowa Persian Gulf Study Group (1997) also surveyed deployed and nondeployed Gulf War veterans from a restricted geographic area to ascertain the prevalence of skin cancer. Compared with nondeployed veterans, Gulf War veterans had a significantly increased prevalence rate difference for skin cancer (Cochran-Mantel-Haenszel rate difference 0.8, 95% CI 0.4-1.3, $p \leq 0.05$).

In the Kang et al. (2000b) study, the population prevalence of self-reported skin cancer was estimated to be 1.5% in Gulf War veterans and 1.4% in Gulf War-era veterans for a statistically significant increased rate difference of 0.15 (95% CI 0.11-0.19, $p \leq 0.05$). Steele (2000) looked at skin cancer in Gulf War-deployed and nondeployed Kansas veterans in 1998. On the basis of a structured telephone interview in which veterans were asked whether they had ever received a physician's diagnosis of or treatment for a medical condition and when it had developed, the OR for skin cancer occurring after 1990 in deployed veterans was 1.17 (95% CI 0.47-2.90). As noted in the discussion of this study above, its limitations include a restricted geographic area, lack of verification of medical conditions by medical record or examination, and poor exposure data.

PTSD and Cancer

Few studies have assessed cancer in Vietnam War and Gulf War veterans who have PTSD. The committee identified only one primary study: Boscarino (2005) examined excess postservice mortality from cancer in Vietnam veterans by using data from the VES 16 years after the war. Mortality was assessed in Vietnam veterans who were known to be alive in 1983 and who completed a telephone interview at that time on PTSD symptoms and health status; 7924 Vietnam-theater and 7364 Vietnam-era veterans completed the telephone interview. Vital status was assessed for the period January 1985-December 2000 with the VA Beneficiary Identification Record Locator Subsystem (BIRLS) Death File, the Social Security Administration Death Master File, and the National Death Index Plus. Cause of death was coded according to *ICD*. During the telephone interview, veterans were asked about 15 PTSD-related symptoms and their frequency; in 1985-1986, PTSD was diagnosed in a subsample of the veterans (2490 theater veterans and 1972 era veterans) on the basis of personal interviews with the Diagnostic Interview Schedule Version III (DIS-III). With DIS-III, 377 veterans were diagnosed with lifetime PTSD on the basis of combat exposure, which was assessed with the Combat Exposure Scale. Boscarino reported that in the telephone interview there was a clear dose-response relationship between low, moderate, high, and very high combat exposure and whether the criteria for PTSD were met. The Cox proportional-hazards ratio for cancer mortality (188 total deaths) was 1.9 for PTSD-positive Vietnam-theater veterans (95% CI 1.1-3.3, $p = 0.018$) and 0.9 (95% CI 0.3-3.1) for Vietnam era veterans with the model adjusted for race, Army volunteer status, Army entry age, Army discharge status, Army illicit drug use, age at interview, intelligence, and pack-years of cigarette-smoking. Strengths of this study include a large sample, a sufficient latent period (17 years) for death from cancer, the use of an in-person structured interview to diagnose PTSD, and an assessment of combat exposure; limitations include lack of specification as to cancer type.

The committee identified several secondary studies that assessed the risk of cancer in veterans of Vietnam (Boscarino 1997) or veterans of any war (Schnurr et al. 2000; Spiro et al. 2006) who had PTSD. Boscarino (1997) found no increase in the presence of cancer in Vietnam veterans who had combat-related lifetime PTSD (n = 1067) compared with those without PTSD (n = 332) (OR 0.87, 95% CI 0.25-2.96, p = 0.817) after adjustment for a variety of demographic, social, and Army characteristics. Schnurr et al. (2000) assessed the prevalence of physician-diagnosed medical disorders and combat-related PTSD in 605 veterans of World War II and the Korean War. Veterans were screened for PTSD with the Mississippi Scale for Combat-Related PTSD. The hazard ratio for cancer was a nonsignificant 1.05 (95% CI 0.90-1.21) adjusted for age, smoking, alcohol consumption, and body-mass index (BMI) at study entry. Similar results were seen by Spiro et al. (2006), who examined the association between self-reports of PTSD and health conditions in 2425 veterans who participated in the Veterans Health Study conducted on outpatients at VA ambulatory-care clinics in 1993-1995. PTSD was assessed with the PTSD Checklist, measures of exposure to traumatic events were obtained, and a medical-history interview was conducted that asked about 22 conditions. An OR for cancer of 1.16 (95% CI 0.82-1.65) was seen in veterans with PTSD compared with veterans with depression and veterans with neither depression nor PTSD adjusted for age and for depression. The OR for skin cancer was an insignificant 1.24 (95% CI 0.85-1.79) for veterans with PTSD vs those without PTSD with or without comorbid depression.

Summary and Conclusions

In general, the three primary studies of male Vietnam veterans considered by this committee did not find statistically significant increases in cancer associated with deployment to Vietnam. The exception is the 50% increase in the risk of NHL in Vietnam veterans compared with era veterans; however, this risk does not appear to correlate with exposure to combat (Selected Cancers Cooperative Study Group 1990a). Two studies of cancer in female Vietnam veterans also failed to find an increased risk of all cancers or gynecologic cancers associated with serving in Vietnam. With respect to the specific question of concern in this review, studies of Vietnam veterans found no evidence that serving in a combat unit increases cancer risk. The studies included a sufficient observation period to detect most cancers that might result from deployment-related stressors experienced in Vietnam. The committee did not identify any secondary studies of cancer in Vietnam veterans.

There is no consistent evidence of a higher overall incidence of cancer in Gulf War veterans than in nondeployed veterans based on the four primary studies and nine secondary studies considered by the committee. Only one study found an increased (but nonsignificant) risk of any cancer in Gulf War veterans (McCauley et al. 2002b), but the sample was small, and there was no verification of the self-reported diagnoses. The other three primary studies and the secondary studies were all negative for an increased risk of cancer in Gulf War veterans. However, many of the Gulf War veterans are young for cancer diagnosis, and for most cancers the followup period after the Gulf War has probably been too short to expect their onset.

The incidence of and mortality from cancer in general and testicular cancer in particular have been assessed in cohort studies. Results regarding testicular cancer from three primary studies of Gulf War veterans were mixed: one study concluded that there was no evidence of an excess risk, a small registry-based study suggested that there may be an increased risk, and a third study of DoD hospitalization records found a slight increase in the first 5 months immediately after the war, but not in the following 2 years. Although the results are inconsistent, the committee believes that followup is warranted to see whether such an association exists when more time has passed, inasmuch as it is still early for the development of most cancers in Gulf War veterans. In the three primary and two secondary studies considered by the committee, the prevalence of skin cancer does not appear to be increased in deployed veterans of either the Vietnam War or the Gulf War when skin cancer is assessed by dermatologic examination.

Boscarino (2005) found an increase in the risk of death from cancer in veterans with PTSD, specifically Vietnam veterans who had participated in the CDC VES. Three secondary studies that assessed the risk of cancer in veterans of other wars, including World War II and the Gulf War, found no increase in the prevalence of any cancer in veterans with combat-related PTSD compared with veterans without PTSD.

In general, the studies reviewed by the committee for cancer did not indicate an increased risk of any cancer in Vietnam or Gulf War veterans with the possible exceptions of testicular cancer in Gulf War veterans and NHL in Vietnam veterans. However, the committee emphasizes that given the latent period of most cancers, a sufficient amount of time has not elapsed since deployment for cancer to develop. Furthermore, many of the studies of Gulf War veterans, but not of Vietnam veterans, did not look for cancer as a health effect. The assessment of cancer as a result of deployment is also complicated by other potential exposures, such as to Agent Orange and other environmental contaminants, during both the Vietnam War and the Gulf War.

The committee concludes that there is inadequate/insufficient evidence to determine whether an association exists between deployment to a war zone and cancer.

TABLE 6-1 Cancer

Reference	Study Design	Population	Outcomes	Results	Adjustments	Comments
All cancers						
CDC 1988b VES	Retrospective cohort, prevalence, population-based, telephone interview followed by screening medical examination	2490 Vietnam-theater veterans, 1972 Vietnam-era veterans randomly selected from 7924 theater veterans and 7364 era veterans who had entered Army in 1965-1971	Cancer (unspecified) diagnosed with medical examination	OR 1.4, 95% CI includes 1.0, NS	Age at enlistment, race, year of enlistment, enlistment status (volunteer vs draftee), score on general technical test, primary military occupational specialty	Low participation rate in control group, CI not given
SCCSG 1990a	Case-control	1157 male Vietnam-theater veterans with NHL, 1776 Vietnam-era controls frequency-matched by age	Cancer diagnoses from eight city or state cancer registries	NHL OR 1.52, 95% CI 1.00-2.32	Registry, age group in 1968, ethnicity, education, other covariates, including reported exposures to pesticides, reported medical history and drugs, smoking, marital status, being raised Jewish	Possible exposure to Agent Orange considered although dioxin in blood not measured
SCCSG 1990b	Case-control	342 male Vietnam-theater veterans with soft-tissue or other sarcomas, 1776 Vietnam-era controls frequency-matched by age	Cancer diagnoses from eight city or state cancer registries	Soft-tissue or other sarcomas OR 0.74, 95% CI 0.39-1.41, NS	Registry, age group in 1968, ethnicity, education, other covariates, including reported exposures to pesticides, reported medical history and drugs, smoking, marital status, being raised Jewish	Limited power to detect rare outcome

TABLE 6-1 Cancer

Reference	Study Design	Population	Outcomes	Results	Adjustments	Comments
SCCSG 1990c	Case-control	310 male Vietnam-theater veterans with Hodgkin's disease, 48 with nasal carcinoma, 80 with nasopharyngeal carcinoma, 130 with primary liver cancer; 1776 Vietnam-era controls frequency-matched by age	Cancer diagnoses from eight city or state cancer registries	Hodgkin's disease OR 1.23, 95% CI 0.65-2.32; nasal carcinoma OR 0.31, 95% CI 0.04-2.20; primary liver cancer OR 0.53, 95% CI 0.14-1.94, all NS	Registry, age group in 1968, ethnicity, education, other covariates, including reported exposures to pesticides, reported medical history and drugs, smoking, marital status, being raised Jewish, occupational exposure	Limited power to detect differences
Watanabe and Kang 1995	Cross-sectional	10,716 Vietnam Marine veterans, 9346 non-Vietnam Marine veterans	Cancer mortality	All cancers RR 1.20, 95% CI 0.93-1.55, NS; lung cancer RR 1.33, 95% CI 0.84-2.10; all cancers rate ratio 1.08, 95% CI 0.84-1.39; larynx rate ratio 2.60, 95% CI 0.27-25.0; lung rate ratio 1.12, 95% CI 0.71-1.76; lymphosarcoma and reticulosarcoma rate ratio 1.21, 95% CI 0.27-5.41; all cancer rate ratios NS	Race, education, year of birth, adjusted for latent period less than or more than 16 years of followup	Did not adjust for other risk factors for cancer, possibly insufficient followup period for some cancers, limited statistical power for rare causes of death
Kang et al. 2000c	Cohort	4140 female Vietnam-theater veterans, 4140 Vietnam-era veteran controls	Gynecologic cancers (breast, ovary, uterus, cervix)	Any gynecologic organ OR 1.14, 95% CI 0.94-1.40; breast OR 1.18, 95% CI 0.91-1.51; ovary OR 1.83, 95% CI 0.72-4.61; uterus OR 1.00, 95% CI 0.61-1.61; cervix OR 1.11, 95% CI 0.74-1.66; all NS	Age, race, branch of service, pay grade, marital status, nursing occupation, smoking, drinking, family history of cancer, use of birth-control pills, postmenopausal estrogen, progestin	85% statistical power if RR had been at least 1.30 for gynecologic cancers

TABLE 6-1 Cancer

Reference	Study Design	Population	Outcomes	Results	Adjustments	Comments
Dalager et al. 1995	Cross-sectional	4586 female Vietnam-theater veterans, 5325 female Vietnam-era veterans	Cancer mortality	All cancers RR 1.00, 95% CI 0.75-1.34, NS	Rank, nursing status, duration of military service, age at entry into followup	Limited statistical power, small sample, insufficient latent period for outcome, did not adjust for other risk factors for cancer
McCauley et al. 2002b	Cross-sectional	GW veterans: 653 Khamisiyah veterans and 610 non-Khamisiyah veterans, 516 nondeployed veterans	Cancer; all deployed vs nondeployed	OR 3.0, 95% CI 1.0-13.1	Age, sex, race, region of residence	Possible recall and selection bias, limited generalizability, did not adjust for other risk factors for cancer
Macfarlane et al. 2003	Cohort	51,721 UK GW-deployed veterans, 50,755 nondeployed veterans; random samples	Cancers identified from National Health Service Central Register	Any cancer RR 0.99, 95% CI 0.83-1.17	Sex, age, service branch, rank	Followup was from April 1991 to diagnosis of cancer, emigration, death, or July 2002, too short for most cancers to develop
Gray et al. 1996	Retrospective cohort, hospitalization	547,076 active-duty GW veterans, 618,335 non-GW veterans	Hospital-discharge diagnoses for neoplasms in DoD facilities	Standardized rate ratio ~1.10 (exact value not given), 95% CI 1.0-1.2 for last 5 months of 1991; rate ratio 0.92, 95% CI ~0.87-1.0 in 1992; rate ratio 0.94, 95% CI ~0.87-1.1); testicular cancer rate ratio 2.12, 95% CI 1.11-4.02 in 1991, no difference in 1992 and 1993	Prewar hospitalization, sex, age, race, branch of service, marital status, rank, length of service, salary, occupation	ORs are statistically significantly below 1, but no values given; no separation of specific illnesses

TABLE 6-1 Cancer

Reference	Study Design	Population	Outcomes	Results	Adjustments	Comments
Gray et al. 2000	Retrospective cohort, hospitalization	652,979 GW veterans, 652,922 randomly selected non-GW-deployed veterans	Hospital-discharge diagnoses for neoplasms in three hospital systems: DoD, VA, COSHPD	DoD PMR 0.98, 95% CI 0.94-1.01; VA PMR 0.88, 95% CI 0.78-0.98; COSHPD PMR 0.86, 95% CI 0.61-1.1	Age, sex, race	Able to assess only illnesses that resulted in hospitalization; possible undetected confounders
Testicular cancer						
Knoke et al. 1998 (Followup of Gray et al. 1996)	Cohort, hospitalization	517,223 active-duty male GW-deployed veterans, 1,291,323 nondeployed active-duty veteran controls	First diagnosis of testicular cancer at U.S. military hospitals worldwide July 31, 1991-April 1, 1996	Rate ratio 1.05, 95% CI 0.86-1.29	Race or ethnicity, age, occupation, rank, salary, length of service, branch of service, marital status	Short followup time but right age range, no specific exposures evaluated, military hospitals only, only active-duty personnel evaluated
Levine et al. 2005	Cohort, cancer registry	621,902 GW veterans vs 746,248 nondeployed veteran controls	Diagnosis of testicular cancer from cancer registries of New Jersey and District of Columbia	Proportional incidence ratio 2.33, 95% CI 0.95-5.70	Age (and age squared), state of residence, deployment status, race	Possible confounding by occupational exposures to chemicals in gulf
Skin cancer						
CDC 1988b VES	Retrospective cohort, prevalence, population-based	2490 Vietnam-theater veterans, 1972 Vietnam-era veterans	Skin cancer diagnosed via screening medical examination	OR 0.8, 95% CI 0.4-1.7, NS	Age at enlistment, race, year of enlistment, enlistment status (volunteer vs draftee), score on general technical test, primary military occupational specialty	Low participation rate in control group, CI not given
Kelsall et al. 2004a	Cross-sectional, mailed questionnaire	1456 Australian GW veterans, 1588 nondeployed veterans	Skin cancer determined with self-reported diagnosis assessed by medical practitioner	OR 1.0, 95% CI 0.7-1.3	Service type, rank, age, education, marital status	Low participation in control group possibly leading to participation bias

TABLE 6-1 Cancer

Reference	Study Design	Population	Outcomes	Results	Adjustments	Comments
PTSD and cancer						
Boscarino 2005 VES	Cross-sectional, mortality in subset of VES	7924 Vietnam-theater veterans (836 with PTSD), 7364 Vietnam-era veterans (214 with PTSD)	Cancer mortality about 30 years after war; mortality and vital status determined with VA BIRLS database, SSA Master Beneficiary Record database, NDI Plus	Vietnam-theater veterans with PTSD HR 1.9, 95% CI 1.1-3.3; Vietnam-era veterans with PTSD HR 0.9, 95% CI 0.3-3.1	Race, Army volunteer status, Army entry age, Army discharge status, Army illicit-drug abuse, intelligence, age, pack-years of cigarette-smoking	Risk factors based on self-reports, PTSD status determined with nonvalidated questionnaire

NOTE: BIRLS = Beneficiary Identification Record Locator Subsystem Death File, CI = confidence interval, COSHPD = California Office of Statewide Health Planning and Development, GW = Gulf War, HR = hazard ratio, IPSG = Iowa Persian Study Group, NDI = National Death Index, NHL = non-Hodgkin's lymphoma, NS = not significant, OR = odds ratio, PMR = proportional morbidity ratio, PTSD = posttraumatic stress disorder, RR = relative risk, SCCSG = Selected Cancers Cooperative Study Group, SSA = Social Security Administration, VA = Department of Veterans Affairs, VES = Vietnam Experience Study.

ENDOCRINE DISEASES

Endocrine diseases include disorders of the adrenals, pituitary, thyroid, parathyroids, pancreas, gonads, and bone. The most common endocrine disorders are diabetes mellitus and disorders of the thyroid, such as hypothyroidism and hyperthyroidism. Hypothyroidism is characterized by deficient secretion of thyroid hormones either primarily because of a defect in the thyroid or secondarily because of a defect in the pituitary's production of thyroid-stimulating hormone (TSH, also called thyrotropin). There are two types of diabetes mellitus: type 1, a marked deficiency of pancreatic insulin secretion, and type 2, a combination of insulin resistance and decreased insulin secretion; both types lead to increased serum glucose concentrations.

In primary papers that evaluated those health effects in veterans, the committee required that an appropriate laboratory test be used to confirm the presence of diabetes or any thyroid disease or that veterans be receiving medication for the conditions. Papers that relied solely on self-reports of the conditions, even if they were self-reports of a physician's diagnosis, were considered to be secondary papers. None of the primary or secondary studies of deployed veterans considered below described diseases of the adrenals, pituitary, or parathyroids. Therefore, the committee assumed that those diseases were not looked for in the population or were so uncommon, even in the studies of large populations of veterans, that they could not be evaluated. The primary studies of diabetes and thyroid disease are summarized in Table 6-2.

Diabetes

Primary Studies

CDC (1988b) completed the VES in 1988, about 15-20 years after the Vietnam War. From a nationally representative random sample of 7924 theater veterans and 7364 era veterans who completed a telephone interview, 2490 of the theater veterans and 1972 of the era veterans also completed physical- and psychologic-health screening examinations in 1985-1986. The prevalence of diabetes in the theater and era veterans was 1.7% and 1.5%, respectively, on the basis of examination by a physician for a nonsignificant OR of 1.1 ($p > 0.05$) adjusted for age at enlistment, race, year of enlistment, enlistment status, score on general technical tests, and primary military occupational specialty.

The committee identified only one primary study that looked at diabetes among U.S. Gulf War veterans (Eisen et al. 2005). In a cross-sectional prevalence study conducted in 2001, 1061 Gulf War-deployed veterans and 1128 nondeployed veterans received physical examinations at 16 VA medical centers. The study was conducted as part of the National Health Survey of Gulf War Era Veterans and Their Families. Study participants were randomly selected for a physical examination from among the 11,441 deployed and 9476 nondeployed veterans who had participated in the 1995 phase of the survey by completing a mail or telephone questionnaire about their health. Diabetes mellitus, defined as a fasting glucose concentration of at least 7.0 mmol/L at examination or as taking a hypoglycemic medication, was found in 4.2% of the deployed and 3.5% of the nondeployed veterans for a nonsignificant OR of 1.52 (95% CI 0.81-2.85, $p = 0.19$) adjusted for age, sex, race, cigarette-smoking, duty type, service branch, years of education, and rank. The study is limited by the relatively low participation rate (53% deployed and 39% nondeployed), which may have introduced participation bias.

Secondary Studies

Two secondary studies that assessed the association of diabetes with having served in Vietnam were identified. Eisen et al. (1991) used the Vietnam Era [1965-1975] Twin Registry of male-male (monozygotic and dizygotic) twins born in 1939-1957 to assess the prevalence of self-reported diabetes in 2260 pairs of male monozygotic twins who were discordant for the disease. Twins were surveyed by mail or telephone interview in 1987 and asked whether they had ever had diabetes (or 12 other health conditions). Of the twins with and without current diabetes, 50% and 55%, respectively, had served in Southeast Asia for an insignificant OR of 0.8 (95% CI 0.2-3.4). When twins were surveyed as to whether they had ever had diabetes since service in Southeast Asia (as opposed to currently having diabetes), there was still an insignificant OR of 3.0 (95% CI 0.6-14.9), indicating that service in Vietnam was not associated with an increased frequency of diabetes. The study had a high response rate, 74.4%, but is limited by the lack of a physical examination to confirm the presence of diabetes.

In the only study that attempted to associate self-reports of diabetes with combat stress, O'Toole et al. (1996b) found that the risk of diabetes did not appear to be linked to increasing combat exposure in Australian Vietnam veterans. A random sample of 641 Australian Army veterans posted to Vietnam in 1964-1972 was interviewed with a health survey questionnaire and a combat-exposure index 20-25 years after the war. Combat-exposure responses were divided into severity quartiles. The ORs for diabetes compared with combat exposure were 1.00, 0.56, 0.92, and 0.61 for each quartile of increase in combat score ($p = 0.557$); the lowest score quartile was used as the referent.

Five secondary studies looked at the presence of diabetes among Gulf War veterans, on the basis of self-reports, and found no significant increase in the prevalence of diabetes in Gulf War veterans compared with their nondeployed counterparts. Gray et al. (2002) surveyed members of the U.S. Naval Mobile Construction Battalions (Seabees) in 1997-1999 by mail questionnaire about medical conditions for which they had received a physician's diagnosis. Seabees deployed to the gulf region ($n = 3831$) were compared with Seabees deployed elsewhere ($n = 4933$) and not deployed ($n = 3104$). Diabetes mellitus was reported by 1.04% of Gulf War-deployed Seabees, 0.91% of those deployed elsewhere, and 1.61% of nondeployed Seabees. The OR for having a diagnosis of diabetes among Gulf War Seabees compared with nondeployed Seabees was 0.77 (95% CI 0.49-1.23) adjusted for age, sex, active-duty or reserve status, race and ethnicity, current smoking, and current alcohol drinking.

Similar results were seen by McCauley et al. (2002b), who conducted a telephone survey of Gulf War veterans from Oregon, Washington, California, North Carolina, and Georgia to assess the prevalence of self-reported medical conditions or hospitalizations 9 years after the war. Veterans were categorized as having been within 50 miles of the Khamisiyah munitions bunker in Iraq ($n = 653$) with possible exposure to chemical-warfare agents, in the Gulf War region but not in the Khamisiyah area ($n = 610$), and not deployed to the gulf region ($n = 516$). The frequency of self-reported diagnoses of diabetes with onset after Gulf War service was 2.3% in all deployed veterans, whether or not they were near Khamisiyah, and 2.5% in nondeployed veterans for a nonsignificant OR of 1.0 (95% CI 0.5-2.4) adjusted for age, sex, race, and region of residence.

In 1998, Steele (2000) assessed the prevalence of self-reports of physician-diagnosed or treated diabetes in 1548 Gulf War-deployed veterans and 482 veterans who served elsewhere. All veterans were living in Kansas at the time of the telephone survey; disease onset must have occurred during 1990-1998. The incidence of diagnosis in this time period was 1% in both groups for a nonsignificant OR of 1.22 (95% CI 0.45-3.30) adjusted for sex, age, income, and education level.

Simmons et al. (2004) surveyed all 51,581 male UK veterans who served in the Gulf War and a demographically similar comparison cohort of 51,688 UK male veterans who were not deployed to the gulf. Among the 23,358 deployed men who responded, 0.2% reported having diabetes with onset after 1990, as did 0.4% of 17,730 nondeployed men who responded, for a nonsignificant OR of 0.7 (95% CI 0.5-1.0) adjusted for age at the time of the survey, service and rank at the time of the Gulf War, serving status at the time of the survey, alcohol consumption, and smoking.

Kang et al. (2000b) conducted a mail and telephone survey to assess the health status of a stratified random sample of Gulf War-deployed veterans compared with veterans who were in the military at the time of the Gulf War but were not deployed to the region. On the basis of 15,817 mail responses and 5,100 telephone responses of self-reports of medical conditions during the preceding 12 months, the authors estimated the population prevalence of diabetes to be 0.8% in Gulf War veterans and 0.9% in Gulf War-era veterans (significant decreased rate difference -0.08, 95% CI -0.11 to -0.05). The authors further estimated that 1.7% of the deployed veterans and 1.5% of the nondeployed veterans had some other endocrine disorder (statistically significant increased rate difference 0.2, 95% CI 0.16-0.24). The response rate in the study was 70%.

Thyroid Disease

Primary Studies

Only one primary study looked at endocrine function in Vietnam veterans. The VES (CDC 1988b) discussed above also assessed thyroid-hormone concentrations in deployed and nondeployed Vietnam veterans 15-20 years after the war. Deployed and nondeployed veterans had the same mean TSH concentration (1.6 mU/L) and the same mean free-thyroxine (free-T4) index (2.2). Of the deployed veterans, 1% had TSH outside the reference range (reference range defined as $\leq$ 10 mU/L for both cohorts combined) compared with 0.6% of the nondeployed veterans for an OR of 2.0 (95% CI 0.9-4.3); 5.4% of the deployed veterans were outside the reference range of the free-triiodothyronine (T3) index ($\geq$ the fifth percentile for the combined cohorts) compared with 4.6% of the nondeployed vets for an OR of 1.2 (95% CI 0.9-1.5). The ORs were adjusted for age at enlistment, race, year of enlistment, enlistment status, score on general technical test, and primary military occupational specialty.

In the Eisen et al. study (2005) discussed above, thyroid function was assessed in the Gulf War-deployed and nondeployed veterans. Hypothyroidism was defined as an untreated TSH concentration of 10.0 mU/mL or greater or as taking medication for hypothyroidism. Hyperthyroidism required an untreated TSH concentration of less than 0.1 mU/mL or as taking medication for hyperthyroidism. Of the deployed Gulf War veterans, 1.6% had hypothyroidism compared with 1.2% of nondeployed veterans for a nonsignificant OR of 1.70 (95% CI 0.75-3.87, p = 0.2) adjusted for age, sex, race, cigarette-smoking, duty type, service branch, and rank. Of the deployed veterans, 0.3% had hyperthyroidism compared with 0.1% of the nondeployed veterans for a nonsignificant OR of 4.86 (95% CI 0.68-34.58, p = 0.11) adjusted for age, sex, race, cigarette-smoking, years of education, and duty type.

Two retrospective cohort studies by Gray et al. (1996, 2000) looked at hospitalizations of Gulf War veterans for "endocrine, nutritional, and metabolic diseases" (*ICD-10* E00-E99). In the first study, DoD hospital-discharge diagnoses by *ICD* category were determined for 1991, 1992, and 1993, and Gulf War veterans (n = 547,076) were compared with other veterans from the same period (n = 618,335); all were regular active-duty personnel in the Army, Navy (including Marines), and Air Force during the war. All data were obtained from the DMDC. The multivariate ORs for each year were all about 0.9 (exact values not given) adjusted for prewar hospitalizations, sex, age, race or ethnic group, branch of service, marital status, rank, length of service, salary, and occupation; thus deployed Gulf War veterans were not at increased risk for hospitalizations for endocrine, nutrition, or metabolic disorders. In the second study, hospital-discharge records of three hospital systems—DoD (n = 182,164), VA (n = 16,030), and the California Office of Statewide Health Planning and Development (n = 5185)—for 1991-1994 were examined. PMRs of hospital-discharge diagnoses by *ICD-9* category were compared for Gulf War veterans and veterans not deployed to the gulf. The PMRs were 0.99 (95% CI 0.93-1.06) for DoD, 1.08 (95% CI 0.92-1.24) for VA, and 0.81 (95% CI 0.48-1.14) for California Office of Statewide Health Planning and Development; all were nonsignificant. All PMRs were adjusted for age and sex, and the DoD PMR was also adjusted for race. Limitations of the studies include the use of hospital-discharge diagnoses and the fact that most endocrine diseases do not require hospitalization.

Secondary Studies

Several secondary studies assessed thyroid function in Gulf War veterans on the basis of self-reports. A mail survey of the entire Canadian military contingent of 2924 male veterans who served in the Gulf War and 3241 Canadian veterans who were in the military but had not been posted to the gulf region asked about the presence of goiter (a form of thyroid disease) or thyroid trouble. Positive responses were reported by 0.9% of the Gulf War veterans and 0.7% of the nondeployed veterans 20-44 years old and by 2.0% of deployed and 1.3% of nondeployed veterans 45-64 years old; the median age of the deployed was 36 years, and that of the nondeployed was 37 years (Goss Gilroy Inc. 1998).

In the Gray et al. (2002) study discussed above for diabetes, 1.15% of the deployed Seabee veterans reported having a thyroid condition, as did 0.69% of the Seabees deployed elsewhere and 0.97% of the nondeployed Seabees. Comparing thyroid conditions in deployed Seabees and nondeployed Seabees yielded a nonsignificant OR of 1.49 (95% CI 0.89-2.5) adjusted for age, sex, active-duty or reserve status, race or ethnicity, current smoking, and current alcohol-drinking.

As with diabetes, Steele (2000) conducted telephone interviews of 1545 Gulf War-deployed and 435 nondeployed veterans living in Kansas that elicited self-reports of physician-diagnosed or treated thyroid conditions; the condition must have first occurred in 1990-1998. The prevalence of a new thyroid condition was 2% in the deployed group and 1% in the nondeployed group for a nonsignificant OR of 2.32 (95% CI 0.81-6.67) adjusted for sex, age, income, and education level.

Morgan et al. (2000) attempted to determine the effects of military stress on a small group of 72 soldiers undergoing survival training, a realistic simulation of combat. Subjects provided serum samples before the field phase of their training, immediately after a highly intense interrogation phase, and at recovery a day after the end of the experience. During the stress of interrogation, total T3 and free T3 were suppressed. Total and free T4 were slightly increased during interrogation but were decreased at recovery, possibly because of conversion to T3. The authors found an unexplained increase in TSH from baseline to recovery with an intermediate increase at interrogation. The findings do not represent an endocrine disease entity and are similar to other changes in the endocrine system that may occur after acute stress.

Posttraumatic Stress Disorder and Endocrine Diseases

Several secondary studies of veterans have examined the association between PTSD and endocrine diseases, such as diabetes or thyroid conditions, but the populations have generally been small and the conclusions based on self-reports of PTSD or medical conditions. In an analysis of VES data collected in 1985-1986 on a random sample of 2490 Vietnam-theater veterans, Boscarino (1997) found that 9.0% of 332 veterans with lifetime PTSD and high combat exposure also had an endocrine-nutritional-metabolic disease compared with 4.0% of 1067 veterans without PTSD and low or no combat exposure. Comparison of the two groups for endocrine-nutritional-metabolic disease yielded a nonsignificant OR of 1.58 (95% CI 0.92-2.73, p = 0.100) adjusted for numerous military, demographic, and socioeconomic variables.

Boscarino (2004) further assessed the prevalence of autoimmune diseases in the VES cohort of 2490 Vietnam-theater veterans. The author assessed 178 veterans with any of 9 autoimmune diseases for the presence of PTSD: 54 veterans were characterized as having PTSD within the last 30 days on the basis of a DIS and meeting the full *Diagnostic and Statistical Manual of Mental Disorders-III (DSM-III)* criteria and 124 veterans were characterized as having comorbid PTSD (PTSD concurrent with psychopathology on the basis of the main Minnesota Multiphasic Personality Inventory scales and considered by the author to be a more severe type of PTSD). Of the 178 veterans with an autoimmune disease and PTSD, six had type 1 diabetes mellitus, four had hypothyroidism, and two had Graves disease (the most common form of hyperthyroidism). The OR for veterans with PTSD compared with veterans without PTSD was 2.9 (95% CI 0.9-8.9, p = 0.066) for diabetes, 8.5 (95% CI 1.9-37.9, p = 0.005) for hypothyroidism, and 3.2 (95% CI 0.6-16.5, p = 0.157) for Graves disease. The ORs were adjusted for age, education, race, intelligence, income, geographic region, Army volunteer status, number of times married, and history of antisocial personality, alcohol abuse, drug abuse, and cigarette-smoking. The study had the advantage of using laboratory tests to confirm the presence of disease, but the number of cases was small.

The Veterans Health Study assessed the prevalence of PTSD, depression, and several medical conditions in a sample of 2425 male ambulatory-care patients at a VA medical facility in the Boston area (Spiro et al. 2006). PTSD was screened for based on responses to the PTSD Checklist for Civilians, reported exposure to traumatic events was assessed with the Laufer Combat Exposure Scale, and health status was based on the self-administered 36-item Medical Outcomes Study Short-Form (SF-36), an instrument to measure physical and mental health, physical and social functioning, and general well-being. Data were collected in 1993-1995; the response rate was 57.2%. The screening criteria for PTSD were met by 20.2% of the patients; when they were compared with those who did not meet the criteria for either PTSD or depression, the OR for type 2 diabetes was a nonsignificant 0.81 (95% CI 0.59-1.11). For thyroid disease, the risk associated with having PTSD was again nonsignificant (OR 1.27, 95% CI 0.58-2.79). ORs were adjusted for age and depression.

Schnurr et al. (2000) failed to find an association in veterans between combat-related PTSD and physician-diagnosed medical conditions. Of 605 combat veterans of World War II and the Korean War assessed for PTSD with the Mississippi Scale for Combat-Related PTSD in 1990, only six were positive for PTSD. Endocrine disease was found in 92 (15%) of the veterans on medical examination. The hazard ratio for having both PTSD and an endocrine disorder was a nonsignificant 1.06 (95% CI 0.88-1.27) adjusted for age, smoking, alcohol consumption, and BMI at study entry.

Female veterans who attended a VA Puget Sound medical facility in 1996-1998 participated in a cross-sectional survey to determine any association between PTSD (screened for with the PTSD Checklist-Civilian Version) and medical conditions as reported on the veteran version of SF-36 (Dobie et al. 2004). Of the 1259 eligible veterans, 266 were positive for PTSD, and 8.9% of the latter had diabetes and 7.7% of those who were negative for PTSD had diabetes, for a nonsignificant OR of 1.51 (95% CI 0.90-2.52) adjusted for age.

Several small studies have examined the association between thyroid hormones and combat-related PTSD in veterans of various wars. Mason et al. (1994) conducted serum radioimmunoassays for total T4, free T4, total T3, free T3, T4-binding globulin, and TSH in 96 male Vietnam veterans who had PTSD and were patients at VA inpatient treatment groups. Veterans with PTSD were compared with 24 demographically similar community controls who did not have PTSD (11 with combat exposure). The PTSD group had moderately higher total T4, total T3, free T3, and T3:T4 ratios, but not free T4. There was also an increase in T4-binding globulin in the PTSD group but no difference between the groups in TSH. Similar TSH in the two groups suggests that there was no significant difference in thyroid metabolic disease between them.

A second study to investigate serum thyroid-hormone concentrations in 65 male Vietnam veterans with PTSD was conducted by Wang et al. (1995). PTSD symptom severity was rated with the Clinician-Administered PTSD Scale (CAPS). Increased CAPS scores correlated positively with free T3, total T3, and total T4, but not free T4 or T4-binding globulin.

When serum thyroid hormones were studied in 12 World War II veterans with PTSD and 18 without PTSD, similar correlations were seen between total and free T3 and PTSD severity (particularly hyperarousal symptoms), but significant differences were not found in total T4, free T4, T4-binding globulin, or TSH between the groups, although there was a slight trend toward higher TSH in the PTSD group (Wang and Mason 1999).

Obesity

Exposure to stressors may affect eating behavior and theoretically might predispose to obesity or eating problems (see Chapter 4 for a discussion of the effects of stress on obesity). No primary studies of obesity in veterans were identified.

A few secondary studies that examined small, selected samples, such as David et al. (2004), or used only self-report measures suggest that PTSD may be associated with an increased frequency of obesity and eating disorders. Dobie et al. (2004) screened female veterans who received care at a VA medical facility in 1996-1998 with a mail questionnaire that included the PTSD Checklist-Civilian Version and SF-36. A comparison of 940 veterans who were negative for PTSD and 266 who were positive for PTSD found that 60 and 66 of them, respectively, were also positive for an eating disorder (OR 5.00, 95% CI 3.37-7.38). Obesity (defined as a BMI over 30) was reported by 35.3% of those without PTSD and 47.0% of those with PTSD, respectively (OR 1.78, 95% CI 1.34-2.35).

Vieweg et al. (2006) examined 144 male Vietnam veterans with PTSD who were 50-59 years old and were patients at a VA medical center. Their mean BMI was 30.2, and 82.8% of them were overweight or obese, far exceeding the current general U.S. population rate of 64.5%.

Other studies, such as Stretch et al. (1995), which had substantial limitations, did not report such an association. Fielder et al. (2006) looked at the 12-month prevalence of bulimia and anorexia nervosa in 892 male and 75 female Gulf War-deployed veterans 10 years after the war and found no evidence of either eating disorder.

Summary and Conclusions

Acute stress and chronic stress activate the endocrine system and thereby influence the immune system, as described in Chapter 4, but it is unclear whether these interactions produce endocrine diseases. Stress also increases caloric intake, and the hormones released by acute and chronic stress, such as cortisol, can accentuate obesity and lead to insulin resistance, a central feature of type 2 diabetes (see Chapter 4). There are several reports that stress with or without comorbid depression has increased the incidence of type 2 diabetes in nonmilitary populations (Kawakami et al. 1999; Mooy et al. 2000; Eaton et al. 1996).

Two primary studies examined the association between deployment and diabetes in Vietnam War veterans (CDC 1988b) and Gulf War veterans (Eisen et al. 2005) and found no increase in the risk of diabetes in deployed veterans of either war. Several secondary studies, one of Vietnam veterans and five of Gulf War veterans, supported the lack of association between deployment to either the Vietnam War or the Gulf War and the presence of diabetes, and one study (O'Toole et al. 1996b) in Vietnam veterans also showed no increase in diabetes with increasing combat exposure.

Furthermore, there were no significant associations between the presence of thyroid diseases and deployment to a war zone, whether in Vietnam or in the Persian Gulf. The four primary studies, one of Vietnam veterans and three of Gulf War veterans, showed no evidence of increased or decreased thyroid function in deployed veterans compared with their nondeployed counterparts. The four secondary studies, all of Gulf War veterans, also showed no association between deployment and thyroid disease. The prevalence of thyroid disease of about 1-2% was slightly lower in both deployed and nondeployed veterans than in the general population—5% for hypothyroidism and 1% for hyperthyroidism (Hollowell et al. 2002). That finding may reflect a male-dominated military inasmuch as thyroid disease is much more common in women than in men.

Five secondary studies that compared endocrine diseases in veterans with PTSD and those without PTSD did not show any significant changes in diabetes or thyroid disease in the two groups, except that one study, by Boscarino (2004), found that Vietnam veterans with PTSD had a greater risk of hypothyroidism. Two studies were of Vietnam veterans, one of veterans of World War II and the Korean War, one of a general veteran population in Boston, and one of a general female veteran population. Many case-control studies of nonmilitary populations have reported a significant relationship between stressful events and the onset of Graves disease, the most common form of hyperthyroidism (Mizokami et al. 2004).

In the three small thyroid-hormone studies of veterans, changes in serum thyroid-hormone concentrations were found in veterans with PTSD compared with veterans without PTSD (Mason et al. 1994; Wang and Mason 1999; Wang et al. 1995) and in men experiencing military survival training (Morgan et al. 2000). However, that no differences in TSH concentrations were seen in those groups suggests that they had no hyperthyroidism or hypothyroidism.

No primary studies of obesity in veterans were identified. One secondary study of male Vietnam veterans found that veterans with PTSD were more overweight than the general U.S. population, a second found that female veterans with PTSD were more likely to have an eating disorder than those without PTSD, and a third found no evidence of eating disorders in Gulf War veterans.

The committee concludes that there is inadequate/insufficient evidence to determine whether an association exists between deployment to a war zone and diabetes mellitus. The committee also concludes that there is inadequate/insufficient evidence to determine whether an association exists between deployment to a war zone and thyroid disease.

TABLE 6-2 Endocrine Diseases

Study	Study Design	Population	Outcomes	Results	Adjustments	Comments
CDC 1988b VES	Retrospective cohort, prevalence, population-based, telephone interview with screening medical examination at followup	2490 Vietnam-theater veterans, 1972 Vietnam-era veterans randomly selected	Screening medical examination, standard hematologic assays, serum chemistry assays	Diabetes OR 1.1, 95% CI includes 1.0; out of TSH reference range OR 2.0, 95% CI 0.9-4.3; out of reference range for free-T3 index OR 1.2, 95% CI 0.9-1.5	Age at enlistment, race, year of enlistment, enlistment status (volunteer vs draftee), score on general technical test, primary military occupational specialty	Low participation rate in control group
Eisen et al. 2005 NHSGWEVTF (Derived from Kang et al. 2000b)	Cross-sectional, prevalence, population-based	1061 GW-deployed veterans, 1128 nondeployed veterans	Diabetes, hypothyroidism, hyperthyroidism	Diabetes OR 1.52, 95% CI 0.81-2.85; hypothyroidism OR 1.70, 95% CI 0.75-3.87; hyperthyroidism OR 4.86, 95% CI 0.68-34.58; all NS	Age, sex, race, cigarette-smoking, duty type, service branch, education, rank (hyperthyroidism not adjusted for service branch or rank)	Low participation rates, deployed (53%), nondeployed (39%)
Gray et al. 1996	Retrospective cohort, hospitalization	547,076 active-duty GW veterans, 618,335 non-GW veterans	Hospital-discharge diagnoses for endocrine-nutritional-metabolic disease	OR about 0.9 (exact value not given), 95% CI < 1.0 for all 3 years	Prewar hospitalization, sex, age, race, branch of service, marital status, rank, length of service, salary, occupation	ORs are statistically significantly below 1, but no values given; no separation of specific illnesses
Gray et al. 2000	Retrospective cohort, hospitalization	652,979 GW-deployed veterans, 652,922 randomly selected nondeployed veterans	Hospital-discharge diagnoses for endocrine, nutritional, and metabolic disease in three hospital systems: DoD, VA, COSHPD	DoD PMR 0.99, 95% CI 0.93-1.06); VA PMR 1.08, 95% CI 0.92-1.24 ; COSHPD PMR 0.81, 95% CI 0.48-1.14	Age, sex, race	Able to assess only illnesses that resulted in hospitalization; possible undetected confounders

NOTE: CI = confidence interval, COSHPD = California Office of Statewide Health Planning and Development, DoD = Department of Defense, GW = Gulf War, NHSGWEVTF = National Health Survey of Gulf War Era Veterans and Their Families, NS = not significant, OR = odds ratio, PMR = proportional morbidity ratio, PTSD = posttraumatic stress disorder, T3 = triiodothyronine, TSH = thyroid-stimulating hormone, VA = Department of Veterans Affairs, VES = Vietnam Experience Study.

PSYCHIATRIC DISORDERS

Numerous investigators have suggested that psychiatric disorders may occur as a consequence of serving in the military during wartime. There are reports associating war-zone trauma with mental illnesses as far back as the Civil War (Pizarro et al. 2006; Wessely 2005), even though the terminology used to classify war-related psychiatric traumatic events has changed considerably. Despite these changes in terminology, there is a substantial literature on the psychiatric effects of war in general, mainly in the context of trauma. There are reports on the prevalence of a wide array of psychiatric disorders and their association with being a veteran (for example, Beebe 1975; Robins et al. 1974; Snow et al. 1988) and with specific combat experiences, including witnessing death and atrocities (Archibald and Tuddenham 1965; Grinker and Spiegel 1945; Kardiner and Spiegel 1947). This section focuses on assessing the evidence of a relationship between deployment-related stress and psychiatric disorders. Substance-use disorders are discussed in the next section.

The challenge for the committee in understanding the plethora of studies available on several potentially diverse cohorts of veterans was first to distinguish clearly between the primary and secondary studies and then to identify studies that explicitly used deployment to a war zone as the exposure of interest in contrast with studies that used serving in the military during wartime, but not necessarily deployment to a war zone, as an overall indicator of risk of development of any psychiatric disorder. As described in Chapter 1, the committee agreed that studies that used PTSD as a presumed marker for deployment-related trauma would also be included in this analysis.

Primary studies provided the basis of the committee's findings on the relationship between deployment-related stress and psychiatric effects. Primary studies were those in which exposure status was determined according to whether subjects had been deployed, not deployed, or deployed to a nonwar zone (for example, Germany) or that used a diagnosis of PTSD as a marker of war-zone trauma. To diagnosis psychiatric disorders and PTSD, primary studies also included an in-person interview and used either the Structured Clinical Interview for *DSM-III-R* (SCID); the Composite International Diagnostic Interview (CIDI), a comprehensive and standardized diagnostic interview designed for assessing mental disorders according to the definitions of the Diagnostic Criteria for Research of *ICD-10* and *DSM-III-R*; or the *DIS*, a research diagnostic interview that assesses psychiatric disorders according to *DSM-III-R* criteria but is designed to be administered by trained lay interviewers; or the CAPS. Primary studies are summarized in Table 6-3.

The secondary studies reviewed and evaluated the same functional domains of interest—such as depression, anxiety, and substance use—and add supplementary information that may increase or decrease confidence in the conclusions drawn from the primary studies.

Primary Studies

The committee identified 11 citations for 7 primary studies (CDC 1988a; Dohrenwend et al. 2006; Fiedler et al. 2006; Ikin et al. 2004; Jordan et al. 1991; Koenen et al. 2003a,b; Kulka et al. 1990; Proctor et al. 2001; Toomey et al. 2007; Wolfe et al. 1999).

The VES was a major study of U.S. Army Vietnam veterans that began with a postservice mortality study (CDC 1987). CDC (1988a) used the cohort to identify and recruit a subsample for phase I of 7924 U.S. Army Vietnam-theater veterans and 7364 Vietnam-era veterans. In phase I, the veterans participated in telephone interviews about their psychosocial health, physical health, and reproductive outcomes. In phase II conducted in 1985-1986, 3317 of the theater veterans and 3126 of the era veterans were invited to participate in a comprehensive health examination to determine the effects of war-zone deployment on psychosocial characteristics (CDC 1988a). Of the theater and era veterans, 2490 (75%) and 1972 (63%), respectively, were enrolled in phase II, which included an examination of psychologic health. The investigators used the DIS and the Minnesota Multiphasic Personality Inventory to assess the veterans for PTSD, alcohol abuse, drug abuse, generalized anxiety, and depression. Six characteristics were controlled for: age at entry into the Army, race, score on the enlistment general technical test (a measure of mental aptitude), enlistment status (drafted or volunteered), year of entry into the Army, and primary military occupational specialty (tactical or nontactical). Vietnam veterans were significantly more likely than era veterans to meet the DIS criteria for generalized anxiety (OR 1.5, 95% CI 1.1-2.1) and depression (OR 2.0, 95% CI 1.4-2.9) in the month prior to examination. Only 2.2% of the theater veterans met the full DIS criteria for combat-related PTSD in the previous month (current), although 14.7% had ever met the criteria (lifetime); results for era veterans were not given.

The congressionally mandated NVVRS constituted nationally representative cohorts of male and female Vietnam theater veterans, era veterans, and civilians; the veteran cohorts were randomly chosen from among all military personnel who had served on active duty during the Vietnam War and who had left service as of September 1987 (Kulka et al. 1990; Weiss et al. 1992). All study participants were interviewed in November 1986-February 1988. The NVVRS was created to determine the prevalence of specific psychiatric disorders and other adjustment problems, both during the course of life (as a measure of predisposing factors) and at the time of the interview. It also included self-reports of war-zone stressor exposures used to create a war-zone stress index to characterize theater veterans as having been subjected to "high exposure" or "low or moderate exposure." A sample of veterans and civilians was obtained from the National Personnel Records Center, the DMDC, and a list developed by VA of all female theater veterans. The NVVRS conducted a total of 3016 interviews, in what was called the National Survey of the Vietnam Generation, with 1200 male theater veterans, 412 male era veterans, 448 male civilians, 432 female theater veterans, 304 female era veterans, and 218 female civilians. The NVVRS also included a preliminary validation component for the survey-based PTSD measures and a clinical-interview component. Response rates were over 83% for Vietnam-theater veterans, 76% for Vietnam-era veterans, and 70% for civilians of those sampled and eligible. Detailed reviews and analyses of military data records were conducted to identify potential differences between veteran respondents and nonrespondents. Although no significant differences were identified, the investigators weighted the data for all the analyses to account for interview-level nonresponse and different probabilities of selection in the civilian cohort. The investigators also controlled for age, race or ethnicity, and female veteran occupation. The occupation of the female veterans was important because many of them were likely to be nurses and therefore to have different exposures to war-zone stressors than their male counterparts (Kulka et al. 1990). Although the DIS was used to interview both veterans and civilians, only a subsample of 260 veterans underwent a semistructured clinical interview by experienced mental-health professionals to also diagnose PTSD and to validate the use of the interview instrument for PTSD used by the researchers. A composite PTSD diagnosis for the subsample was made based on the interviews, the Mississippi Scale for Combat-Related PTSD, the SCID, and the PTSD Scale of the Minnesota Multiphasic Personality Inventory.

The estimated prevalence of current PTSD was 15.2% in all male theater veterans and 8.5% in female theater veterans (Kulka et al. 1990). The prevalence of current (6-month) PTSD was 2.5% in male and 1.1% in female era veterans and 1.2% and 0.3%, respectively, in civilians. The prevalence of lifetime PTSD was 30.6% in male theater veterans and 26.9% in female theater veterans. High levels of war-zone stress, including exposure to at least one traumatic event, were reported by 75.2% of the male theater veterans and 9.2% of the era veterans, and 32.9% of the veterans reporting low or moderate war-zone stress also reported definite traumatic experiences. The prevalence estimate of PTSD among veterans with high war-zone exposure was 35.8% in men and 17.5% in women. The likelihood of having PTSD was increased in men who were in the Army or Marine Corps, were in junior enlisted pay grades, were 17-19 years old when they entered Vietnam, had served on active duty for more than 4 but less than 20 years, had ever been wounded or injured in combat, or had received a combat medal. Women who had more war-zone stress, were younger, or had been on active duty for more than 4 but less than 20 years had increased prevalence of PTSD. PTSD was highly comorbid with other psychiatric disorders: 75% of men with PTSD had a lifetime diagnosis of alcohol abuse or dependence, 44% had generalized anxiety disorder (GAD), and more than 20% had another psychiatric disorder.

The NVVRS has been criticized for overestimating the lifetime rate of PTSD. To address that issue, Dohrenwend et al. (2006) reanalyzed the NVVRS data from the military records of 1200 Vietnam theater veterans with a records-based military-history measure (MHM) of exposure to war-zone stressors. They found that 96.5% of veterans categorized as probably having had low exposure with the MHM had reported their exposure as low or moderate in the NVVRS, and 72.1% of those categorized as having had very high exposure with the MHM had reported their exposure as high. Over 86% of the veterans with war-related PTSD described events judged by the blind raters to have been personally life-threatening or to have involved witnessing death of or physical harm to others. A diagnosis of PTSD was based on the SCID and included a functional assessment with the Global Assessment of Functioning scale. The military records of the clinical subset of 260 veterans examined for the NVVRS were re-examined for this study. A dose-response relationship between PTSD and exposure to war-zone stressors was established. Current (as of 1988) war-related PTSD was diagnosed in 0.3% of low-exposure veterans, 14.4% of moderate-exposure, 27.0% of high-exposure, and 28.1% of very high-exposure. Lifetime war-related PTSD prevalence was 22.5%, and current war-related PTSD prevalence 12.2%. When Dohrenwend et al. adjusted the diagnoses for impairment of functioning and documentation of exposure to war-related traumatic events, the prevalence of lifetime and current war-related PTSD dropped to 18.7% and 9.1%, respectively, in the veteran subset.

Jordan et al. (1991) used the NVVRS data to determine that the most prevalent current disorders among male theater veterans were alcohol abuse or dependence (11%) and GAD (5%); these rates were not different from those of Vietnam-era veterans or civilians. The most prevalent current disorders in female Vietnam-theater veterans were depression and GAD (both 4%). Although the rate of depression was higher in female theater veterans than in female era veterans or civilians, that was not the case for GAD, which did not differ significantly among the groups.

Overall, Jordan et al. (1991) found that the NVVRS showed few differences in the prevalence and distribution of psychiatric disorders among veterans who saw combat in Vietnam and veterans who did not. The major differences appear to be related to the level of combat stress. Of male theater veterans exposed to high war-zone stress, 43% met the criteria for a specific psychiatric disorder other than alcohol abuse or dependence. That was significantly higher than rates found for either low or moderate war-zone stress in male theater veterans (21.1%), era veterans (25.6%), or civilians (18.1%). Because the use of self-reported war-zone stress-exposure information was found to correspond well with the information found in the military records, such as receipt of combat medals, this is one of the few early studies that differentiated between the types of stress encountered in a war zone. Among male veterans with high war-zone stress exposure, 63.1% had at least one lifetime psychiatric disorder and 29.8% had a current diagnosis. Compared with the 783 male veterans with low war-zone stress, the 406 with high war-zone stress had more GAD (10.8% vs 24.4%, $p < 0.05$), dysthymia (1.4% vs 12.3%, $p < 0.001$), major depression disorder (MDD) (3.1% vs 11.1%, $p < 0.01$), obsessive-compulsive disorder (0.5% vs 5.5%, $p < 0.01$), and antisocial personality disorder (7.1% vs 16.6%, $p < 0.01$). Female veterans had fewer psychiatric disorders associated with high war-zone stress, although 22.3% had lifetime major depression and 9.9% had lifetime dysthymia, and these rates were significantly higher than in female veterans exposed to low war-zone stress.

Two primary studies were included that used data from the Vietnam Era Twin Registry study, a longitudinal twin study. Koenen et al. (2003b) used the Combat Exposure Index and the DIS-III-R to measure PTSD and other psychiatric outcomes in monozygotic twin pairs. The cohort consists of male-male twin pairs born in 1937-1957 in which both members of the pair served in the military during the Vietnam era (Eisen et al. 1991). Zygosity was determined by a questionnaire and blood-group typing methods that achieved 95% accuracy. Thirty-seven male twin pairs were identified in which one twin was a Vietnam-theater veteran with combat-related PTSD and a score of at least 7 on the Combat Exposure Index, and 76 male twin pairs were identified in which one twin was a Vietnam-theater veteran without lifetime PTSD and score of at least 7 on the Combat Exposure Index; all co-twins were not deployed to Vietnam. Deployed twins with PTSD were more likely than twins without PTSD to have any mood disorder (OR 8.89, 90% CI 3.66-21.59), MDD (OR 6.32, 90% CI 2.57-15.55), dysthymia (OR 3.80, 90% CI 1.09-13.28), any anxiety disorder (OR 8.63, 90% CI 2.20-33.83), or panic disorder (OR 4.48, 90% CI 1.04-19.41). Twins with PTSD were also more likely than their co-twins to have any mood disorder (OR 4.00, $p < 0.05$) or MDD (OR 2.50, $p < 0.05$) but not other comorbid disorders. Combat-exposed twins that had diagnoses of any of the comorbid psychiatric disorder above also reported more PTSD symptoms in all three symptom clusters (see Chapter 5), including symptoms that had no diagnostic overlap with the comorbid disorders, than did veterans without these disorders.

In another study of the same Vietnam Era Twin Registry cohort, Koenen et al. (2003a) used the entire sample of all 1874 monozygotic twin pairs from the Vietnam Era Twin Registry on whom complete DIS-III-R diagnostic information was available. The study focused on five lifetime diagnoses: MDD, alcohol dependence, drug dependence, cannabis dependence, and tobacco dependence. (Information on substance dependence from the study is discussed in the next section of this chapter.) Measures used were a four-level index of combat exposure (Janes et al. 1991) and a structured psychiatric interview administered to the Vietnam Era Twin Registry twins by telephone with DIS-III-R. Participants were given a diagnosis of combat PTSD (C-PTSD) if they reported combat as a traumatic event and met *DSM-III-R* criteria for PTSD in relation to the event. Conditional logistic regression was used to account for the paired structure of the data and to calculate the matched pairs' ORs and 95% CIs. Premilitary trauma history, age at entry into the military, and education level at the time of entry into the military were controlled for in three models for each psychiatric diagnosis. Combat exposure unadjusted for C-PTSD was found to be significantly associated with MDD (OR 1.22, 95% CI 1.03-1.44) but it was insignificant when adjusted for C-PTSD (OR 1.10, 95% CI 0.92-1.33). C-PTSD unadjusted for combat exposure was also significantly associated with MDD (OR 3.04, 95% CI 1.48-6.24); however, after adjustment for combat exposure, the OR for the association between C-PTSD and MDD was substantially reduced (OR 2.55, 95% CI 1.16-5.61). The investigators suggest that C-PTSD is a mediator of the relationship between combat exposure and MDD. Although the study design using monozygotic twins eliminates the confounding effects of genetic and shared environmental risk factors in the relationships examined, it remains unclear whether other, unmeasured factors might increase the risk of C-PTSD and other mental disorders.

Ikin et al. (2004) conducted in-person interviews of 1381 Australian Gulf War veterans using the CIDI for psychiatric disorders as part of a cross-sectional survey of all Australian veterans deployed to the Gulf War and 1377 comparison veterans not deployed to the gulf. They found that the prevalence of any psychiatric disorder (first present after the Gulf War) was 30.8% in Gulf War veterans and 21.1% in the comparison group (OR 1.6, 95% CI 1.3-1.9) controlled for service type, rank, age, education, and marital status. Deployed veterans were almost 4 times as likely to meet criteria for PTSD (OR 3.9, 95% CI 2.3-6.5) and also were at increased risk for MDD (OR 1.6, 95% CI 1.3-2.0).

Proctor et al. (1998) selected stratified random samples of two demographically heterogeneous Gulf War cohorts from Fort Devens, Massachusetts (n = 2313) and New Orleans (n = 928) that were being studied longitudinally. The resulting subcohorts (Fort Devens, n = 186; New Orleans, n = 66) were compared to a small comparison population of Germany-deployed veterans from the Maine National Guard (n = 48). This study met the criteria for a primary study in that the in-person CAPS was used for PTSD and the SCID was used for other psychiatric disorders. Data were collected in 1994-1996. The samples were selected to produce equal representation of high and low symptom veterans. After adjustment for oversampling of women, participation bias, and age, sex, and education differences, both gulf-deployed groups had higher symptom prevalence of the items that make up the body-system symptom scores in the SF-36 than the Germany-deployed group. Approximately 5% of the Fort Devens cohort, 7% of the New Orleans cohort, and none of the Germany cohort were diagnosed with current PTSD and those with PTSD scored higher on the Expanded Combat Exposure Scale. Compared with the Germany-deployed group, significant differences were found for both gulf-deployed groups in reporting of frequent periods of anxiety or nervousness: OR 7.1 for the Fort Devens cohort and 5.3 for the New Orleans cohort (95% CI excludes 1.0 for both ORs). Self-reported symptoms of frequent periods of feeling depressed were significant only for the Fort Devens cohort (OR 6.0, 95% CI excludes 1.0).

Using the same well-characterized Fort Devens, New Orleans, and Germany-deployed subcohorts as Proctor et al., Wolfe et al. (1999) used the SCID to examine the relationship of psychiatric disorders to health problems. The prevalences of panic disorder, agoraphobia, social phobia, simple phobia, obsessive-compulsive disorder, GAD, and somatoform disorder did not differ between the gulf-deployed and Germany-deployed cohorts. There were slight but significant differences in the rates of current and lifetime PTSD between each of the gulf-deployed groups (5.4% and 6.5%, respectively, in the Fort Devens group and 7.2% and 8.2% in the New Orleans group) and the Germany-deployed group (no PTSD). The largest differences were seen in MDD: all three groups had 2.5-3 times more lifetime MDD than current MDD, and the Fort Devens group had twice the prevalence of lifetime MDD as the New Orleans group (22.5% Fort Devens, 10.2% New Orleans, and 4.2% Germany-deployed). The investigators found a small but significant association between increased health-symptom reports and the diagnosis of PTSD or MDD for the combined deployed groups. However, almost two-thirds of gulf participants reporting moderate to high health symptoms were found to have no axis I (major psychiatric) disorders. The rates of most psychiatric disorders were lower than national comorbidity estimates except PTSD, MDD, and dysthymia, which had rates similar to those in the National Comorbidity Survey (NCS) (Kessler et al. 1995). The Wolfe et al. study had a participation rate of 62% for the Fort Devens cohort and 85% for the Germany-deployed unit, but budget constraints limited participation by the New Orleans cohort to 37%.

Fiedler et al. (2006) compared the prevalence of MDD, panic attacks, social phobia, obsessive-compulsive disorder, GAD, and any psychiatric disorder in random samples of 967 Gulf War-deployed veterans and 784 era veterans. The sample was obtained from the DMDC. Study participants were administered the 12-month version of the CIDI using the *DSM-IV* criteria to assess PTSD and the CIDI-Short Form/*DSM-IV* for the remaining psychiatric disorders by telephone interview with computer-assisted technology. Deployed veterans had a significantly greater prevalence of any psychiatric disorder than nondeployed veterans (26.1% vs 16.1%, $p < 0.05$) including MDD (15.1% vs 7.8%), panic attack (1.6% vs 0.5%), social phobia (3.6% vs 1.7%), obsessive-compulsive disorder (2.8% vs 1.1%), PTSD (3.4% vs 0.9%), GAD (6.0% vs 2.7%) and any anxiety disorder (16.0% vs 9.7%). After control for demographic variables and other psychiatric disorders, deployed veterans were found to have higher risks of MDD (OR 2.07, 95% CI 1.50-2.85) and any anxiety disorder (OR 1.81, 95% CI 1.34-2.45). Lower rank, female sex, and divorced-single status all were significant independent predictors of psychiatric disorder. The study is limited in that the response rate was suboptimal (55%) and responders differed from nonresponders in that a greater proportion of whites and officers volunteered for the study.

In a recent study by Toomey et al. (2007), 1061 veterans deployed to the Gulf War were compared with 1128 Gulf War-era veterans. They used the randomly selected subset of 11,441 deployed and 9476 nondeployed veterans who have been followed since 1995 for the National Health Survey of Gulf War Era Veterans and Their Families (Eisen et al. 2005). The study used structured clinical interviews for all psychologic examinations conducted in 1998-2001; PTSD was diagnosed with the CAPS, and the CIDI was used to diagnose the other axis I psychiatric disorders. The investigators calculated the prevalence of mental disorders beginning during the deployment period and evaluated their prevalence 10 years later. They found that 10 years after the end of the Gulf War, those deployed to that region had a persistent increased prevalence of mental disorders, especially PTSD (OR 5.78, 95% CI 2.62-12.74), all anxiety disorders (OR 4.43, 95% CI 2.49-7.88), and MDD (OR 1.81, 95% CI 1.03-3.32). The multiple-regression model was adjusted for age, sex, ethnicity (white vs other), years of education (less than 12 vs 12 or more), duty type (active vs reserve or Guard), service branch (Army or Marines vs Navy or Air Force) and rank (enlisted vs officer) unless otherwise noted. The participation rates in the study were 53% for the deployed veterans and 39% for the nondeployed; the authors examined possible participation bias and determined that, overall, participation bias was independent of deployment status.

Secondary Studies

Secondary studies were based primarily on retrospective or cross-sectional study designs with self-reported information whose major limitations were poor response rates and the potential for recall bias. The number and types of psychiatric disorders reported varied widely from study to study and included current (those occurring in the preceding month or week), 12-month, and lifetime reports mainly of MDD, GAD, alcohol abuse or dependence, specific phobias, and PTSD. Although many of the studies used different case definitions or different screening instruments, one (Eisen et al. 2004) assessed the test-retest reliability of the DIS-III-R interviews used. The investigators found that in general test-retest reliability of the lifetime prevalence of most of the *DSM-III-R* psychiatric diagnoses was acceptable (Kappa statistics 0.54-0.76); however, reliability was poor (Kappa statistic < 0.40) for panic disorder and GAD.

Eleven secondary studies on nine veteran populations used self-reported data to consider whether deployed veterans differed from nondeployed veterans for a wide variety of psychiatric disorders (Black et al. 2004a; Dlugosz et al. 1999; Erickson et al. 2001; Forman-Hoffman et al. 2005; Goss Gilroy Inc. 1998; Gray et al. 2002; Grieger et al. 2006; Hoge et al. 2004, 2006; O'Toole et al. 1996a; Simmons et al. 2004). O'Toole et al. (1996a) studied Australian Vietnam veterans, and Hoge et al. (2004, 2006) studied U.S. troops returning from OEF and OIF; the other eight studies studied Gulf War veterans.

In 1997, Goss Gilroy Inc. (1998) mailed a health-status questionnaire to all Canadian military personnel who had deployed to the Gulf War (n = 4262) and a comparison group of Canadian military personnel who had served elsewhere (n = 5699), matched on age and gender. The response rates were 73% (n = 3113) and 60.3% (n = 3439), respectively. The major self-reported health outcomes found to be significantly increased in deployed Gulf War veterans, compared with nondeployed veterans, were health provider-diagnosed PTSD (OR 3.34, 95% CI 2.13-5.26), anxiety (OR 2.20, 95% CI 1.55-3.12), MDD (OR 3.67, 95% CI 3.04-4.44), and symptoms of PTSD (OR 2.69, 95% CI 1.69-4.26).

Gray et al. (2002) conducted a cross-sectional survey in 1997-1999 of 3831 active-duty and reserve Navy Seabees who had served in the Gulf War and 3104 Seabees who had remained in the United States. The mailed survey gathered self-reports on prewar medical history, war exposure, symptoms, geographic service during the war, PTSD, depression, and anxiety. For deployed vs nondeployed Seabees, risks were significantly increased for depression (OR 1.77, 95% CI 1.41-2.27), PTSD (OR 4.23, 95% CI 2.59-6.92), and suicidal thoughts (OR 2.16, 95% CI 1.64-2.84) when adjusted for age, sex, active-duty or reserve status, race or ethnicity, current smoking, and current alcohol drinking.

Using the Iowa Persian Gulf cohort, Black et al. (2004b) administered a telephone survey to a population-based sample of 4886 members of the military in Iowa who were enlisted at the time of the Gulf War. Subjects were randomly selected from Gulf War regular military and National Guard or reserves and non-Gulf War regular military and National Guard or reserves. Medical and psychiatric disorders were assessed in 3695 of those selected, with a final participation rate of 76%. Deployed military personnel (n = 1896) were twice as likely as nondeployed military personnel (n = 1799) to report having a current anxiety disorder (estimated prevalence 4.0% [SE 1.0] vs 1.8% [SE 0.4]) or any anxiety disorder (estimated prevalence 5.9% [SE 0.6] vs 2.8% [SE 0.5]). In a multivariate model, predeployment psychiatric difficulties—which included predeployment psychiatric treatment and predeployment diagnosis of PTSD, depression, or anxiety—were independently associated with current anxiety disorder; this suggested that predeployment precursors were associated with development of anxiety (OR 4.4,

95% CI 2.2-8.9). Participation in combat was strongly associated with the development of various manifestations of anxiety: PTSD (OR 2.1, 95% CI 1.7-4.2), panic disorder (OR 6.2, 95% CI 3.0-13.0), and GAD (OR 2.1, 95% CI 1.2-3.5).

Using self-reports of symptoms occurring after 1990 from 1296 male UK veterans deployed to the Gulf War compared with 12,364 male UK veterans who were fit for duty but not deployed to the gulf, Simmons et al. (2004) found significantly ($p < 0.001$) increased risks of depression (OR 16.1, 95% CI 12.7-20.4); anxiety, stress, or sleep disturbance (OR 10.8, 95% CI 8.7-13.5); mood swings, aggression, or irritability (OR 16.1, 95% CI 13.2-19.7); and PTSD and associated symptoms (OR 34.9, 95% CI 20.8-58.7). ORs were adjusted for age at the time of the survey, service and rank at the time of the war, serving status at the time of the survey, alcohol consumption, and smoking. The questionnaire for the study focused on reproduction and child health but included open-ended questions about new medical problems or changes in health experienced by the veterans since 1990. However, confidence in the findings is weakened by the retrospective nature of the study and the relatively poor response rate (53% of Gulf War veterans and 42% of non-Gulf War veterans).

Dlugosz et al. (1999) examined risk factors for hospitalization for a mental disorder after service in the Gulf War. In active-duty men ($n = 1,775,236$) and women ($n = 209,760$) in the U.S. Army, Air Force, Navy, and Marine Corps, the investigators identified 30,539 initial postwar hospitalizations with a principal discharge diagnosis of a mental disorder by using the DMDC hospitalization database grouped into 10 *ICD-9* codes. A sample of the military hospital charts was reviewed to assess reliability of the diagnoses in the large database files. Using Cox proportional-hazards regression models, the investigators examined the association between Gulf War deployment and hospitalization for mental disorders. Adjusted incidence risk ratios showed that being deployed in combat or combat support units but not being in the ground war in Iraq or Kuwait in February 1991 was associated with an increased risk of hospitalization because of acute reactions to stress (risk ratio 1.57, 95% CI 1.11-2.22). Veterans who had served in combat troops or combat support troops during the ground war were not at increased risk for hospitalizations for mood, neurotic disorders, personality disorders, adjustment disorders, or acute stress reactions. Moreover, Gulf War veterans were not significantly different from their nondeployed counterparts with regard to psychiatric comorbidities at the time of initial hospitalization.

Patterns of comorbid psychiatric disorders in veterans of the Gulf War were also reported by Forman-Hoffman et al. (2005). In Phase I, data were obtained from the Iowa Gulf War Study conducted in 1995-1996 on a stratified random sample of 3695 Gulf War-deployed and elsewhere-deployed military personnel who resided in Iowa and participated in a telephone survey. In Phase II, 374 veterans from Phase I who had symptoms of cognitive dysfunction, depression or chronic widespread pain and 228 veterans who did not have any of these conditions, received in-person assessments in 1999-2002. Assessment included administration of the Anxiety Sensitivity Index for depressive and anxious symptoms, the Mini-Mississippi Index for PTSD, the Barsky Amplification Scale for social support and somatization symptoms, and the SF-36 for personality traits, pain, and health-related quality of life and the SCID-IV. Mental-health comorbidity was based on a diagnosis of at least two current mental disorders from the SCID-IV and independent psychiatrist review in which the psychiatrist was blinded to case and deployment status. Of the 602 surveyed veterans, 32% had a current mental disorder, primarily anxiety disorders (22.4%), depressive disorders (14.2%), and substance-use disorders (5.9%). Over 35% of veterans with a current mental disorder had at least one other co-occurring mental disorder, mostly depressive and anxiety disorders; and this comorbidity was associated with significant impairment of health-related quality of life in this population of veterans.

O'Toole et al. (1996a) studied a random sample of 641 Australian Army Vietnam veterans using a battery of self-reporting instruments to assess psychologic status. Vietnam-related PTSD was assessed by the PTSD module of the SCID and the DIS. The most prevalent lifetime psychiatric conditions in Australian Vietnam veterans were alcohol abuse or dependence (42.6%), PTSD (18.7%), somatoform pain disorder (16.5%), social phobias (14.8%), and simple phobias (10.2%); somatoform pain disorder emerged as one of the most prevalent and enduring disorders. The most prevalent 6-month psychiatric conditions were also alcohol abuse or dependence (20.1%), somatoform pain disorder (12.6%), social phobias (11.3%), and simple phobias (7.8%); PTSD was not diagnosed. Furthermore, PTSD, alcohol abuse or dependence, and phobias were all related to combat exposure (a combat self-report scale was contained in the SCID) but not to being posted to a combat unit. The risk of a diagnosis of each of those and other psychiatric disorders increased with increasing combat exposure. When the prevalence of lifetime or current PTSD was compared with responses to a 21-item combat index, there was a linear dose-response relationship with increasing combat exposure. The OR for each combat-score quartile for lifetime PTSD was 1.00, 3.03, 5.36, and 9.18; for current PTSD, the ORs were 1.00, 2.11, 6.97, and 10.33 for each quartile increase in combat exposure. For lifetime alcohol abuse or dependence, the ORs were 1.00, 1.07, 1.56, and 1.86 ($p = 0.002$); for GAD, the ORs were 1.00, 0.91, 1.81, and 3.14 ($p = 0.003$); for social phobia, the ORs were 1.00, 1.24, 1.80, and 2.18 ($p = 0.012$); for panic disorder, the ORs were 1.00, 3.20, 3.27, and 10.10 ($p = 0.001$); and for dysthemia, the ORs were 1.00, 0.98, 1.67, and 2.58 ($p = 0.009$).

A number of secondary studies were cross-sectional surveys of diverse populations of veterans, including two of veterans returning from deployments to OEF and OIF (Hoge et al. 2004, 2006). In January 2003, Hoge et al. (2004) surveyed 2530 soldiers from one Army infantry brigade for mental-health problems before a year-long deployment to Iraq. In 2003, they also surveyed 1962 soldiers returning from a 6-month deployment in Afghanistan, 894 soldiers returning from an 8-month deployment to Iraq, and 815 Marines returning from a 6-month deployment to Iraq; the second group of soldiers and the Marines had been in the forefront of ground-combat operations in Iraq. PTSD was assessed with the 17-item PTSD Checklist from VA; MDD and GAD were assessed with a questionnaire that included questions about functional impairment. Compared with the prevalence of mental-health problems in the Army group before deployment, MDD was significantly increased in the Army groups after deployment to Afghanistan (OR 1.33, 95% CI 1.03-1.71, $p < 0.05$) or to Iraq (OR 1.53, 95% CI 1.12-2.08, $p < 0.01$), but not in the Marines. PTSD was not significantly increased in the soldiers deployed to Afghanistan but was in those deployed to Iraq (OR 2.84, 95% CI 2.17-3.72, $p < 0.01$) and in the Marines (OR 2.66, 95% CI 2.01-3.51, $p < 0.01$). GAD was not increased in any of the groups after deployment. This study is limited because different groups of soldiers were surveyed before and after deployment, no Marines were surveyed before deployment, and the mental-health assessments were based on screening instruments.

Similar results were seen in a later study by Hoge et al. (2006), who surveyed 303,905 Army soldiers and Marines returning from deployments mainly in Iraq and Afghanistan. All returning veterans were required to complete a brief postdeployment health assessment (PDHA). The PDHA includes two questions for depression modified from the two-item patient health questionnaire and the four-item screen for PTSD developed by the National Center for PTSD, both of which are intended for use in primary care settings; and four questions related to suicide, interpersonal relationships, and interest in receiving care. The PDHA also included three questions about combat experiences, including whether the solider had seen anyone wounded, killed, or dead; had engaged in direct combat and discharged a weapon; or felt in great danger of being killed. The investigators did not assess for prior trauma. Of the veterans returning from Iraq (n = 222,620), Afghanistan (n = 16,318), or deployment elsewhere (Bosnia, Turkey, Uzbekistan, Kosovo, on a ship, or other; n = 64,967), 19.1%, 11.3%, and 8.5%, respectively, met the risk criteria for a mental-health problem. The 8.5% for the deployed-elsewhere soldiers was similar to the prevalence of mental-health problems reported by soldiers prior to their first deployment to OIF or OEF. The OR for OIF veterans compared to those deployed elsewhere was 2.72 (95% CI 2.63-2.80, $p < 0.001$). Mental-health problems were associated with combat exposure. Almost 10% of the OIF veterans, 4.7% of the OEF veterans, and 2.1% of those deployed elsewhere screened positive for PTSD.

Erickson et al. (2001) surveyed a cohort of 2949 Army veterans from Fort Devens, Massachusetts, immediately after their return from the Gulf War (time 1) and then 18-24 months later (time 2) to examine the temporal relationship between depression and PTSD. The Mississippi Scale for Combat-Related PTSD and the Brief Symptom Inventory were administered to all participants, and results were analyzed at time 2. A latent-variable, cross-lag panel model found evidence of a reciprocal relationship between PTSD and depression, which means the best-fit model includes both the progression from PTSD to depression and from depression to PTSD. Essentially, it provides some support for Kessler's notion that each outcome could be antecedent to the other (Kessler et al. 1995). The committee notes that the use of latent variables required that an index be developed both for the measurement of PTSD and for the measurement of depression; thus, the results are not tied strictly to diagnosis, but rather to separate symptom clusters. Moreover, after adjustment for military and demographic characteristics, the results suggest that the reciprocal relationship only held up on followup at time 2 for re-experiencing and avoidance-numbing symptoms.

Grieger et al. (2006) examined the influence of battle injury on combat-related PTSD or of depression on PTSD in 243 soldiers hospitalized after serious combat injury, including life-threatening or seriously disfiguring injuries (n = 613). The longitudinal cohort was evaluated at 1, 4, and 7 months with the PTSD Checklist; depression was assessed with the Patient Health Questionnaire. Soldiers who did not meet the criteria for PTSD or depression at 1 month but who did at 7 months were compared with soldiers who remained below the diagnostic threshold for PTSD or depression at 7 months. The investigators noted that most of the soldiers with PTSD or depression at 7 months did not meet criteria for either condition at 1 month. Moreover, at 1 month, 4.2% of the soldiers had probable PTSD and 4.4% had depression; at 4 months, 12.2% had PTSD and 8.9% had depression; and at 7 months, 12.0% had PTSD and 9.3% had depression. After controlling for demographic characteristics (age, marital status, and sex), early severity of physical problems was strongly associated with later PTSD or depression. Of those contacted, fewer than 0.5% refused to participate. The investigators note that there were no differences at 1 month in the rates of probable depression, probable PTSD, or either condition between soldiers who completed all three assessments and those who did not complete the followup assessments.

Suicide ideation was not included in this section as a psychiatric outcome itself, but, as in depression, there are consistent reports that ideation is greater in deployed veterans than in nondeployed veterans (Fontana and Rosenheck 1995a; Fu et al. 2002; Gray et al. 2002). Suicide ideation is also briefly discussed in the section "Suicide and Accidental Death."

Summary and Conclusions

The committee considered 11 citations on seven primary studies: three on veterans of the Vietnam War and four on veterans of the Gulf War. Three of the publications on Vietnam veterans were based on the NVVRS, one on the VES, and two on the Vietnam Era Twin Registry. Of the publications on Gulf War veterans, two studies analyzed datasets from well-defined cohorts from Louisiana, Massachusetts, and Maine; one used a subset of veterans from the National Health Survey of Gulf War Era Veterans and Their Families; one used a random sample of veterans; and one study looked at Australian Gulf War veterans. All the studies, regardless of the veteran population or the techniques of ascertainment, found that veterans who were deployed to war zones had a greater prevalence of psychiatric disorders—particularly PTSD, other anxiety disorders, and MDD—than did veterans who served in the military at the same time but were not deployed to a war zone. PTSD was also found to be highly comorbid with other psychiatric disorders, particularly GAD and MDD. Furthermore, both the prevalence and the severity of those disorders were associated with the level of combat experienced. The 11 secondary studies, most of them of Gulf War veterans, also showed an association between deployment and PTSD, other anxiety disorders, and MDD, as well as other psychiatric disorders.

The committee concludes that there is sufficient evidence of an association between deployment to a war zone and the development of psychiatric disorders, including PTSD, other anxiety disorders, and depressive disorders.

TABLE 6-3 Psychiatric Disorders

Study	Study Design	Population	Outcomes	Results	Adjustments	Comments
CDC 1988a VES	Retrospective cohort, prevalence, population-based, telephone interview with screening medical examination at followup	2490 Vietnam-theater veterans, 1972 Vietnam-era veterans	Screening medical-health examination and psychologic evaluation with DIS and MMPI	Generalized anxiety OR 1.5, 95% CI 1.1-2.1; depression OR 2.0, 95% CI 1.4-2.9	Age at entry into Army, race, score on enlistment general technical test, enlistment status, year of entry, primary military occupational specialty	Low participation of control group
Kulka et al. 1990 NVVRS	Cross-sectional, NSVG	1200 Vietnam-theater men and 432 women, 412 Vietnam-era men and 304 women, 668 nationally representative civilians; subset of 344 theater veterans also underwent clinical interview with mental-health professional	DIS for psychiatric disorders, self-reported levels of exposure to war-zone stress; composite diagnoses of 260 theater veterans with MCRPS, SCID, and PTSD Scale of the MMPI Detailed reviews and analyses of military data records to identify potential differences between veteran respondents and nonrespondents	Current combat-related PTSD: 15.2% men, 8.5% women Lifetime combat-related PTSD: 30.6% men, 26.9% women	Weighting of data for all analyses to account for interview-level nonresponse and different probabilities of selection in civilian cohort; control for age, race or ethnicity, female veteran occupation	Response rates over 83% of Vietnam-theater veterans, 76% of Vietnam-era veterans, 70% of civilians Because use of self-reported war-zone stress exposure information corresponded well with information in military records, such as receipt of combat metals, this is one of few early studies that differentiated between types of stress encountered in a war zone

TABLE 6-3 Psychiatric Disorders

Study	Study Design	Population	Outcomes	Results	Adjustments	Comments
Dohrenwend et al. 2006 NVVRS	Cross-sectional, NSVG	1200 Vietnam theater men; subset of 260 who underwent clinical interview	Reanalyzed data from NSVG and compared self-reports of war-zone stress with military and other records; used SCID to diagnose PTSD	Current: 12.2 (9.1% adjusted for both impairment and documentation) Lifetime: 22.5% (18.7% adjusted for both impairment and documentation)	Global Assessment of Functioning, documentation of exposure to traumatic experiences in war zone	PTSD prevalence rates were determined only for subset of 260 theater veterans Good verification of reported level of war-zone stress exposure with military and other records
Jordan et al. 1991 NVVRS	Cross-sectional, NSVG	1200 Vietnam-theater men and 432 women, 412 Vietnam-era men and 304 women, 668 nationally representative civilians	DIS for psychiatric disorders, self-reported levels of exposure to war-zone stress Detailed reviews and analyses of military data records to identify potential differences between veteran respondents and nonrespondents	Prevalence rates for any lifetime psychiatric disorder other than alcohol abuse or dependence in male veterans 43% for high war-zone stress, 25.6% for moderate war-zone stress, 21% for low war-zone stress, and 18.1% for civilians Prevalence of low-war-zone-stress veterans vs high-war-zone stress-veterans—major depression 3.1% vs 11.1%, $p < 0.01$; dysthymia 1.4% vs 12.3%, $p < 0.001$; obsessive-compulsive disorder 0.5% vs 5.5%, $p < 0.01$; GAD 10.8% vs 24.4%, $p < 0.05$; alcohol abuse and dependence 37.2% v 45.6%, $p < 0.05$; antisocial personality disorder 7.1% vs 16.6%, $p < 0.01$	Weighting of data for all analyses to account for interview-level nonresponse and different probabilities of selection in civilian cohort; control for age, race or ethnicity, female veteran occupation	Response rates over 83% of Vietnam-theater veterans, 76% of Vietnam-era veterans, 70% of civilians Because use of self-reported war-zone stress exposure information corresponded well with information in military records, such as receipt of combat metals, this is one of few early studies that differentiated between types of stress encountered in a war zone

TABLE 6-3 Psychiatric Disorders

Study	Study Design	Population	Outcomes	Results	Adjustments	Comments
Koenen et al. 2003a VET Registry	Co-twins control study	1874 male monozygotic twin pairs; both twins served in military during Vietnam War	CEI, DIS-III-R	Major depression comorbidity: combat adjusted for PTSD OR 1.10, 95% CI 0.92-1.33; PTSD adjusted for combat OR 2.55, 95% CI 1.16-5.61	Conditional logistic regression; premilitary, trauma history, age at entry into military, level of education	Study eliminates genetic and shared environmental factors as confounders of comorbidity of combat exposure and combat-related PTSD and other psychiatric disorders
Koenen et al. 2003b VET Registry	Co-twins control study	Twins in VET Registry; 37 male twin pairs with one twin being a Vietnam veteran with PTSD, 76 male twin pairs with one twin being a Vietnam veteran without PTSD; all co-twins served in the military but were not deployed to Vietnam	CEI, DIS-III-R	Lifetime PTSD vs non-PTSD for: any mood disorder OR 8.89, 90% CI 3.66-21.59; major depression OR 6.32, 90% CI 2.57-15.55; dysthymia OR 3.80, 90% CI 1.09-13.28; any anxiety disorder OR 8.63, 90% CI 2.20-33.83; panic disorder OR 4.48, 90% CI 1.04-19.41; ORs also increased for all symptoms comparing PTSD with co-twins or PTSD co-twins with non-PTSD co-twins		
Ikin et al. 2004	Cross-sectional survey of all Australian GW-deployed veterans	1381 GW-deployed veterans, 1377 nondeployed comparison veterans	CIDI	PTSD OR 3.9, 95% CI 2.3-6.5; major depression OR 1.6, 95% CI 1.3-2.0	Service type, rank, age, education, marital status	GW veterans were younger, more likely in Navy, and lower-ranked than comparison group

TABLE 6-3 Psychiatric Disorders

Study	Study Design	Population	Outcomes	Results	Adjustments	Comments
Proctor et al. 2001	Cohort study, part of larger longitudinal GW cohort study	Fort Devens cohort (n = 186) and New Orleans cohort (n = 66) of GW-deployed veterans, small comparison population of Germany-deployed veterans from Maine National Guard (n = 48)	CAPS used for PTSD, SCID used for other psychiatric disorders	Both gulf-deployed groups reported higher individual symptom prevalence on items that make up body system symptom scores compared with Germany-deployed group; report of frequent periods of anxiety or nervousness OR 7.1 (Fort Devens) and OR 5.3 (New Orleans); self-reported symptoms of frequent periods of feeling depressed significant only for Fort Devens cohort (OR 6.0); 95% CI excludes 1.0 for all comparisons	Adjustment for oversampling of women, participation bias, age, sex, education	Health symptoms are all self-reports
Wolfe et al. 1999	Cohort study as part of larger longitudinal GW cohort study (same cohorts as used by Proctor et al. 2001)	Fort Devens cohort (n = 148) and New Orleans cohort (n = 56) of GW-deployed veterans, small comparison population of Germany-deployed veterans from Maine National Guard (n = 48)	SCID to examine relationship of psychiatric disorders with health problems	Rates of current and lifetime PTSD: 5.4% and 6.5% (Fort Devens), 7.2% and 8.2% (New Orleans), 0% and 0% (Germany-deployed) Rates of current and lifetime MDD: 6.6% and 22.5% (Fort Devens), 4.5% and 10.2% (New Orleans), 0% and 4.2% (Germany-deployed)	Adjustment for over-sampling of females, participation bias, age, sex, education	
Fiedler et al. 2006	Cross-sectional	967 GW-deployed and 784 era veterans (67% active duty, 15% National Guard, 18% reserve); 1765	Telephone interview using CIDI based on the *DSM-III-R*	Deployed vs nondeployed had significantly ($p < 0.05$) greater prevalence in preceding 12 months: major depression 15.1% vs 7.8%, panic attack 1.6% vs	Self-reports 10 years after conflict	Response rate 55%, differences in demographics between respondents and nonrespondents

TABLE 6-3 Psychiatric Disorders

Study	Study Design	Population	Outcomes	Results	Adjustments	Comments
		deployed and 1832 GW-era veterans		0.5%, social phobia 3.6% vs 1.7%, obsessive-compulsive disorder 2.8% vs 1.1%, PTSD 3.4% vs 0.9%, GAD 6.0% vs 2.7%, any anxiety disorder 16.0% vs 9.7%, any psychiatric disorder 26.1% vs 16.1% Depression OR 2.07, 95% CI 1.50-2.85 Any anxiety disorder OR 1.81, 95% CI 1.34-2.45		relatively small
Toomey et al. 2007 NHSGWEVTF (Derived from Kang et al. 2000b)	Longitudinal, cross-sectional	1061 GW-deployed, 1128 GW-era veterans; used subset of veterans followed since 1995	CIDI used to diagnose axis I mental disorders, CAPS used to diagnose PTSD, CES	10 years after GW, persistent increased prevalence of mental disorders: war-onset current PTSD OR 5.78, 95% CI 2.62-12.74; all anxiety disorders OR 4.43, 95% CI 2.49-7.88; anxiety disorders other than PTSD OR 3.79, 95% CI 1.80-7.99; MDD OR 1.81, 95% CI 1.03-3.32; pain disorder OR 91.66, 95% CI 10.52-798.21; at least one mental disorder OR 2.12, 95% CI 1.44-3.11	Age, sex, ethnicity, years of education, duty type (active-duty vs reserve or National Guard), service branch, rank	Participation rate 53% of deployed veterans, 39% of nondeployed; possible participation bias although authors report that degree of bias was independent of deployment status

NOTE: CAPS = Clinician-Administered PTSD Scale, CEI = Combat Exposure Index, CI = confidence interval, CIDI = Composite International Diagnostic Interview, DIS = Diagnostic Interview Schedule, DIS-III-R = Diagnostic Interview Schedule for *DSM-III*, *DSM-III* = *Diagnostic and Statistical Manual for Mental Health Disorders*, third edition, GAD = generalized anxiety disorder, GW = Gulf War, MDD = major depressive disorder, NHSGWEVTF = National Health Survey of Gulf War Era Veterans and Their Families, NSVG = National Survey of the Vietnam Generation, NVVRS = National Vietnam Veterans Readjustment Study, OR = odds ratio, PTSD = posttraumatic stress disorder, SCID = Structured Clinical Interview for *DSM-III-R*, VES = Vietnam Experience Study, VET Registry = Vietnam Era Twin Registry.

SUBSTANCE-USE DISORDERS

DSM-IV defines substance-use disorders as dependence (characterized by tolerance, withdrawal, needing increasing amounts, persistent desire, and unsuccessful efforts to cut down) or abuse (characterized by recurrent use causing domestic, work, interpersonal, or legal problems, or use in physically hazardous situations) of drugs or alcohol. The lifetime and 12-month prevalences of substance-use disorders in the NCS were about 15% and about 4%, respectively (Kessler et al. 2005a,b). Those rates can be 2-3 times higher in men than in women, depending on the substance. The most reliable method for determining a history of substance-use disorders is the diagnostic interview. In treated populations, current drug use is validated with urine screens. In community and military populations in general, current alcohol problems are often assessed with a screening questionnaire. Two well-validated screening tools that were used in several military studies are the CAGE—a four-item scale to assess cutting down [C], feeling annoyed by people criticizing your drinking [A], feeling guilty about drinking [G], and using alcohol as an eye-opener in the morning [E])—and the Alcohol Use Disorders Identification Test (AUDIT)—a 10-item scale developed by the World Health Organization.

A primary study for substance-use disorders is defined as one that had a generalizable sample of deployed and nondeployed veterans, an indicator variable for combat stress, and reliable ascertainment of a substance-use disorder or a problem with alcohol or drugs. Secondary studies failed to fulfill all of those criteria or focused on other populations of interest, such as peacekeepers. Primary studies of substance-use disorders are summarized in Table 6-4.

Primary Studies

The committee identified six primary studies on the relationship of deployment stress to substance-use disorders: three of veterans of the Vietnam War and three of veterans of the 1991 Gulf War. The two studies with the richest sources of evidence were the VES conducted by CDC (1988a) and the congressionally mandated NVVRS (Jordan et al. 1991). Designs characteristics of those studies were provided in the preceding section on psychiatric disorders; information specifically related to substance-use disorders is discussed below.

The VES involved a cohort of 2490 Vietnam-theater veterans and a comparison group of 1972 Vietnam-era veterans, who participated in a face-to-face structured diagnostic interview, the DIS, to assess substance-use disorders in 1985-1986. After adjustment for the six baseline characteristics of age at entry into the Army, race, score on an enlistment general technical test, enlistment status (drafted or volunteer), year of entry into the Army, and primary military occupational specialty (tactical or nontactical), CDC (1988a) found that the current (1-month) prevalence of alcohol disorders was significantly higher in the theater veterans (13.7%) than in the era controls (9.2%) (OR 1.5, 95% CI 1.2-1.8). The rates of drug disorders were not significantly different between the groups (0.4% for theater veterans and 0.5% for era veterans; OR 0.9, 95% CI 0.4-2.0). Analysis of the 1-year prevalence data from the VES, however, did not find significant differences in rates of alcohol or drug-use disorders between the theater veterans (14% and 4%, respectively) and the era veterans (16% and 4%, respectively) (Boscarino 1995). There was no significant relationship between severity of combat exposure and either alcohol or drug-use disorders.

Examining lifetime and current (6-month) prevalence of several psychiatric disorders in the NVVRS, Jordan et al. (1991) found significantly higher rates of alcohol and drug abuse or dependence in Vietnam-theater veterans (1200 men and 432 women) than in Vietnam-era veterans (412 men and 304 women) or civilian controls (450 men and 218 women). The most prevalent disorder among male veterans was alcohol abuse or dependence: 39.2% lifetime and 11.2% current for theater veterans and 37.9% lifetime and 9.2% current for era veterans. The prevalence of lifetime and current alcohol abuse or dependence in female theater veterans was 9.1% and 4.9%, respectively, and in female era veterans 4.2% and 1.1%, respectively. The prevalence of lifetime and current drug abuse or dependence was 5.7% and 1.8% in male theater veterans, respectively, and 5.3% and 1.0% in male era veterans. For women, the prevalence of lifetime and current drug abuse or dependence was 1.0% or less for all groups. However when the theater group was dichotomized by level of war-zone stress—high (406 men and 170 women) and low or moderate (783 men and 262 women)—the investigators found that the men and women exposed to high war-zone stress did have significantly higher rates of both lifetime and current alcohol and drug abuse or dependence than the other groups. The 6-month prevalence of alcohol disorders among men was 17.2% in the high group, 8.8% in the low or moderate group, 9.2% in the era controls, and 7.8% in the civilian sample, and 3.4%, 1.6%, 1.0%, and 0.9%, respectively, for women. The lifetime prevalence was 45.6%, 37.2%, 37.9%, and 27.1%, respectively, for men and 10.6%, 8.2%, 4.6%, and 1.5%, respectively, for women. For drug disorders, the current prevalence among men were 3.9%, 1.1%, 1.0%, 0.9%, respectively; the prevalence among female veterans was 0.0% for all groups. The lifetime prevalence of drug disorders was 8.4%, 4.9%, 6.0%, and 3.4%, respectively, for men, and 2.57%, 0.0%, 0.6%, and 0.9%, respectively, for women. Thus, an association of problems with substance use was demonstrated with exposure to combat stress, but not with deployment to a war zone.

Goldberg et al. (1990) used the Vietnam Era Twin Registry to assess alcohol-drinking patterns in Vietnam-theater veterans. They analyzed 2169 monozygotic twin pairs. Veterans who served in Vietnam had a higher consumption of alcohol than those who did not serve (17.0% vs 21.4%), and the degree of combat exposure was related to higher daily alcohol consumption. For example, the prevalence of high average daily consumption increased from 15.3% in theater veterans with no combat exposure, to 20.7%, 24.5% and 24.7% in veterans with low, medium, and high combat exposure, respectively (χ^2 trend = 6.625, p = 0.010). The authors noted that they did not control for alcohol consumption before military service because of the potential for recall bias. McLeod et al. (2001) also used data from the Vietnam Era Twin Registry and found that combat exposure was associated with alcohol consumption.

Koenen et al. (2003a) also used telephone interview data from the 1993 Vietnam Era Twin Registry study to assess severity of combat exposure, alcohol consumption, and substance-use disorders in 1874 male-male monozygotic twin pairs. As in the NVVRS, severity of combat exposure was significantly associated with alcohol dependence (OR 1.16, 95% CI 1.02-1.31), drug dependence (OR 1.34, 95% CI 1.03-1.48), and cannabis dependence (OR 1.36, 95% CI 1.09-1.71). After adjustment for combat-related PTSD (diagnosed with the DIS-III-R), combat exposure was significantly associated only with alcohol dependence (OR 1.15, 95% CI 1.01-1.30) and cannabis dependence (OR 1.31, 95% CI 1.04-1.66).

In the Gulf War, stress appears to have increased the risk of substance-related conditions. In the large Iowa cohort of regular military, National Guard, and reservists surveyed by telephone in 1995-1996 (1896 deployed and 1799 nondeployed military personnel), the prevalence of symptoms of alcohol abuse as determined with CAGE was 17.0% and 19.4% in

Gulf War-deployed regular military and reserve/National Guard veterans, respectively, and 12.2% and 16.8% in nondeployed regular military and reserve controls, respectively, for a statistically significant prevalence difference of 2.4 (95% CI 0.4-4.5, $p \leq 0.05$) (Iowa Persian Gulf Study Group 1997). The response rate for the telephone interview (76%) was relatively high.

The CIDI was administered in Australia as part of a two-phase study of 1381 Gulf War veterans and 1377 nondeployed controls (Ikin et al. 2004). Health professionals conducted interviews in clinics throughout the country. The prevalence of alcohol and drug abuse or dependence before the Gulf War was similar in the deployed and nondeployed groups (23.7% and 27.9%, respectively, for alcohol dependence or abuse and 2.8% and 2.3%, respectively, for drug dependence or abuse). The incidence rates for the disorder being first present after the war were significantly higher in deployed veterans than nondeployed veterans for both alcohol disorders (19.8% vs 12.6%, $p = 0.001$) and drug disorders (3.7% vs 1.8%, $p = 0.015$) for ORs of 1.5 (95% CI 1.2-2.0) for alcohol and 1.9 (95% CI 1.1-3.2) for drugs adjusted for service type, rank, age, education, and marital status. Significantly more deployed than nondeployed veterans also met criteria for alcoholism in the year before the interview (4.3% vs 2.5%, $p = 0.011$) for an adjusted OR of 1.8 (95% CI 1.1-2.8) but not the criteria for drug dependence or abuse (0.7% vs 0.6%, $p = 0.863$, OR 0.8, 95% CI 0.3-2.5).

Fiedler et al. (2006) conducted telephone interviews 10 years after the Gulf War with a national sample of 967 U.S. military personnel deployed to the Gulf and 784 nondeployed controls using the 12-month version of the CIDI. They found similar rates of alcohol disorder in the two groups (4.6% in deployed and 3.1% in nondeployed veterans), but the deployed had significantly higher rates of drug dependence (1.2% vs 0.1%, $p < 0.05$) and "any dependence" (5.1% vs 3.2%, $p < 0.05$) than the nondeployed.

Thus, the preponderance of the evidence from the six primary studies suggests that deployed Vietnam and Gulf War veterans, particularly personnel exposed to greater war-zone stress, have higher rates of alcohol or drug disorders than nondeployed controls.

Secondary Studies

Secondary studies are those with inadequate or no comparison groups, studies of treated populations or nonmilitary populations, and studies that used alcohol or drug measures of unknown reliability and validity. Four studies of Vietnam veterans are in this category. Helzer (1984) interviewed 943 Vietnam veterans in 1972, of whom 605 were eligible for a 2-year followup; at the time of followup, 571 were reinterviewed (94% response rate). The original sample included 470 respondents chosen at random from all enlisted personnel who returned from Vietnam in September 1971 and 495 others identified as illicit drug users on the basis of a urine screening test at the time of departure from Vietnam. The interview schedule was not described in detail, but problem use of alcohol was defined as having regular use of alcohol plus one or two alcohol-abuse symptoms; alcoholism was defined having regular use of alcohol plus three or more alcohol-abuse symptoms or at least one hospitalization because of drinking. At the first interview, 42% of combatants (those who were on combat patrols or dangerous duties, were under enemy fire, or were surrounded by the enemy) were problem drinkers or alcoholics compared with 28% of noncombatants ($p < 0.001$); a similar pattern was found at followup (45% vs 29%, $p < 0.001$). In the subsample of 297 veterans with no preservice alcohol problems, 24% of combat veterans and 19% of noncombat veterans were problem drinkers at the first interview, and 31% and 21% at the followup ($p < 0.05$ for both comparisons). After additional analyses, however, the author concluded that the effects of combat were small and that preservice alcohol and antisocial problems were stronger predictors.

Reifman and Windle (1996) conducted a secondary analysis of VES data on illicit drug use on the basis of self-reports from 2490 Vietnam veterans. The VES was conducted in 1985-1986. They found that combat exposure severity was significantly related to drug use in the preceding year (OR 1.01, 95% CI 1.01-1.02); the relationship remained even after controlling for PTSD.

Prigerson et al. (2002) conducted a secondary analysis of data from the 1990-1992 NCS, a national survey of mental health and substance abuse in the general population (Kessler et al. 1995). They found that combat exposure, mostly in the Vietnam war, contributed significantly and directly to 12-month substance abuse with an estimated relative risk of 2.22 (8.0% attributable to combat exposure; 95% CI 1.06-4.15) adjusted for age, race, urbanicity, and low socioeconomic status in the family of origin. An analysis of 641 Australian Vietnam veterans also found that severity of combat exposure based on a combat exposure scale developed for the study was significantly associated ($p = 0.007$) with current (1-month) alcohol abuse or dependence with ORs of 1.00, 1.21, 1.42, and 2.21 for increasing quartiles of combat exposure; no association with drug abuse or dependence was seen with ORs of 1.00, 2.83, 1.21, 1.74, respectively (O'Toole et al. 1996a).

Four surveys of Gulf War veterans also included items on alcohol and drug-abuse symptoms. In telephone interviews with 1545 Gulf War-deployed and 435 nondeployed veterans living in Kansas in 1998, Steele (2000) included "alcohol or drug dependence" as one of 37 conditions on a checklist. Veterans indicated whether they had been diagnosed or treated by a physician for any condition with new onset during 1990-1998. Prevalence was similar in the deployed (3%) and nondeployed (2%) groups for a nonsignificant OR of 1.47 (95% CI 0.65-3.31) adjusted for sex, age, income, and education level.

In 2002, Jones et al. (2006) mailed questionnaires to 1382 UK armed forces personnel that included three items from AUDIT (how often the person drank in the preceding 12 months, how many drinks are usually consumed when the person drinks, and whether a relative, friend, or doctor was ever concerned or suggested that the person cut down). They found that being deployed to more than one country (as opposed to never or to one country) within the preceding 5 years was significantly related to excessive alcohol intake (OR 2.3, 95% CI 1.5-3.6, $p < 0.001$).

McCauley et al. (2002b) conducted a telephone survey of 653 Gulf War-deployed troops who had been near the Khamisiyah munitions site in Iraq in March 1991, 610 troops deployed elsewhere in the gulf, and 516 troops not deployed to Southwest Asia. The questionnaire focused on medical conditions that had been diagnosed by a physician since the Gulf War. The comparison of deployed with nondeployed veterans was not significant for combined alcohol or substance abuse (OR 1.7, 95% CI 0.9-3.4).

Dlugosz et al. (1999) examined risk factors for hospitalization for a mental disorder after service in the Gulf War. In active-duty men ($n = 1,775,236$) and women ($n = 209,760$) in the U.S. Army, Air Force, Navy, and Marine Corps, the investigators identified 30,539 initial postwar hospitalizations. Adjusted incidence risk ratios showed that service in the Gulf War in a combat occupation was associated with an increased risk of hospitalization for alcohol-related disorders (risk ratio 1.13, 95% CI 1.04-1.23) although being in a combat support occupation was not (risk ratio 1.00, 95% CI 0.91-1.11). However, being in the war in a support occupation was associated with an increased risk of drug-related hospitalization (risk ratio 1.42, 95% CI 1.03-1.96), although being in a combat occupation was not (risk ratio 1.16, 95% CI 0.82-1.65).

Moreover, Gulf War veterans were not significantly different from their nondeployed counterparts with regard to psychiatric comorbidities at the time of initial hospitalization.

In 2003, Hoge et al. (2004) administered an anonymous survey to Army and Marine troops 1 week before a year-long (Army) or 6-month (Marines) deployment to Iraq or Afghanistan (n = 2530) and 3-4 months after return from combat duty (n = 3671). The survey asked two questions about problems related to the use of alcohol. The rates of alcohol misuse were lower before deployment than after. Specifically, before deployment to Iraq, 17.2% of the soldiers indicated using alcohol more than they meant to, after deployment to Iraq 24.2% did (OR 1.5, 95% CI 1.3-1.9) as did 24.5% after deployment to Afghanistan (OR 1.6, 95% CI 1.4-1.8). In addition, before deployment to Iraq, 12.5% of the soldiers said that they felt a need to cut down on their drinking, after deployment to Iraq, 20.6% indicated a need to cut down (OR 1.8, 95% CI 1.5-2.2) as did 18.2% after deployment to Afghanistan (OR 1.6, 95% CI 1.3-1.9). Although the before and after findings were not matched by individual, these results are consistent with greater problem drinking being associated with deployment to a war zone.

Thus, the findings from the Vietnam War, Gulf War, and OEF and OIF surveys that included screening measures of alcohol or drug problems are somewhat mixed, but the majority of studies point in the direction of increased substance problems as a function of deployment.

Posttraumatic Stress Disorder and Substance-Use Disorders

It is well established that alcohol use and drug use are comorbid with PTSD and other psychiatric conditions in clinical and nonclinical populations of veterans and nonveterans (Jacobsen et al. 2001; Kessler et al. 1995; Mellman et al. 1992; Sutker et al. 1993a). It has been suggested that the high rates of comorbidity between PTSD and substance-use disorders show that they may be functionally related to each other (Jacobsen et al. 2001). O'Toole et al. (1998) found that Australian Vietnam veterans with PTSD were at higher risk for alcohol abuse or dependence (OR 1.6, 95% CI 1.2-2.1) and for drug abuse and dependence (OR 5.4, 95% CI 1.9-15.5) than era veterans. Koenen et al. (2003a), in a study of Vietnam veterans from the NVVRS, found that combat-related PTSD unadjusted for combat exposure was significant only for drug dependence (OR 2.26, 95% CI 1.05-4.88) but not for alcohol or cannabis dependence (OR 1.39, 95% CI 0.76-2.56 and OR 2.24, 95% CI 0.95-5.31, respectively).

An analysis of data from the Fort Devens Gulf War cohort (n = 1006) indicated that alcohol and drug use were significantly associated with the cardinal PTSD symptoms of avoidance, re-experiencing, and hyperarousal (Shipherd et al. 2005). A 1999 study of 1101 Canadian male peacekeepers using AUDIT and the PTSD Checklist-Military Version found significantly more alcohol problems in those with PTSD and a significant trend for AUDIT scores to increase with level of PTSD (none, subthreshold, and full) (Yarvis et al. 2005). Furthermore, Ouimette et al. (1996) found a positive correlation between severity of PTSD symptoms and severity of substance-abuse symptoms in 52 women who served overseas during the Vietnam era.

Summary and Conclusions

Studies of troops deployed to Vietnam and the Persian Gulf have consistently found higher rates of substance-use problems than in nondeployed controls. Of the six primary studies, three are of Vietnam veterans and three are of Gulf War veterans. Data from the VES and the NVVRS showed that deployment was associated with alcohol use, although only the NVVRS found a significant association of drug abuse with deployment. The Vietnam Twin Registry study also found an association of deployment with alcohol abuse and with drug abuse. Two of the three studies of Gulf War veterans, one in an Iowa population and one in Australian veterans, found a higher prevalence of alcohol-use disorders in deployed veteran; a third conducted 10 years after the war, did not. The two studies that assessed drug-use disorders in Gulf War veterans both found an increased prevalence of such disorders in deployed veterans. Results from the secondary studies were also mixed: five of the seven studies found a positive association between alcohol abuse or dependence and deployment, but two studies did not. For drug-use disorders, the results were similarly mixed: two studies showed a positive association, but three did not.

Combat exposure has also been associated with an increased likelihood of substance-related problems. The evidence is reasonably consistent for an association with alcohol abuse/dependence but was considered limited but suggestive for drug abuse for two reasons. First, studies of veterans did not adjust for predeployment substance abuse when analyzing postdeployment prevalences. Second, unlike alcohol, drug use is an illegal behavior, and studies of combat soldiers did not screen for drug abuse.

The determinations of drug abuse were based on self-reports, without independent corroboration. Most of the recent studies of Gulf War veterans relied on screening measures or telephone interviews. The studies were cross-sectional, and the findings are based entirely on self-reports. Because substance-use disorders involve externalizing behaviors, corrobation by other sources would have enhanced the validity of information. An important limitation of those studies that might be corrected in the future is the lack of comprehensive, direct assessments of substance disorders that include age-of-onset information.

The committee concludes that there is sufficient evidence of an association between deployment to a war zone and alcohol abuse. The committee also concludes that there is limited but suggestive evidence of an association between deployment to a war zone and drug abuse.

TABLE 6-4 Substance-Use Disorders

Study	Study Design	Population	Outcomes	Results	Adjustments	Comments
CDC 1988b VES	Retrospective cohort, prevalence, population-based, telephone interview with screening medical examination at followup	2490 Vietnam-theater veterans, 1972 Vietnam-era veterans randomly selected from 7924 theater veterans and 7364 era veterans who had entered Army in 1965-1971	DIS-III-R, preceding month alcohol and drug abuse or dependence	Alcohol prevalence 13.7% vs 9.2%, OR 1.5, 95% CI 1.2-1.8; drugs prevalence 0.4% vs 0.5%, OR 0.9, 95% CI 0.4-2.0, NS	Age at enlistment, race, year of enlistment, enlistment status (volunteer vs draftee), score on general technical test, primary military occupational specialty	Low participation rate in control group; actual confidence interval not given
Boscarino 1995 VES	Cross-sectional, used subset of VES	2490 Vietnam-theater veterans, 1972 Vietnam-era veterans randomly selected from 7924 theater veterans and 7364 era veterans who had entered Army in 1965-1971	DIS-III-R, preceding year substance abuse or dependence	Alcohol: prevalence 16% vs 14% era (NS); drugs: 4% in both groups	Age at Army entry, enlistment status, Vietnam volunteer status	Predictors of alcohol abuse: childhood delinquency, illicit Army drug use, not being married, low social support; predictors of drug abuse: delinquency, Army drug; combat exposure in Vietnam not associated with alcohol or drug abuse
Jordan et al. 1991 NVVRS	Cross-sectional, NSVG	1200 Vietnam-theater men and 432 women 412 Vietnam-era men and 304 women, 688 nationally representative civilians	DIS for lifetime and 6-month (current) psychiatric disorders, self-reported levels of exposure to war-zone stress Detailed reviews and analyses of military data records to identify potential differences between	Prevalence of alcohol or drug abuse or dependence for high war-zone stress, low war-zone stress, era, and civilians: Alcohol (men) lifetime 46%, 37%, 38%, 27%; 6 months 17%, 9%, 9%, 8%; Drugs (men) lifetime 8%, 5%, 6%, 3%; 6 months 4%, 1%, 1%,	Data weighted to account for interview-level nonresponse and different probabilities of selection in civilian cohort; control for age, race or ethnicity, female veteran occupation	Response rates were greater than 83% for Vietnam-theatre veterans, 76% for Vietnam-era veterans and 70% for civilians. Because the use of self reported war zone stress exposure information was found to correspond well with military records, such

TABLE 6-4 Substance-Use Disorders

Study	Study Design	Population	Outcomes	Results	Adjustments	Comments
			veteran respondents and nonrespondents	1%; Alcohol (women) lifetime 11%, 8%, 5%, 2%; 6 month 3%, 2%, 1%, 1% Drugs (women) lifetime 3%, 0%, 1%, 1%; 6 months all 0%		as receipt of combat metals, this is one of the few early studies that differentiated between the types of stress encountered while in a war zone
Goldberg et al. 1990 VET Registry	Vietnam Era Twin registry; telephone survey in early 1987	2169 male monozygotic twin pairs both serving active duty military during Vietnam War, 829 theater veterans, 1340 era veterans	5-level alcohol index; high alcohol consumption = ~5 drinks/day; 5-level combat exposure index	Average daily alcohol consumption greater in twins who served in SE Asia (21.4%) vs no SE Asia service (17%). Prevalence of heavy alcohol consumption increased with combat exposure: no 15.3%, low 20.7%, medium 24.5%, and high 24.7% ($\chi^2 = 6.625$)	Co-twin alcohol drinking measures Demographic and service variables tested and found not to be confounders	Response rate 74%; no control for alcohol consumption prior to military service
Koenen et al. 2003a VET Registry	Co-twins control study	1874 male monozygotic twin pairs in which both twins served in military during Vietnam War	Combat Exposure Index, DIS-III-R	Combat exposure associated with alcohol dependence OR 1.16, 95% CI 1.02-1.31; drug dependence OR 1.34, 95% CI 1.03-1.48; cannabis dependence OR 1.36, 95% CI 1.09-1.71; adjusted for PTSD, combat exposure associated with alcohol dependence OR 1.15, 95% CI 1.01-1.30 and cannabis dependence OR 1.31, 95% CI 1.04-1.66	Education, age at entry to military, premilitary trauma, co-twin, PTSD	Temporality not considered for association of combat-related PTSD with alcohol and substance use outcomes

TABLE 6-4 Substance-Use Disorders

Study	Study Design	Population	Outcomes	Results	Adjustments	Comments
Iowa Persian Gulf Study Group 1997	Cross-sectional, prevalence	1896 GW veterans, 1799 nondeployed veterans	CAGE	Prevalence of alcohol abuse 17.4% in deployed vs 12.6% in nondeployed ($p = 0.02$); prevalence difference 2.4, 95% CI 0.4-4.5	Age at enlistment, race, year of enlistment, enlistment status (volunteer vs draftee), score on general technical test, primary military occupational specialty	No information on CAGE cut-point; 76% response rate
Ikin et al. 2004	Cross-sectional, mailed questionnaire followed by health assessment at clinic	1381 GW-deployed Australian veterans, 1377 nondeployed comparison veterans	CIDI for disorders pre-Gulf War, post-Gulf War, preceding 12 months	Alcohol dependence or abuse OR 1.5, 95% CI 1.2-2.0; drug dependence or abuse OR 1.9, 95% CI 1.1-3.2	Service type, rank, age, education, marital status	GW veterans were younger, more likely to be in Navy, and lower ranked; response rate was 50%
Fiedler et al. 2006	Cross-sectional, prevalence study, telephone interview, 10 years after conflict	967 GW-deployed vs 784 era veterans (67% active duty, 15% National Guard, 18% reserve); random sample from 1765 deployed and 1832 GW-era veterans	Telephone interview with CIDI based on the *DSM-III-R*	Deployed vs nondeployed had greater 12-month prevalence of following psychiatric disorders in previous 12 months: alcohol dependence 4.6% vs 3.1% (NS); drug dependence 1.2% vs 0.1% ($p < 0.05$) ; any dependence 5.1% vs 3.2% ($p < 0.05$)		Response rate was 59% deployed and 51% nondeployed; differences in demographics between respondents and nonrespondents was relatively small; being deployed to places other than the Gulf was a risk factor for alcohol/drug dependence

NOTE: CAGE = *c*utting down, feeling *a*nnoyed by people criticizing your drinking, feeling *g*uilty about drinking, and using alcohol as an *e*ye-opener in the morning, CI = confidence interval, CIDI = Composite International Diagnostic Interview, DIS = Diagnostic Interview Schedule, DIS-III-R = Diagnostic Interview Schedule for *DSM-III, DSM-III = Diagnostic and Statistical Manual for Mental Health Disorders*, third edition, GW = Gulf War, NS = not significant, NSVG = National Survey of the Vietnam Generation, NVVRS = National Vietnam Veterans Readjustment Study, OR = odds ratio, PTSD = posttraumatic stress disorder, VES = Vietnam Experience Study, VET Registry = Vietnam Era Twin Registry.

NEUROBEHAVIORAL AND NEUROCOGNITIVE EFFECTS

This section focuses on neurobehavioral performance as measured by tests of cognition and in some cases sensory integrity or motor speed and coordination. For the purposes of this section, in addition to the criteria for primary and secondary studies established in Chapter 2, the committee required that primary studies of neurobehavioral effects have used data derived from neurobehavioral tests rather than relying on self-reports of neurobehavioral deficits. Secondary studies had additional methodologic limitations or did not include combat veterans (see Chapter 2). The secondary studies were reviewed and included in the discussion because they evaluated the same functional domains, such as attention and memory, and in some cases used the same neurobehavioral tests as did primary studies; they therefore provide valuable supplementary information that helps to increase or decrease confidence in the conclusions drawn from the primary studies. Confidence in a study is substantially reduced if its statistical analysis did not adjust for confounders or if individually administered neurobehavioral tests were given by examiners not blinded to the status of cases and controls; blinding is of less concern if tests were administered on a computer. Summaries of the primary studies are given in Table 6-5.

Primary Studies

The committee identified three primary studies that compared deployed veterans with those deployed elsewhere or not deployed. David et al. (2002) compared the neurobehavioral-test performance of 209 UK soldiers deployed to the Persian Gulf, 54 UK Bosnia peacekeeping soldiers, and 78 UK Gulf War-era nondeployed soldiers. Study participants were a random sample of a larger cohort that had responded to an earlier mailed survey about symptoms, illnesses, and exposures (Unwin et al. 1999). A broad array of neurobehavioral tests were administered to all participants. The results of the data analysis were incompletely reported, so evaluation was limited by the lack of standard deviations of the mean test scores. No differences were reported among the groups after correction for age, education, intelligence (according to the National Adult Reading Test), and Beck Depression Inventory score.

Proctor et al. (2003) studied 143 Gulf War veterans and 72 nondeployed veterans of the Danish military; participants were randomly selected from among the 916 Gulf War deployed veterans and 236 nondeployed veterans studied by Ishoy et al. (1999). Deployed veterans served in the gulf region during August 1990-December 1997 as peacekeepers and thus had no direct combat exposure. Neuropsychologic tests addressing mood, attention, executive function, motor skills, visuospatial abilities, verbal memory, and visual memory were administered. The self-reports of Danish Gulf War veterans suggested a significantly higher prevalence of eight of 16 neuropsychologic symptoms than their nondeployed counterparts, but no significant differences between the deployed and the nondeployed were found by thorough analyses of the data from the neurobehavioral tests.

In the Neurocognition Deployment Health Study, Vasterling et al. (2006) determined the effects of war-zone deployment on neuropsychologic health. A cohort of 654 active-duty Army soldiers were examined before deployment to Iraq in 2003 as part of OIF and on return from Iraq deployment in 2005 and were compared with 307 soldiers who were similar in military characteristics but not deployed overseas. After adjustment for deployment-related head injury, stress, and depression, deployment to Iraq was associated with statistically significant neuropsychologic effects: lower scores on tests of attention, working memory, executive function, verbal learning, and visual memory retention; more distress from confusion and tension, but higher proficiency in simple reaction time.

Secondary Studies

Four secondary studies addressed whether Gulf War-deployed veterans differed from nondeployed veterans (Axelrod and Milner 1997; Lindem et al. 2003; Vasterling et al. 2003; White et al. 2001), and a further study examined cognitive function in exercises designed to simulate the stress of combat (Lieberman et al. 2005b). Only Axelrod and Milner (1997) found reliable differences in neurobehavioral test performance between the groups after correction for age and education.

Lindem et al. (2003) found that Gulf War-deployed veterans who scored poorly on the Test of Memory Malingering (TOMM), which assesses motivation to perform well, had lower scores on neuropsychologic tests of attention, executive function, and memory. Their study is part of a larger study begun by McEwen (2004) to compare veterans recruited from three cohorts: Fort Devens and New Orleans (n = 58), and 19 Germany-deployed veterans from a Maine National Guard unit. There were no significant differences in mean TOMM scores between the Gulf War-deployed and the Germany-deployed groups. Those who scored lower on the TOMM had a greater prevalence of lifetime PTSD (13.6%) than those with higher scores (1.8%). White et al. (2001) used a larger sample of the McEwen study cohorts from Fort Devens and from New Orleans (total n = 193) and compared them to 47 Germany-deployed veterans. No differences in neuropsychologic test performance were seen between the Gulf War-deployed and Germany-deployed troops, but poorer performance on cognitive tests in Gulf War-deployed veterans was associated with self-reports of exposure to chemical-warfare agents. Similar results were seen in a small study by Vasterling et al. (2003), who found that Gulf War-deployed veterans reported more concerns about cognitive functioning than nondeployed veterans, but those concerns were not confirmed by neurocognitive measures. A study by Lieberman et al. (2005a) found significant ($p < 0.001$) decrements in cognitive function, vigilance, reaction time, attention, memory, and reasoning during stressful combat-like training compared with baseline prestress performance in 31 U.S. Army officers who had volunteered for an intense training exercise.

Posttraumatic Stress Disorder and Neurocognitive and Neurobehavioral Effects

The committee identified three analyses of Vietnam veterans drawn from the CDC VES and seven secondary studies that examined the relationship between PTSD and neurocognitive and neurobehavioral outcomes. Barrett et al. (1996) used information from the VES to compare cognitive impairment from PTSD and other psychiatric diagnoses in Vietnam veterans. The 2441 veterans were categorized as to whether they had lifetime PTSD and whether the PTSD was comorbid with a current diagnosis of another psychiatric disorder, using the DIS. Several neurobehavioral tests—the California Verbal Learning Test (CVLT), the Rey-Osterrieth Complex Figure Drawing Test, the Wisconsin Card Sorting Test (WCST), and the Wechsler Adult Intelligence Scale-Revised (WAIS-R)—were administered to all participants. Results indicate that PTSD alone was not associated with impairment in cognition; however, veterans with PTSD and current depression, anxiety, or substance use (n = 128) had lower scores on all tests of cognitive functioning than veterans with PTSD alone (n = 236), veterans with only another psychiatric diagnosis (n = 242), and veterans with no psychiatric diagnoses (n = 1835). After adjustment for military and demographic characteristics, results suggest that cognitive deficits might be associated with concomitant diagnoses of PTSD and another psychiatric disorder.

Crowell et al. (2002) examined the influence of combat-related PTSD on neurocognitive functioning in a randomly selected subsample of middle-aged Vietnam Army veterans from the VES. Veterans were categorized as having current PTSD (n = 80), having PTSD in the preceding year but without current symptoms (n = 80), psychiatric controls with a *DSM-III* diagnosis but not PTSD (n = 80), and normal controls (n = 80). PTSD was diagnosed with the DIS-III-A. All veterans completed the WAIS-R, CVLT, Rey-Osterrieth Complex Figure Drawing Test, the Paced Auditory Serial Addition Test (PASAT), the Word List Generation Tasks, the WCST, and the Grooved Pegboard Test. After control for demographic characteristics and comorbid psychiatric conditions, the four groups showed no appreciable differences in cognitive functioning.

Zalewski et al. (1994) also used data from the VES to compare neuropsychologic performance in 241 Vietnam veterans with PTSD, those with GAD (n = 241), those with no history of psychiatric illness (n = 241). Comorbid psychiatric disorders—primarily substance abuse or dependence—were present in 80% of the PTSD group and 72% of the GAD group. Cognitive functioning was measured with the WAIS-R block design subtest, the CVLT, the Rey-Osterrieth Complex Figure Drawing Test, and the PASAT. A one-way multivariate analysis of variance revealed no significant differences among the three groups on independent measures of cognitive function.

The secondary studies addressed whether veterans with PTSD differed from veterans without a PTSD diagnosis. Findings were inconsistent; when results were positive in the numerous studies described below, the domains that were most often affected pertained to attention and memory.

In a small study of 32 Vietnam combat veterans, Gilbertson et al. (2001) found that although veterans with PTSD demonstrated poorer performance on most of the neurocognitive tests, only attention and memory were significant ($p = 0.003$) predictors of PTSD status in combat veterans. Similarly, Koso and Hansen (2006) found cognitive impairments with large effect sizes pertaining to attention, working memory, executive function, and memory in 20 Bosnian male combat veterans with PTSD, age- and intelligence-matched to veterans without PTSD.

Uddo et al. (1993) found that Vietnam veterans with PTSD had memory and attention deficits, and two studies by Vasterling et al. found attention and memory deficits to be associated with PTSD in Gulf War veterans (Vasterling et al. 1998) and in Vietnam veterans (Vasterling et al. 2002) even when they controlled for combat exposure. Yehuda et al. (1995) demonstrated that combat veterans with PTSD have specific deficits in memory related to retroactive interference and a decrement in retention although they have normal abilities in initial attention, immediate memory, and cumulative learning and active inference from previous learning.

Finally, Vasterling et al. (2000) sought to determine whether dysfunction of the frontolimbic system of the brain was implicated in PTSD. They compared 51 Vietnam-combat veterans with and without PTSD (n = 26 and n = 25, respectively) with 17 Vietnam-era veterans without a psychiatric disorder. The University of Pennsylvania Smell Identification Test, the Continuous Performance Test, the Auditory-Verbal Learning Test, and the WCST were used to determine cognitive functioning. Olfactory identification was used to assess orbitofrontal integrity. PTSD-diagnosed veterans had more performance deficits in odor identification and verbal learning, but not on the other cognitive tests, than veterans without PTSD; this suggested frontolimbic dysfunction in PTSD (see Chapter 5 for further discussion of the neurobiology of PTSD).

Summary and Conclusions

Three primary studies of the association of deployment to a war zone, whether OIF or the Persian Gulf, with neurobehavioral performance had mixed results. David et al. (2002) and Proctor et al. (2003) found only slight differences in cognitive functioning in UK troops deployed to the Gulf War and in Danish peacekeepers deployed to the Gulf after the conflict ended, respectively. Vasterling et al. (2006) found significant neurocognitive and neurobehavioral impairments in veterans deployed to OIF. In conclusion, primary studies of deployed veterans and veterans not deployed to a war zone do not clearly demonstrate differences in cognitive and motor measures as determined with neurobehavioral testing. Results of secondary studies also are mixed.

Primary studies specifically of PTSD and neurocognitive performance found that PTSD alone was not associated with deficits on tests of cognition. However, the studies do not appear to have included specific tests for memory, such as explicit memory. Secondary studies of PTSD were not uniform in their findings; however, when test results were positive, the most common findings were deficits in attention and memory.

The committee concludes that there is inadequate/insufficient evidence to determine whether an association exists between deployment to a war zone and neurocognitive and neurobehavioral effects.

TABLE 6-5 Neurobehavioral and Neurocognitive Effects

Reference	Study Design	Population	Outcomes	Results	Adjustments	Comments
David et al. 2002	Case-control, clinical evaluations	209 male UK GW-deployed, 54 Bosnia-deployed, 78 era nondeployed soldiers randomly selected from larger cohort of UK veterans who participated in earlier mailed survey (see Unwin et al. 1999)	WAIS-R scaled scores: vocabulary, digit span, arithmetic, similarities, picture arrangement, block design, object assembly, digit symbol, PASAT, sustained attention to response task, Stroop Trailmaking A and B WMS: logical memory (immediate and delayed recall), verbal paired associates (immediate and delayed recall), Camden recognition memory test, Purdue pegboard; individually administered tests, blinded examiners	Only difference between groups was lower score in Purdue pegboard for GW-deployed group	ANCOVA adjusted for education, age, NART, BDI; multiple comparison adjustment for least significant difference procedure and Bonferroni	Careful treatment of potential confounders, such as depression, mood, intelligence, education
Proctor et al. 2003	Cross-sectional	143 male Danish GW-deployed veterans, 72 male nondeployed troops randomly selected from 84% and 58% of total Danish armed forces deployed and nondeployed, respectively, at time of GW	WAIS-R Information subscale, continuous performance test, trail-making, WCST, Purdue pegboard, WAIS-R block design, CVLT, WMS visual reproductions, TOMM; individually administered tests except in computer-based NES; blinded examiners	No overall differences in neuropsychologic domains, significant test differences in domains ($p \leq 0.05$) for CVLT and WCST	MANCOVA by neuropsychologic domain, adjusted for age	Response rate 75%

TABLE 6-5 Neurobehavioral and Neurocognitive Effects

Reference	Study Design	Population	Outcomes	Results	Adjustments	Comments
Vasterling et al. 2006	Cohort-controlled, prospective	961 male and female active-duty Army soldiers: 654 Iraq-deployed, 307 nondeployed	MOS-CF, POMS, trail-making Parts B and A, NES3, CPT, WMS3, Verbal Paired Associates I and II, WMS Visual Reproductions I and II, ANAM simple reaction time, code substitution and learning, code substitution and delay, matching to sample, logical relations, mathematical processing, running memory, tapping (right and left)	Deployment associated with compromise on sustained attention ($ß = 0.11$, $p < 0.001$), verbal learning ($ß = -1.51$, $p = 0.003$), visual spatial memory ($ß = -3.82$, $p < 0.001$); deployment associated with negative state affect on measures of confusion ($ß = 1.40$, $p < 0.001$), tension ($ß = 1.24$, $p < 0.001$); deployment associated with improved simple reaction time ($ß = 4.30$, $p = 0.003$)	Multiple linear regression analyses adjusted for battalion membership, deployment-related head injury, stress, depression	Response rate 94% predeployment, 75% postdeployment
Barrett et al. 1996 (Derived from VES)	Cross-sectional, neuropsychologic examination	2,441 Vietnam veterans: 236 with PTSD, 242 with other psychiatric disorders, 128 with PTSD and another psychiatric diagnosis, 1835 with no psychiatric diagnosis	CVLT, Rey-Osterrieth complex figure test, WCST, WAIS-R (information and block design); PTSD diagnosed with DIS	Veterans with PTSD and concurrent psychiatric disorder demonstrated impairment in cognitive functioning compared with other groups	ANOVA	
Crowell et al. 2002 (Derived from VES)	Cross-sectional	Vietnam veterans with current PTSD ($n = 80$), PTSD in preceding year but no active symptoms ($n = 80$), psychiatrically	DIS-III-A and MMPI used to determine presence of combat stressors and diagnosis of PTSD WAIS-R (information and block design),	No statistically significant differences among the four groups on neuropsychologic measures	ANOVA, MANOVA, matched with respect to age, education, race, premilitary measures of	Participants include only male Vietnam-era Army veterans exposed to combat-related stressors

TABLE 6-5 Neurobehavioral and Neurocognitive Effects

Reference	Study Design	Population	Outcomes	Results	Adjustments	Comments
		matched control group without PTSD (n = 80), normal control group (n = 80)	CVLT, Rey-Osterreith Complex Figure, PASAT, Word List Generation Task, WCST, Grooved Pegboard Test		cognitive functioning, income level	
Zalewski et al. 1994 (Derived from VES)	Cross-sectional	723 Vietnam veterans: 241 with PTSD, 241 with GAD, 241 with no history of psychiatric diagnosis	WAIS-R block design, CVLT, Rey-Osterreith Complex Figure, PASAT	No differences in cognitive functioning among groups	MANOVA	Data collected in 1985-1986, high levels of comorbid psychiatric disorders in groups with PTSD and GAD

NOTE: ANAM = Automated Neuropsychological Assessment Matrices, ANCOVA = analysis of covariance, ANOVA = analysis of variance, BDI = Beck Depression Inventory, CPT = Continuous Performance Test, CVLT = California Verbal Learning Test, DIS = Diagnostic Interview Schedule, GAD = generalized anxiety disorder, GW = Gulf War, MANOVA = multivariate analysis of variance, MDD = major depressive disorder, MMPI = Minnesota Multiphasic Personality Inventory, MOS-CF = Medical Outcomes Study Cognitive Functioning Scale, NART = National Adult Reading Test, NES = Neurobehavioral Evaluation System, PASAT = Paced Auditory Serial Addition Test, PTSD = posttraumatic stress disorder, R = revised, POMS = Profile of Mood States, TOMM = Test of Memory Malingering, VES = Vietnam Experience Study, WAIS = Wechsler Adult Intelligence Scale, WCST = Wisconsin Card Sorting Test, WMS = Wechsler Memory Scale.

CHRONIC FATIGUE SYNDROME

Many veterans returning from the Gulf War and other wars have reported experiencing chronic fatigue (McCauley et al. 2002a). Unexplained chronic fatigue, experienced by both the general public and veterans, has been the subject of much discussion by clinicians and researchers alike (Buskila 2000; Straus 1991), but its etiology and course are still unclear. The prevalence of chronic fatigue in the general adult population appears to be less than 2% (Buskila 2000). CDC developed a case definition of chronic fatigue syndrome (CFS), first published in 1988 and revised in 1994 (Box 6-1). It is characterized by the presence of severe fatigue with related functional impairment and the occurrence of at least four of eight other defining symptoms over at least 6 months (Freeman et al. 2005; Fukuda et al. 1994). The most commonly reported symptoms are headache, postexertional malaise, impaired cognition, and muscle pain (Wills et al. 2003). McCauley et al. (2002a) found that 103 of 799 veterans deployed to the Gulf War in 1990-1991 fulfilled the case definition in 1998. The committee notes that fatigue, but not symptoms of fatigue sufficient to meet the CDC definition, is one of the most widely reported symptoms in surveys of Gulf War veterans (Cherry et al. 2001a; Engel et al. 2000; Gray et al. 1999; Ishoy et al. 1999; Kang et al. 2000b; Kelsall et al. 2004a; Simmons et al. 2004; Steele 2000; Unwin et al. 1999).

As in fibromyalgia and chronic pain (discussed later in this chapter), no laboratory tests or pathologic physical signs are widely accepted or provide a definitive diagnosis. The CDC criteria require that three elements be completed as part of a comprehensive evaluation. The first element, determining whether the symptom criteria for CFS are present, requires that a person be queried specifically about length and severity of fatigue and about eight ancillary symptoms. The second, determining whether other medical conditions are present, mandates a complete physical examination, a battery of specified laboratory tests, and a medical history. The third is an assessment of exclusionary conditions (such as lupus, mononucleosis, depression, and multiple sclerosis) (Fukuda et al. 1994; McEwen 2002).

BOX 6-1 Case Definition of Chronic Fatigue Syndrome

CDC criteria for CFS require the presence of both the following:

Clinically evaluated, unexplained persistent or relapsing chronic fatigue that is of new or definite onset (that is, not lifelong), is not the result of ongoing exertion, is not substantially alleviated by rest, and results in substantial reduction in previous levels of occupational, educational, social, or personal activities.

The concurrent occurrence of four or more of the following symptoms: substantial impairment in short-term memory or concentration; sore throat; tender lymph nodes; muscle pain; multi-joint pain without swelling or redness; headaches of a new type, pattern, or severity; unrefreshing sleep; and post-exertional malaise lasting more than 24 hours. These symptoms must have persisted or recurred during 6 or more consecutive months of illness and must not have predated the fatigue.

SOURCE: CDC (2007a).

A primary study for CFS requires that it be diagnosed by a health professional. A secondary study is one in which a CFS-like condition has been documented and a comparison is made between deployed and nondeployed veteran populations. Self-reports of CFS and self-reports of a physician diagnosis of CFS were included in the secondary studies. The primary studies of CFS are summarized in Table 6-6.

Primary Studies

The only primary study identified by the committee is that of Eisen et al. (2005), a cross-sectional prevalence study of 12 health measures in 1061 Gulf War-deployed and 1128 nondeployed veterans conducted in 2001 as part of the National Health Survey of Gulf War Era Veterans and Their Families. All randomly selected study participants had participated in the 1995 phase of the survey by completing a mail or telephone questionnaire about their health. CFS was diagnosed by clinical examination on the basis of the International Chronic Fatigue Syndrome Study Group case definition (Fukuda et al. 1994) by VA clinicians who were blind to the deployment status of the veterans. Veterans with psychiatric disorders were excluded from the sample. Eisen et al. (2005) found that only three of the 38 deployed veterans who self-reported CFS met the criteria on examination and only two of the eight nondeployed veterans who self-reported CFS received this diagnosis, so the authors concluded that self-reports of CFS in both deployed and nondeployed veterans are unreliable. Clinically diagnosed CFS, however, had the largest OR of the 12 medical illnesses or symptoms addressed. CFS was more prevalent in deployed veterans (1.6%) than in nondeployed veterans (0.1%) giving an OR of 40.6 (95% CI 10.2-161.15, $p < 0.001$) after adjustment for age, sex, race, cigarette-smoking, duty type, service branch, and rank. The strengths of this large study are its population-based design, stratified sampling method, analysis of participation bias, comprehensive examination, and use of computer-based algorithms by researchers who were blinded to deployment status. One limitation is the low response rates: 53% of the eligible deployed veterans and 39% of the eligible nondeployed veterans.

Secondary Studies

The committee identified six secondary studies that explored the relationship between deployment to a war zone and CFS. In all six, a diagnosis of CFS was self-reported, CFS was determined on the basis of self-reports of symptoms similar to those of CFS, or the presence of CFS was based on criteria other than those of CDC. Gray et al. (2002) found an OR of 7.60 (95% CI 4.76-12.13) for self-reports of physician-diagnosed CFS in Gulf War-deployed Seabees vs nondeployed Seabees; the OR was adjusted for age, sex, active-duty or reserve status, race or ethnicity, current smoking, and current alcohol-drinking. The prevalence of CFS was 5.17% in the Gulf War-deployed Seabees ($n = 3831$) who reported such a diagnosis, 0.79% in Seabees deployed elsewhere ($n = 4933$), and 0.68% in nondeployed Seabees ($n = 3104$).

In a survey of UK military personnel deployed to the Gulf War or to Bosnia or on active duty but not deployed, Reid et al. (2001) found that the prevalence of CFS was not statistically different between the Gulf War-deployed and nondeployed troops (2.1% vs 1.8%), but both groups had a greater prevalence of CFS than did the group deployed to Bosnia (0.7%). CFS was determined by the researchers on the basis of responses to a fatigue questionnaire combined with the SF-36 questionnaire for functional disability to meet the CDC criteria for CFS. The OR for CFS in the gulf vs Bosnia groups was 2.3 (95% CI 1.2-4.3) and in the gulf vs era veterans 1.2

(95% CI 0.8-1.8) adjusted for sex, age, marital status, education, rank, and employment status. CFS was associated with reported exposures to combat-related injury (OR 4.1, 95% CI 2.2-7.7), explosions of Scuds (OR 2.6, 95% CI 1.5-4.6) or artillery (OR 2.4, 95% CI 1.4-4.1), hearing chemical alarms (OR 2.5, 95% CI 1.2-5.3), witnessing a person's death (OR 2.2, 95% CI 1.3-3.8), seeing maimed soldiers (OR 2.0, 95% CI 1.2-3.6), and burning rubbish or feces (OR 2.0, 95% CI 1.0-3.4).

In a telephone survey of Iowa veterans of the Gulf War, a greater prevalence of chronic fatigue symptoms was reported by regular military (1.0%, n = 985) and National Guard/reserve (2.9%, n = 911) veterans than by nondeployed regular (0.2%, n = 968) and National Guard/reserve veterans (1.1%, n = 831) (Iowa Persian Gulf Study Group 1997). The statistically significant increased prevalence rate difference between deployed and nondeployed veterans was 1.4 (95% CI 0.9-2.0) after adjustment for age, sex, race, branch of military, and rank. The presence of a CFS-like condition was based on a combination of symptoms given in the CDC criteria (Freeman et al. 2005) and scores on the Chalder fatigue scale, a widely used scale to measure physical and mental fatigue in CFS patients (Putnam et al. 2006). The overall response rate was high (76%).

Canada deployed about 4500 troops to the gulf region in 1991 to provide naval operations and medical support. In 1997, a survey of the health status of the entire Canadian Gulf War forces was undertaken, comparing Gulf War-deployed troops with Canadian forces deployed elsewhere at the time (Goss Gilroy Inc. 1998). The assessment was based on a mailed survey that used the same questions as were used by the Iowa Persian Gulf Study Group (1998). Deployed veterans were more than 5 times as likely as nondeployed veterans to report symptoms of CFS (OR 5.27, 95% CI 3.95-7.03). Veterans who had served with land units had a slightly higher risk of CFS than those who served in air or sea units (OR 1.56, 95% CI 1.15-2.12). The response rate of the Gulf War veterans was 73%.

A cross-sectional mailed survey by Unwin et al. (1999) of three cohorts of UK veterans—3284 deployed to the gulf, 1815 deployed to Bosnia, and 2408 nondeployed—found that self-reported CFS (or myalgic encephalitis) was more strongly associated with deployment to the gulf than with deployment to Bosnia (OR 2.1, 95% CI 1.1-4.0) or no deployment (OR 2.7, 95% CI 1.6-4.6). ORs were adjusted for age, smoking, alcohol consumption, marital status, education, rank, employment, military or civilian status on followup, and a general health questionnaire. The prevalence of CFS (or myalgic encephalitis) was low in all the cohorts—3.3% in the gulf, 0.8% in the Bosnia, and 0.8% in the era cohort—although reports of symptoms of fatigue were relatively common: 50.7%, 26.3%, and 27.7%, respectively. Fatigue was associated with belief of exposure to chemical attack.

Zhang et al. (1999) reported that Gulf War veterans with CFS have several immune-function abnormalities in lymphocyte subpopulations not seen in healthy veterans or in civilians with CFS.

Posttraumatic Stress Disorder and Chronic Fatigue Syndrome

Only one secondary study examined the relationship between CFS and PTSD in Gulf War veterans. Kang et al. (2003) sent a self-administered 48-item questionnaire in 1995 to a large sample of active-duty, reserve, or National Guard veterans deployed during the Gulf War (n = 11,441) or not deployed (n = 9476). Current CFS-like illness was assessed according to responses to questions based on the CDC criteria for CFS (Fukuda et al. 1994); veterans had to have at least four of eight symptoms for 6 months or longer. The risk of current PTSD was estimated on the basis of responses to the 17-item PTSD Checklist that corresponded to the symptoms in the *DSM-III-R*. No clinical examinations were conducted for either CFS or PTSD. Compared with nondeployed veterans, Gulf War veterans had a greater risk for both PTSD (12.1% vs 4.3%) and CFS (5.6% vs 1.2%). The OR for current PTSD in deployed vs nondeployed veterans was 3.1 (95% CI 2.7-3.4) and 4.8 (95% CI 3.9-5.9) for CFS; ORs were adjusted for age, marital status, rank, and unit component and PTSD was also adjusted for sex. The authors also attempted to determine the effects of deployment stressors on the risk of PTSD and CFS in the reserve and National Guard units that were activated but not deployed and were deployed to the gulf. Although PTSD increased with intensity of stress, a risk of a CFS-like illness did not show a similar relationship and increased from 0.8% of members who were not activated to 1.7% of members who were activated and deployed but not to the gulf. The risk of having CFS was higher in members deployed to the gulf than deployed elsewhere but did not vary significantly with increasing combat stress, ranging from 5.4% to 7.3%. This study did not identify members who had comorbid PTSD and CFS, nor did it attempt to determine how soon after deployment the symptoms of each disorder were apparent. The study had the advantage of a population-based cohort with a relatively high participation rate of 70%, but it is limited by the lack of a physical examination for CFS or a psychiatric interview for PTSD.

Summary and Conclusions

Because the diagnosis of CFS depends entirely on symptoms, not on physical or laboratory findings, its prevalence varies widely from study to study. The only primary study demonstrated a higher prevalence of CFS in Gulf War-deployed veterans than in nondeployed veterans, although the absolute difference in prevalence was very small (1.6% vs 0.1%). Of the five secondary studies comparing Gulf War-deployed veterans with nondeployed veterans or veterans deployed elsewhere, three showed a higher prevalence of self-reports of CFS, CFS symptoms, or CFS-like illnesses; the other two studies did not see a difference in the prevalence of CFS between the two groups. Of the three secondary studies using the CDC definition of CFS, two had a positive association, and one no association. In addition, some of the secondary studies reviewed were not limited to CFS but included fatigue or CFS-like illnesses.

The committee concludes that there is limited but suggestive evidence of an association between deployment to a war zone and chronic fatigue syndrome.

TABLE 6-6 Chronic Fatigue Syndrome

Study	Study Design	Population	Outcomes	Results	Adjustments	Comments
Eisen et al. 2005 NHSGWEVTF (Derived from Kang et al. 2000b)	Population-based, cross-sectional, prevalence, in-person medical and psychiatric evaluations	1061 GW-deployed vs 1128 nondeployed veterans, veterans selected from among those who had participated in 1995 mail and telephone survey	CFS based on in-person interviews according to CDC CFS criteria and exclusionary diagnoses from history, interviews, examinations, laboratory testing	OR 40.6, 95% CI 10.2-161.15	Age, sex, race, cigarette-smoking, duty type, service branch, rank	Low participation rates (53% of deployed and 39% of nondeployed), but analysis of nonparticipants and participants reveals that participants, both deployed and nondeployed, are more likely to report symptoms of CFS

NOTE: CDC = Centers for Disease Control and Prevention, CFS = chronic fatigue syndrome, CI = confidence interval, GW = Gulf War, NHSGWEVTF = National Health Survey of Gulf War Era Veterans and Their Families, OR = odds ratio.

SLEEP DISTURBANCES

Complaints of disturbed sleep are common symptoms of many disorders and have been frequently reported by veterans of the Gulf War (Barrett et al. 2002b) and the Vietnam War (Neylan et al. 1998). Sleep-related problems affect 50-70 million Americans of all ages (National Heart Lung and Blood Institute 2007). Disturbances of sleep are generally assessed in two ways. Most commonly, people are simply asked to report on characteristics of their sleep, such as how long they sleep, whether their sleep is disturbed by nightmares, and whether their sleep is restful. Sleep disturbances and sleep disorders, such as sleep apnea, can also be assessed objectively in a laboratory, usually by recording the electroencephalogram and determining how much time is spent in one of the defined sleep stages and how much time is spent awake. Such laboratory assessments are time-consuming and expensive and therefore are not often used.

This section considers the types of sleep disturbances reported in large surveys of deployed and nondeployed Gulf War veterans. No studies that included objective measures of sleep disturbance or a physician's diagnosis of a sleep problem or disorder in veterans of the Gulf War or any other war, except for those with PTSD as discussed below, were identified. None of the studies reviewed in this section met the committee's criteria for a primary study, so no summary table is included.

Self-Reports of Sleep Disturbance

The committee identified several studies that assessed self-reported information on sleep from deployed and nondeployed veterans of the 1991 Gulf War (Cherry et al. 2001a; Engel et al. 2000; Gray et al. 2002; Ishoy et al. 1999; Kang et al. 2000b; Kelsall et al. 2004a; Proctor et al. 1998; Steele 2000; Unwin et al. 1999). However, none of them supplemented the self-reported data with systematically collected information from a clinical interview or other objective measures.

Several researchers have found increased reports of disturbed sleep among U.S. veterans deployed to the Gulf War. In 1995, the VA used a mailed questionnaire to survey 11,441 U.S. Gulf War-deployed veterans and 9476 nondeployed controls; Kang et al. (2000b) found a higher frequency of sleep problems in the deployed veterans, with several sleep symptoms being significantly more prevalent among the Gulf War veterans than the nondeployed veterans: unrefreshing sleep (47% vs 24%, rate difference 23, 95% CI 22.8-23.2), difficulty in sleeping (37% vs 21%, rate difference 16, 95% CI 15.9-16.1), and excessive sleepiness (30% vs 14%, rate difference 16, 95% CI 15.9-16.1).

Using data from a self-report questionnaire, Proctor et al. (1998) compared the sleep problems of 252 Gulf War-deployed veterans with those of 48 era veterans who had been deployed to Germany; about 30% of the Gulf War veterans and 11% of the comparison group reported an inability to fall asleep (OR 3.4-3.6, 95% CI excludes 1.0). Trouble in sleeping was reported by 14.6% of 527 Gulf War-deployed U.S. Navy Seabees and 4.9% of their nondeployed counterparts for an OR of 3.4 (95% CI 2.3-5.0) 3-4 years after the war (Gray et al. 1999).

In a study of Navy Seabees, Gray et al. (2002) found that the 3832 Seabees deployed to the Persian Gulf had more nightmares and flashbacks (OR 4.58, 95% CI 3.50-6.00) and more trouble in sleeping (OR 3.08, 95% CI 2.71-3.50) than 3104 nondeployed Seabees. In 1998, Steele (2000) assessed symptoms suggestive of Gulf War illness in 1435 deployed and 409 nondeployed veterans, all from Kansas. Deployed veterans reported not feeling rested after sleep and problems in falling or staying asleep significantly more often than nondeployed veterans (OR 2.69, 95% CI 2.04-3.54 and OR 2.98, 95% CI 2.18-4.08, respectively).

A similar pattern was observed among Gulf War veterans from other countries. Unwin et al. (1999) conducted a cross-sectional mailed survey of a random sample of UK veterans: 3284 Gulf War-deployed, 1815 deployed to the Bosnia conflict, and 2408 era veterans. The Gulf War veterans reported a higher frequency of sleeping difficulties than the Bosnia cohort (OR 1.7, 95% CI 1.5-2.0) or the era cohort (OR 1.9, 95% CI 1.7-2.2) adjusted for age, smoking, alcohol consumption, marital status, educational attainment, rank, employment status, civilian or military status on followup, and score on a general health questionnaire. More UK veterans deployed to the Gulf War than nondeployed veterans reported waking up feeling tired and worn out, losing sleep because of worry, and having nightmares (Cherry et al. 2001a). Australian Gulf War veterans also reported more sleep problems than their nondeployed counterparts (Kelsall et al. 2004a). The most frequently reported symptom among the deployed veterans was feeling unrefreshed after sleep (OR 1.7, 95% CI 1.4-2.1). More deployed veterans also reported sleep difficulties (OR 1.8, 95% CI 1.5-2.2). ORs were adjusted for service type, rank, age, education, and marital status. Ishoy et al. (1999) compared the frequency of self-reported sleep difficulties in Danish veterans who had been deployed to the Persian Gulf during 1990-1997 as peacekeepers and age- and sex-matched controls. They found a higher frequency of sleep problems in the deployed subjects. For example, 19.4% of the deployed and 9.1% of the nondeployed controls reported problems in falling asleep.

Posttraumatic Stress Disorder and Sleep

Because difficulty in falling asleep or staying asleep and nightmares are two of the diagnostic criteria for PTSD, it is difficult to distinguish between PTSD and comorbid psychiatric disorders, such as MDD and GAD, many of which are also characterized by sleep disturbances. Nevertheless, several studies have looked at sleep disturbances in veterans with and without PTSD. Using questionnaire data from the NVVRS, Neylan et al. (1998) obtained self-reported information on five items in the Mississippi Scale for Combat-Related PTSD that assess sleep. Three domains of sleep were addressed: difficulties in sleep onset, nightmares, and sleep maintenance disturbance. Subjects were asked about the frequency with which the sleep problems occurred. Vietnam-theater veterans who met the case definition of PTSD at the time of the survey reported more disturbances in all three domains. For example, difficulties in falling asleep at least sometimes were reported by 44.0% of combat veterans with PTSD, 5.5% of combat veterans without PTSD, 9.4% of era veterans, and 5.0% of civilian comparison subjects ($p < 0.0001$). Difficulties in staying asleep occurred in 90.7% of combat veterans with PTSD, 62.5% of combat veterans without PTSD, and 63.1% of era veterans ($p < 0.0001$). Nightmares were reported by 52.4% of the combat veterans with PTSD, 4.8% of those without PTSD, and 5.7% of era veterans. Frequent or very frequent nightmares and difficulties in falling asleep were reported only by subjects with PTSD. Using hierarchic multiple regression, the investigators found that 48% of the variance in frequency of nightmares was accounted for by non-sleep-related PTSD symptoms. Combat exposure accounted for an additional 9% of the variance for nightmares. The weighted Pearson correlation of combat exposure and nightmares was 0.63 ($p < 0.001$). Limitations of this study include its retrospective assessment of combat exposure and that sleep measures were subjective and not standardized.

Engel et al. (2000) assessed physical symptoms in 21,244 Gulf War veterans who enrolled themselves in DoD's Comprehensive Clinical Evaluation Program (CCEP) in 1994-1996. Of the total sample, 23.2% of those with no psychologic condition reported having sleep disturbance compared with 64.5% of those with PTSD and 45.3% of those with a psychologic condition but not PTSD. Only 8.7% of those in the CCEP who considered themselves healthy reported sleep disturbance compared with 34% of those with a medical illness.

Inman et al. (1990) compared 35 Vietnam veterans with PTSD and 37 veterans with insomnia but without PTSD. The researchers found no differences in the severity of the insomnia between the two groups, but the veterans with PTSD had more sleep-related anxiety symptoms, such as talking or shouting during sleep, fear of going to sleep, having disturbing thoughts while lying in bed, waking from a frightening dream, and finding it hard to return to sleep.

Several small studies have used objective sleep measures to assess sleep quality in veterans with PTSD. In 1991-1994, Engdahl et al. (2000) studied 59 combat veterans of World War II and the Korean War (including 30 prisoners of war), 30 of whom had current PTSD (as diagnosed with the SCID). There was no difference between veterans with and without PTSD in any of 18 sleep measures gathered over three nights by polysomnography, except for a small increase in rapid-eye-movement (REM) sleep and fewer arousals per minute from non-REM sleep in the PTSD veterans; the amount of REM-sleep correlated with PTSD severity.

Other studies identified sleep abnormalities in the electrophysiologically monitored sleep of small samples of veterans with PTSD and other psychiatric disorders. Mellman et al. (1995a) found recurrent awakening, increased movement during sleep, and threatening dreams to be more prevalent in 20 Vietnam veterans with combat-related PTSD than in eight noncombat veterans without PTSD; these sleep abnormalities may be associated with nondiminished central noradrenergic activity at night (Mellman et al. 1995b). Dow et al. (1996) compared Vietnam veterans who had PTSD and depression with those who had depression alone; the only significant difference was prolonged sleep latency in the depressed group. Vietnam veterans with combat-related PTSD had less REM sleep and less sleep efficiency than a veteran group with depression; this suggests that sleep maintenance is impaired in PTSD (Mellman et al. 1997; Woodward et al. 2000; see also Chapter 5).

Dagan et al. (1991) found that although veterans with PTSD complained of sleep disturbances, objective measures of sleep obtained using an actigraph to differentiate between sleep and waking were not impaired in those with PTSD. In a small study of 12 veterans with war-related PTSD and 12 controls without PTSD, there were no significant differences in polysomnographic recording between the two groups; however, those with PTSD had significantly higher auditory awaking thresholds and more hostile and aggressive dreams (Lavie et al. 1998). Increased sleep problems in veterans with combat neuroses or PTSD have been reported in veterans of other conflicts (Lavie et al. 1979). One study of over 4 million veterans in the Veterans Health Administration health-care database estimated that 2.9% of the veterans had sleep apnea and that almost 12% of those also had PTSD (Sharafkhaneh et al. 2005).

Nevertheless, as concluded by reviews that were not limited to consideration of PTSD only in veterans (Caldwell and Redeker 2005; Harvey et al. 2003), objective findings regarding sleep disturbance even among people with PTSD are inconsistent. Harvey et al. (2003) reviewed over 25 studies of sleep in combat veterans, primarily from the Vietnam War, and other groups with PTSD and found mixed results. Some of the studies showed that those with PTSD had more disturbed sleep and lower sleep efficiency, but other studies showed that those with PTSD are not outside the normal range of objective sleep measures. Harvey et al. (2003) suggest that people with PTSD may perceive their sleep as more disturbed than it actually is.

Summary and Conclusions

There is consistent evidence that veterans deployed to war zones have a higher frequency of complaints of disturbed sleep than do comparable control groups; however, objective measures of sleep disturbances or diagnoses of sleep disorders, such as narcolepsy and sleep apnea, are lacking in veteran studies. None of the studies comparing deployed with nondeployed veterans of the Gulf War or other wars included objective measures of sleep problems. Because the studies relied solely on self-reports of sleep problems, the committee concludes that there is inadequate evidence to determine whether veterans deployed to a war zone are at increased risk for sleep disturbances.

More research has been conducted on sleep problems in veterans with war-related PTSD. One study examined the relationship between complaints of sleep disturbances and an indicator of exposure to deployment-related stressors. In an examination of data from the NVVRS, Neylan et al. (1998) found a relationship between PTSD and complaints of sleep disturbance, especially nightmares, even after adjusting for the presence of symptoms of sleep disturbance in the diagnostic criteria for PTSD. Those data are consistent in suggesting that deployment to a war zone is associated with increased complaints of disturbed sleep. The committee notes that PTSD is highly comorbid with other psychiatric disorders, such as MDD, that are also characterized by sleep problems. The comorbidity adds to the complexity of assessing sleep disturbance in veterans and others with PTSD.

There are several problems in drawing conclusions about the more general question of the role of deployment-related stress in producing sleep disturbances. The studies of self-reports of sleep disturbances cited in this section did not include information about the relationship between deployment-related stressors and the development of complaints of disturbed sleep, nor did they address the degree to which the sleep disturbances might be part of a syndrome, such as depression or PTSD. An additional limitation is the low response rates that characterize such studies and increase the likelihood of bias in the results.

Objective sleep measures have not been studied in sufficiently large veteran populations to permit generalization about the association between deployment to a war zone and sleep disturbance or disorders or between PTSD and sleep disturbances.

The committee concludes that there is inadequate/insufficient evidence to determine whether an association exists between deployment to a war zone and sleep disorders or objective measures of sleep disturbances.

CARDIOVASCULAR DISEASES

The term *cardiovascular disease* encompasses a wide variety of conditions, the most important of which are related to the development of atherosclerosis in the arteries and high blood pressure; these can lead to coronary heart disease (CHD)—which may be manifested clinically as myocardial infarction (MI), angina, or sudden cardiac death—and to cerebrovascular disease, which may present clinically as a stroke or transient ischemic attack. The three most important risk factors for cardiovascular disease are blood pressure, blood cholesterol, and smoking. All are affected by stress and lifestyle and so could be affected by deployment, particularly to a war zone (in the case of hypertension). Hypertension can be regarded both as a type of cardiovascular disease and as a risk factor for CHD and stroke. This section considers those medical conditions and also considered lesser manifestations of cardiovascular disease, including chest pain and arrhythmia, both of which may be manifestations of CHD but also occur commonly in the absence of any structural disease. Thus, chest pain that occurs in patients without CHD (that is, people who have normal coronary angiograms) tends to occur in younger people who have psychiatric conditions, such as anxiety and depression, which can occur in veterans deployed to a war zone.

That war is stressful and may result in symptoms characteristic of heart disease is documented in the medical literature as Da Costa syndrome after the U.S. Civil War and as soldier's heart in World War I (Jones et al. 2002). The scientific literature on the cardiovascular effects of exposure to wartime stress can be divided into three general categories: first, studies of the acute effects of war, including hospitalization for or death from myocardial infarction in the civilian population; second, studies of the delayed effects, including symptoms and objective findings of cardiovascular disease that persist or emerge after the war is over; and third, studies of changes in acute physiologic reactivity during simulated sounds or sights of war in veterans who have developed PTSD (see Chapter 5).

The following sections review the epidemiologic information available on the cardiovascular effects seen in deployed and nondeployed veterans. No studies reported on cardiovascular effects in terms of quantified or categorized levels of stress experienced by veterans deployed to a war zone, so deployment itself is used as a surrogate for deployment-related stress, as explained in Chapter 1. For cardiovascular effects, primary studies were ones that met the committee's criteria, as given in Chapter 2; however, self-reports of cardiovascular disease and of hypertension were considered to be primary reports if a self-report was part of a thorough interview and specified that the veteran was reporting a previous physician diagnosis or treatment for the condition. Self-reports of cardiovascular disease based on a mail questionnaire or other instrument, such as the SF-36, were considered to be secondary studies if they were otherwise well conducted. Primary studies are summarized in Table 6-7.

As in previous sections, the committee has also looked at the effects of the Gulf War, the Vietnam War, and World War II. PTSD is a well-described outcome of exposure to war and one of PTSD's components is heightened autonomic arousal (for example increased blood pressure), so we also examine the cardiovascular consequences of PTSD.

Cardiovascular Symptoms

A number of studies have examined the array of self-reported cardiovascular symptoms and clinical disease in veterans, primarily after the Gulf War. Gray et al. (2002) administered mailed questionnaires to 3831 Gulf War veterans (Navy Seabees) and 3104 nondeployed Seabees 7 years after the war. The deployed veterans self-reported a significantly higher prevalence of all 33 medical problems, including chest pains, than the nondeployed veterans (OR 3.06, 95% CI 2.52-3.71) in the 12 months before the survey. Proctor et al. (1998) surveyed two stratified random samples of Gulf War veterans (220 from Fort Devens and 71 from New Orleans) and a control group of 50 Gulf War-era veterans who were deployed in Germany from a larger cohort of active-duty, reserve, and National Guard members. Participants completed the Health Symptom Checklist in 1992-1993 and an expanded version in 1994-1996. The authors found nonsignificantly higher prevalences of a wide variety of self-reported symptoms—including chest pain, irregular heart beats, and racing heart—in the Gulf War veterans than in the nondeployed veterans. Another study by McCauley et al. (2002b) consisted of a telephone survey of 1779 Gulf War veterans in three groups: those who were possibly exposed to chemical-warfare agents from the destruction of the Khamisiyah munitions bunker, those who were deployed to Iraq but not exposed, and those who were not sent to Iraq. The deployed veterans reported more physician diagnoses of high blood pressure (OR 1.7, 95% CI 1.3-2.4) and heart disease (OR 2.5, 95% CI 1.1-6.6), but there was no evidence that those who had possibly been exposed to chemical-warfare agents had a higher prevalence of any cardiovascular events.

Stretch et al. (1995) conducted a survey of Gulf War veterans from Hawaii and Pennsylvania 2-3 years after the war and found that significantly ($p < 0.05$) more of the 1524 deployed veterans than the 2524 nondeployed veterans (6.7% vs 2.4%) reported "heart problems" among other symptoms. UK veterans who had been deployed to both Bosnia and the Gulf War (n = 570) complained of more chest pain (25.2%) and rapid heartbeat (15.1%), as 1785 veterans who had not been deployed to either war (13.2% and 8.0%, respectively) or 2049 veterans who had served only in Bosnia (12.4% and 7.5%, respectively) (Hotopf et al. 2003a). The ORs for deployed to both conflicts vs deployed to neither conflict were 2.2 (95% CI 1.7-2.8) and 2.2 (95% CI 1.6-2.9) for chest pain and rapid heartbeat, respectively. Thus, there are consistent findings that deployment to a war zone, particularly the Gulf War, is associated with an increase in self-reports of many physical symptoms, including chest pain and increased heart rate, but these symptoms do not necessarily imply any structural heart disease.

Hypertension

Primary Studies

In epidemiologic studies, hypertension is generally defined on the basis of measuring blood pressure (ideally more than once) or patients reporting that they have received a diagnosis of hypertension and are taking antihypertensive medication. Two primary studies compared deployed with nondeployed veterans for hypertension. In a cross-sectional prevalence study, Eisen et al. (2005) conducted medical examinations of 1061 deployed and 1128 nondeployed Gulf War veterans 10 years after the conflict. Veterans who participated in the study had been part of the larger National Health Survey of Gulf War Era Veterans and Their Families conducted in 1995. Hypertension was defined as a blood pressure greater than 140/90 mm Hg or a history of hypertension and taking antihypertensive medication. The difference in the prevalence of hypertension on clinical evaluation at a VA medical facility between deployed (9.1%) and nondeployed veterans (12.6%) was not significant (OR 0.90, 95% CI 0.60-1.33). ORs were adjusted for differences in age, sex, race, years of education, cigarette-smoking, duty type, service branch, and rank. The study was limited by low participation rates (53% of eligible deployed and 39% of eligible nondeployed) and the number of years that had passed since the war. Blanchard et al. (2006) re-examined the same data as those of Eisen et al. to determine the prevalence of chronic multisymptom illness and came to a similar conclusion: hypertension was not higher in Gulf War-deployed veterans than in their nondeployed counterparts, whether or not the veterans had multisymptom illness.

The VES, conducted by CDC in 1985-1986, looked at cardiorespiratory conditions in 2490 Vietnam-theater Army veterans and 1972 Vietnam-era veterans. In Phase 1 conducted about 15-20 years after the war, a telephone interview was used to assess whether the veterans had any one of a number of health effects; in Phase 2, participants received physical examinations to screen for health status. A diagnosis of hypertension was based on a measured blood pressure above 140/90 mmHg or by patients reporting that they were taking antihypertensive medication. The prevalence of hypertension was not significantly higher in the theater veterans (33.5%) than in the era veterans (31.4%) (OR 1.1, 95% CI 0.9-1.2) after adjustment for age at enlistment, race, year of enlistment, enlistment status, score on a general technical test, and primary military occupation. About 5% of the veterans in each group reported using antihypertensive medication at the time of the study (CDC 1988b).

Secondary Studies

Secondary studies are defined as those in which the diagnosis of hypertension was based only on self-reports. A cross-sectional study of 1456 Australian Gulf War veterans and 1588 nondeployed veterans, surveyed 10 years after the war, found no increase in the prevalence of self-reports of physician diagnoses or of treatment of hypertension after the war in the deployed veterans (OR 1.2, 95% CI 0.9-1.6) after adjustment for service type, rank, age, education, and marital status (Kelsall et al. 2004a). The strength of this study is that a physician assessed and rated the likelihood of each self-reported medical condition during a followup face-to-face interview although a physical examination was not conducted.

Several other cross-sectional studies relied exclusively on self-reports. The largest, conducted by VA (Kang et al. 2000b), was a mailed survey with followup telephone interviews of a population-based sample of 11,441 Gulf War veterans and a stratified random sample of 9476 nondeployed veterans. The study was the first phase of the National Health Survey of Gulf War Era Veterans and Their Families conducted in 1995, which surveyed 30,000 deployed and nondeployed Gulf War veterans for health problems, and was used by Eisen et al. (2005). A slightly higher (but significant because of the large numbers) prevalence of hypertension was reported in the Gulf War veterans than in the nondeployed veterans (11.4% vs 7.6%, rate difference 3.84, 95% CI 3.75-3.93) in the preceding 12 months.

In a cross-sectional study by Hotopf et al. (2003a), a stratified random sample of 2049 UK veterans of the Bosnia peacekeeping mission, 570 veterans who had served in both the Gulf War and Bosnia, and 1785 nondeployed veterans completed a mail questionnaire that asked about a variety of health effects. No difference in the frequency of self-reported hypertension was seen between the groups (6.1% in both the deployed and the nondeployed and 4.2% in those deployed only to Bosnia).

Three other studies reported a statistically significant increase in self-reported hypertension. The Seabee Health Study (Gray et al. 2002), a survey of 3831 Gulf War-deployed Navy Seabees and 3104 nondeployed Seabees in which questionnaires were mailed to the participants 7 years after the Gulf War (1997-1999), found a significantly higher rate of self-reported hypertension in the Seabees who had been deployed than in those who had not (OR

1.82, 95% CI 1.48-2.26) after adjustment for age, sex, active-duty or reserve status, race or ethnicity, current smoking, and current alcohol-drinking. McCauley et al. (2002b) compared the self-reported rates of hypertension in 1263 veterans who were deployed to Iraq (653 within 50 km of Khamisiyah and 610 who were deployed to Southwest Asia but outside a 50-km radius) with rates in 516 nondeployed veterans. Eight years after the war, the incidence of hypertension was higher in the deployed veterans (OR 1.7, 95% CI 1.3-2.4). Finally, in a small study of 141 Gulf War-deployed veterans and 46 veterans deployed to Germany evaluated 4 years after the war, Proctor et al. (2001) found more hypertension in the deployed veterans (13.9% vs 4.4%, $p < 0.05$).

Haley et al. (2004) used 24-hour blood-pressure monitoring, the gold standard for defining hypertension, to determine whether there were abnormalities of the autonomic nervous system that might explain the chronic symptoms experienced by many Gulf War veterans. They found no difference in blood pressure between 22 deployed and 18 nondeployed male Gulf War veterans. The deployed veterans had become ill during or shortly after deployment. Although the study used an appropriate approach to determine hypertension, it is limited by the small number of subjects and the inclusion of veterans who were reported to be ill.

Heart Disease

Primary Studies

The most important form of heart disease that might be related to deployment stress is CHD. It is, however, relatively unlikely to be clinically manifested before the age of 45-50 years; thus, even if deployment did accelerate the development of CHD, it would be difficult to detect such an effect in Gulf War veterans, although not in Vietnam or World War II veterans. Because the average age of military personnel who were deployed in the Gulf War was around 28 years (Eisen et al. 2005), it is not surprising that no studies have reported CHD effects. For the present analysis, primary studies are defined as those in which the diagnoses of CHD were made by physical examination or CHD events (myocardial infarction and cardiac death) were based on hospitalizations or death certificates.

A survey by Kang and Bullman (2001) performed 7 years after deployment found that cardiovascular mortality in male Gulf War veterans was lower (1.30 per 10,000 person-years) than in non-Gulf War veterans (2.05 per 10,000 person-years). The adjusted rate ratio derived from a Cox proportional-hazards model (controlled for age, race, branch of service, unit component, and marital status) was 0.90 for men (95% CI 0.81-1.01) and 0.96 for women (95% CI 0.55-1.69). The vital status of 621,902 Gulf War veterans and 746,248 other veterans was determined from VA and Social Security Administration databases; death certificates were used to establish cause of death. Both veteran groups had significantly lower mortality from cardiovascular disease than the general population.

Two studies by Gray et al. (1996, 2000) looked at hospitalization records of Gulf War era veterans for discharge diagnoses of the *ICD-9-CM* category circulatory system diseases. In the first study, the researchers determined DoD hospital-discharge diagnoses for 1991, 1992, and 1993, comparing 547,076 Gulf War veterans with 618,335 other veterans from the same period. The multivariate ORs for each year were all 0.9-1.1 (exact values not given) adjusted for prewar hospitalizations, sex, age, race or ethnic group, branch of service, marital status, rank, length of service, salary, and occupation. In the second study, they examined hospital-discharge records for 1991-1994 for three hospital systems: 182,164 records from the DoD, 16,030 records from the VA, and 5,185 records from the California Office of Statewide Health Planning and Development. PMRs of hospital-discharge diagnoses of Gulf War veterans and veterans not deployed to the gulf were compared. The PMRs were 0.94 (95% CI 0.91-0.98) for DoD, 0.85 (95% CI 0.76-0.93) for VA, and 0.98 (95% CI 0.82-1.14) for California Office of Statewide Health Planning and Development. All PMRs were adjusted for age and sex, and the DoD PMR was also adjusted for race.

In the CDC VES study, discussed above, the researchers conducted physical examinations for cardiorespiratory conditions (CDC 1988b). Specifically, the 2490 Vietnam-theater and 1972 Vietnam-era veterans were evaluated for problems of the peripheral arterial system with a Doppler instrument, electrocardiograms that were read by cardiologists, and chest x-ray pictures. No significant differences were found between the theater and era veterans in the prevalences of altered peripheral arterial hemodynamics (4.7% vs 3.6%, OR 1.2, 95% CI 0.9-1.7), ischemia (1.9% vs 1.8%, OR 1.1, 95% CI 0.7-1.7), or any electrocardiographic findings (14.3% vs 13.9%, OR 1.1, 95% CI 0.9-1.3), which included bradycardia, tachycardia, extrasystoles, and nonspecific ST- and T-wave changes. A slight increase in risk of left ventricular hypertrophy (1.6% vs 1.0%, OR 1.8, 95% CI 1.0-3.3) was seen in theater veterans. The prevalence of cardiac findings in the chest x-ray pictures did not differ significantly between theater and era veterans (1.0% vs 0.9%, OR 1.3, 95% CI 0.7-2.5). All ORs were adjusted for age at enlistment, race, year of enlistment, enlistment status (volunteer vs draftee), score on a general technical test, and primary military occupational specialty.

As part of the VES, postservice mortality in a cohort of 9324 U.S. Army Vietnam veterans was compared with that in 8989 Army Vietnam-era veterans who served in Korea, Germany, or the United States (CDC 1987, 1988b). Veterans were assessed from discharge through 1983, and vital status was ascertained from files of the Army, VA, Social Security Administration, the Internal Revenue Service, and the National Center for Health Statistics. Death certificates were used to establish cause of death, which was categorized by an experienced nosologist who was blind as to veteran deployment status. During the roughly 12-18 years of followup, the crude mortality from diseases of the circulatory system was 9.4 per 100,000 person-years in Vietnam veterans and 19.0 per 100,000 person-years in era veterans, for a rate ratio of 0.49 (95% CI 0.25-0.99). The study results indicate that Vietnam veterans had a 51% lower mortality from cardiovascular diseases than era veterans; the difference was evident over the entire followup period and for all types of circulatory diseases.

Secondary Studies

Studies that relied on self-reports of heart disease or that combined "hard" measures (for example, myocardial infarction) and "soft" measures (for example, angina) of heart disease were classified as secondary studies. A survey of 11,441 Gulf War veterans and 9476 nondeployed veterans found no difference in the rates of self-reported CHD or stroke (Kang et al. 2000b). Only one study reported any increase in heart disease. McCauley et al. (2002b) conducted telephone interviews with 653 veterans who were deployed near Khamisiyah in Iraq and compared them with 610 who were deployed to Southwest Asia but not near Khamisiyah and 516 who were not deployed. The interviews took place 8 years after deployment. The deployed veterans were more likely to report having a postwar diagnosis of heart disease (OR 2.5, 95% CI 1.1-6.6) although the disease was not specified. This study's positive findings based self-reports may merely reflect increased reporting of all medical conditions or more nonspecific symptoms among Gulf War veterans.

Blood Lipid Concentrations

The Danish Gulf War Study was conducted on 686 of the 821 Danish troops deployed to the Persian Gulf region as UN peacekeepers during 1990-1997 and 231 age- and sex-matched control veterans. Health examinations included blood tests of the veterans 7 years after deployment (Ishoy et al. 1999). Total cholesterol, high-density lipoprotein (HDL), and triglycerides were the same in the two groups.

Other studies have examined lipid concentrations as a function of PTSD. Karlovic et al. (2004) compared blood lipids in 53 Croatian War veterans with PTSD and 49 with combat experience but no PTSD and found that those with PTSD had significantly higher total cholesterol (264 vs 226 mg/dL, $p = 0.001$), low-density lipoprotein (LDL) (169 vs 137 mg/dL, $p = 0.002$), and triglycerides (196 vs 138 mg/dL, $p = 0.001$) and had lower HDL (43 vs 62 mg/dL, $p < 0.001$). There was no difference in BMI between the two groups. Kagan et al. (1999) compared lipids in 73 Vietnam veterans with PTSD and 113 male volunteers admitted into a substance-abuse program who were matched for demographic factors, such as age. The lipid concentrations were compared with those of the general male population in the National Health and Nutrition Examination Survey (NHANES) and with averages of male veterans. Total cholesterol, LDL, and triglycerides were highest in the veterans with PTSD, and HDL was marginally lower.

Solter et al. (2002) compared blood lipids in 103 Croatian veterans with combat-related PTSD and a control group of 92 patients with MDD. Veterans with combat-related PTSD had higher mean concentrations of cholesterol (6.2 vs 5.3 mmol/L, $p < 0.001$), LDL cholesterol (3.9 vs 3.5 mmol/L, $p = 0.005$), and triglycerides (2.9 vs 1.5 mmol/L, $p < 0.001$) and had lower HDL cholesterol (1.0 vs 1.3 mmol/L, $p < 0.001$) than the control group.

Posttraumatic Stress Disorder and Cardiovascular Effects

As discussed in Chapter 5, PTSD is one of the best-established health effects resulting from exposure to traumatic events during deployment to a war zone. It also has profound effects on the autonomic nervous system and other systems that mediate the development of cardiovascular disease, so it is important to examine the state of knowledge of these relationships. Excessive autonomic nervous system arousal in response to trauma-related cues is one of the diagnostic features of PTSD. Two general types of study are relevant here: those of the long-term effects of PTSD on cardiovascular variables and those of the psychophysiologic effects of simulated combat in subjects with and without PTSD.

Heart Rate

A number of studies have performed laboratory testing of veterans with and without PTSD. They have generally involved the measurement of heart rate, blood pressure, and other cardiovascular variables while the subjects were at rest and then compared the changes that occurred during mental-challenge tests. There have been many studies of a generally similar design, and the committee notes that in several of them the subjects with PTSD showed an increase in resting heart rate, which led to the suggestion that PTSD might be a risk factor for hypertension. Buckley and Kaloupek (2001) performed a meta-analysis of 34 studies that gathered indicators of basal cardiovascular activity, including heart rate, systolic blood pressure, and diastolic blood pressure of subjects with diagnosed PTSD and two types of comparison groups: subjects who had been exposed to trauma but did not have PTSD and subjects with no history of exposure. Twenty-five of the studies included veterans whose original traumatic stress was combat-related; the time between the traumatic event and the measurement of cardiovascular activity ranged from 2 months to 29 years. In total, cardiovascular measures of 2670 subjects were analyzed in all the studies. The main finding was that people with a current PTSD diagnosis had a resting heart rate that was 5 beats/minute faster than subjects in the control groups. It has also been observed that an increase in heart rate immediately after a trauma is a predictor of PTSD (Shalev et al. 1998).

Hypertension

Findings that people with PTSD have an increased heart rate are fairly consistent, but results related to blood pressure have been less clear. Some of the epidemiologic studies described above that relied mostly on self-reports for the identification of hypertension also compared its prevalence in veterans with and without PTSD. However, one study that used a more thorough method to assess the prevalence of hypertension in veteran populations with possible PTSD found no increase in hypertension in aging veterans with PTSD. The VA Normative Aging Study was established in 1961 to follow 2280 community-dwelling men in the greater Boston area; more than 90% of the men were veterans at entry in the study. The cohort included 1002 veterans who completed a mailed Mississippi Scale for Combat-Related PTSD in 1990 and 944 veterans who completed the Keane PTSD scale of the Minnesota Multiphasic Personality Inventory in 1986 (Kubzansky et al. 2007). Men with pre-existing angina pectoris, a history of MI, or diabetes were excluded from the study; the mean age of the 1990 study population was 63 years. Study participants receive physical examinations every 3-5 years. A correlation analysis of scores from the Mississippi Scale for Combat-Related PTSD with systolic blood pressure showed no relationship; however, there was a slight correlation ($r = -0.06$, $p = 0.04$) between lower diastolic blood pressure and the score on the Mississippi Scale for Combat-Related PTSD but not on the Minnesota Multiphasic Personality Inventory-2. Veterans with higher PTSD scores were at slightly greater risk for total CHD (RR 1.21, 95% CI 0.93-1.57, adjusted for age, smoking, blood pressures, serum total cholesterol, BMI, family history of CHD, education, and alcohol intake), particularly nonfatal MI (RR 1.30, 95% CI 0.92-1.84, adjusted for coronary risk factors). The associations were slightly strengthened when depression was also controlled for. Several of the studies of deployed veterans described above observed a marked increase of PTSD as a result of deployment without any increase in the prevalence of hypertension (Kelsall et al. 2004a; Kubzansky et al. 2007; McCauley et al. 2002b; Schnurr et al. 2000; Spiro et al. 2006).

A study of 147 Dutch resistance fighters in World War II (82 of whom had PTSD) found that the prevalence of hypertension in those with PTSD was not higher than in those without PTSD (32% vs 31%) (Falger et al. 1992). The authors noted that 56% of the veterans, 60-65 years old at the time of the study, were currently suffering from PTSD diagnosed with the SCID according to *DSM-III-R* criteria. This study is limited by the lack of confirmation by physical examination of the cardiovascular factors reported by participants. A study of Croatian veterans of the Balkan wars (Karlovic et al. 2004) included 43 with PTSD, 37 with PTSD and comorbid MDD, 38 with MDD alone, and 39 healthy controls. Veterans with PTSD (with or without MDD) showed no differences from the other veterans in blood pressure.

One nationally representative study that reported an association between PTSD and hypertension in a civilian population is the NCS (Lauterbach et al. 2005). It compared 429 subjects with PTSD with 5448 subjects without PTSD. Hypertension was reported twice as frequently (14.2%) in those with PTSD as in those without (7.7%). There was no control for other predictors of hypertension, however, such as obesity.

The meta-analysis of Buckley and Kaloupek (2001), discussed in the section above on heart rate, did not find any consistent differences in blood pressure between people with and without PTSD. Although blood pressure was measured much less often as an end point than was heart rate, some of the individual studies found a slight increase of hypertension in people with PTSD. Interpretation of the results is difficult because subjects who had been treated for hypertension were generally excluded, and it is not clear to what extent their hypertension reflected sustained differences, as opposed to an enhanced anticipatory response. A study by Hughes et al. (2006) that was published after the meta-analysis by Buckley and Kaloupek measured heart rate and blood pressure with a beat-to-beat monitor in 80 subjects with PTSD (about one-fourth of whom were combat veterans) and 50 healthy control subjects. They found no difference in resting heart rate or blood pressure between the groups.

One of the most informative methods for studying psychosocial influences on cardiovascular function is 24-hour ambulatory blood-pressure and heart-rate monitoring, which was performed in several small studies. In a study of 11 Vietnam veterans with PTSD and seven without, Muraoka et al. (1998) found that the PTSD group had a significantly higher heart rate (by 9 beats/minute) both when they were awake and when they were asleep and a slightly higher systolic pressure while they were awake, but the difference was not significant. In a study of 117 Vietnam veterans, of whom 61 had PTSD and 56 did not, ambulatory monitoring of heart rate and blood pressure was carried out for 12 hours during the daytime (Beckham et al. 2000, 2003). The blood pressure was the same in the two groups, but there was slightly greater variability in the PTSD group. There was a nonsignificant increase in heart rate (78 vs 75 beats/minute) in the PTSD group. The variability of both blood pressure and heart rate was slightly but significantly higher in the PTSD group. However, there was evidence of an interaction between PTSD and smoking in that smokers who had PTSD had the highest blood pressure (Beckham et al. 2004).

Haley et al. (2004) performed 24-hour monitoring of heart rate, polysomnography, and blood pressure in 22 Gulf War-deployed veterans and 18 nondeployed and found that heart rate declined less during the night in the deployed veterans independent of sleep measures. The heart-rate differences were attributed to differences in vagal control. The nocturnal fall in blood pressure was the same in the two groups.

A more direct way to evaluate resting sympathetic nervous activity is to measure the kinetics of norepinephrine with a radioisotope-dilution technique. In a small study of 12 Vietnam veterans with PTSD and six healthy control subjects, that method failed to show any evidence of increased norepinephrine production (Murburg et al. 1995). It has been reported that 24-hour excretion of urinary catecholamines is increased in patients with PTSD (Yehuda et al. 1992). Plasma catecholamines measured over 24 hours may also be high in PTSD (Yehuda et al. 1998).

The combination of all those findings constitutes fairly strong evidence that resting heart rate is slightly increased in patients with PTSD. In contrast, there is no clear indication that PTSD leads to hypertension. Such changes are of potential significance for the long-term development of heart disease because there is extensive evidence that increased heart rate is a risk factor for both hypertension and cardiovascular events (Palatini and Julius 1997).

Cardiovascular Reactivity

Several studies have established that there is sympathetic hyperreactivity in Vietnam veterans with PTSD as manifested by increases in heart rate, blood pressure, and plasma catecholamines in response to simulated combat (Blanchard et al. 1991; Lindauer et al. 2006; Orr et al. 1998, 2003; Pallmeyer et al. 1986). Beckham et al. (2002) investigated the cardiovascular responses to a relived anger task in 118 male Vietnam combat veterans—62 with PTSD and 56 without it—who were outpatients at a VA medical facility. Current PTSD was diagnosed with the SCID for axis I disorders and the Mississippi Scale for PTSD. Veterans with PTSD reported more combat exposure as measured with the Combat Exposure Scale and had lower socioeconomic status than veterans without PTSD. Participants completed standardized diagnostic measures, hostility measures, and a laboratory session in which they relived a self-chosen anger memory while their heart rate and blood pressure were measured continuously with an Ohmeda Finapres blood-pressure monitor. Baseline diastolic and systolic blood pressure and heart rates did not differ between the two groups; however, veterans with PTSD took less time to feel anger, had greater mean heart rate and greater blood-pressure response during relived anger, and reported greater anger and anxiety during the task. The increased cardiovascular reactivity observed in those studies may be specific to simulated combat.

Orr et al. (1998) also investigated the effects of three stressors on resting heart rate and systolic and diastolic blood pressure in 20 Vietnam veterans with and 15 without combat-related PTSD as diagnosed by the SCID according to criteria of the *DSM-III-R* (all participants were free of drug and alcohol use). Stressors were mental arithmetic and immersion of a hand in icy water for 1 minute. The only difference between the two groups in cardiovascular response was increased diastolic blood pressure in veterans with PTSD, but not those without PTSD; this suggested a reduced autonomic response in PTSD. The findings on mental arithmetic were confirmed by Pallmeyer et al. (1986), who studied heart rate and diastolic and systolic blood pressure in five groups: Vietnam veterans with PTSD ($n = 12$), Vietnam veterans without PTSD but with a comparable level of combat exposure ($n = 10$), Vietnam veterans with other psychiatric disorders ($n = 5$), era veterans without any psychiatric disorders ($n = 5$), and nonveterans with anxiety disorder ($n = 8$); all patients were medication free for the 72-hours prior to testing. Cardiovascular responses were measured during the performance of mental-arithmetic tasks and during repeated exposure to emotionally meaningful combat sounds and music. Veterans with PTSD had higher basal heart rates under all experimental conditions, and they were the only group to show a significant increase in heart rate in response to combat sounds, even at low volume.

Orr et al. (2003) conducted a study of 130 monozygotic twin pairs recruited from the Vietnam Era Twin Registry; in each pair, one twin had served in combat in Vietnam and the other had served in the military but not in Vietnam. PTSD was diagnosed with the CAPS, and each combat-exposed twin completed the Combat Severity Scale and the SCID with *DSM-IV* criteria for other psychiatric disorders. Study participants were exposed to auditory startle stimuli and assessed for heart rate and other skin-conductance and orbicularis oculi electromyographic responses. Twins with PTSD had greater combat severity and greater heart-rate response than twins without PTSD.

Cardiovascular Symptoms

As in studies comparing deployment and nondeployment, PTSD in Gulf War veterans has been found to be associated with an increased prevalence of multiple physical symptoms. Hoge et al. (2007) studied 2863 OIF veterans 1 year after their return from combat duty in Iraq and found that chest pain was reported by 15.1% of veterans who had PTSD but by only 3.5% of those who did not (OR 4.98, 95% CI 3.51-7.05, $p < 0.0001$).

The Veterans Health Study, conducted by the VA at four ambulatory-care medical clinics in the Boston area in 1993-1995, found that veterans with PTSD (n = 351) screened with the PTSD Checklist-Civilian Version were significantly more likely ($p < 0.05$) than veterans without PTSD (n = 1455) to complain of angina (OR 2.09, 95% CI 1.64-2.66) and congestive heart failure (OR 1.64, 95% CI 1.03-2.61) but not high blood pressure (OR 1.24, 95% CI 0.98-1.57) or transient ischemic attacks (OR 1.55, 95% CI 0.88-2.70); ORs were adjusted for age and depression. Health status was assessed with the SF-36 self-administered questionnaire (Spiro et al. 2006).

Falger et al. (1992) found that angina was more common in Dutch World War II resistance fighters than in a control group of men of similar age who had not been in the resistance. About half the resistance fighters had PTSD in 1986, and those with it were more likely to complain of angina (31% vs 14%). An analysis of 605 male veterans of World War II and the Korean War with a followup of about 25 years found no increase in hypertension or CHD in relation to PTSD (Schnurr et al. 2000).

Cardiovascular Disease

Two primary studies assessed the effect of having PTSD on cardiovascular disease, one in Vietnam veterans (Boscarino 2005) and one in World War II and Korean War veterans (Kubzansky et al. 2007).

Boscarino (2005) examined the causes of death among male Vietnam Army veterans about 30 years after their military service and 16 years after they had completed a telephone survey to ascertain their health status. The men were included in a national random sample of veterans from the VES. Cardiovascular mortality was increased in the 836 theater veterans with PTSD but not in the 214 era veterans with PTSD (hazard ratio 1.7, 95% CI 1.0-2.7, p = 0.034).

Kubzansky et al. (2007) analyzed data on two cohorts of 1946 male veterans (average age, 60 and 63 years) who were evaluated for PTSD in 1986 and 1990 and followed for 11-15 years for the Normative Aging Study. Two measures were used to screen for PTSD: the Mississippi Scale for Combat-Related PTSD was administered to 1002 men in 1990 and the Keane PTSD scale was administered to 944 men in 1986. The end points included angina, MI, and death from CHD. Although there was a linear relationship between the severity of PTSD and the incidence of cardiovascular events in both cohorts, it lost significance if there was adjustment for potential confounders (including blood pressure and cholesterol) in both cohorts. Thus, for total CHD events, the RR was 1.19 (95% CI 0.98-1.43) in the Mississippi Scale for Combat-Related PTSD cohort and 1.21 (95% CI 0.99-1.48) in the Keane scale cohort. Adjusting for depression as an additional confounder was attempted in both cohorts. In the Mississippi Scale for Combat-Related PTSD cohort, this was done by using the Center for Epidemiological Studies Depression Scale score, but the relationship between PTSD and total CHD events was still not significant (RR 1.21, 95% CI 0.93-1.57), although it did achieve significance in the Keane scale cohort (RR 1.35, 95% CI 1.03-1.78). However, in the latter case, depression was controlled for by using the Symptom Checklist-90 scale, which is not generally regarded as a robust measure of depression. There was no evidence of any effect of PTSD on mortality.

In a secondary study, Boscarino and Chang (1999) examined the electrocardiograms (ECGs) of 4462 randomly selected male Army veterans: 2490 who were deployed to Vietnam and 1972 who were not. The average interval between deployment and the analysis was 17 years. ECGs, medical examinations, and psychiatric evaluations with the DIS (based on *DSM-III*) were conducted in 1985-1986 at one medical facility. PTSD was present in 54 veterans, anxiety in

186, and depression in 157. All those with PTSD, 66% of those with anxiety, and 71% of those with depression had served in Vietnam. PTSD was associated with increased atrioventricular conduction defects (OR 2.81, 95% CI 1.03-7.66, $p < 0.05$) and MI (OR 4.44, 95% CI 1.20-16.43, $p < 0.05$) adjusted for numerous socioeconomic and health risk factors. Depression was associated with increased arrhythmia (OR 1.98, 95% CI 1.22-3.23, $p < 0.01$). Anxiety disorder was not associated with any ECG abnormalities. The study is limited by the small number of subjects in each psychiatric group.

In another analysis, Boscarino (1997) examined the medical records of 1399 Vietnam veterans from the CDC VES, of whom 332 had PTSD, 17 years after exposure. Circulatory diseases (defined by *ICD-9* codes 401-459) were more common in those with lifetime PTSD than in those without PTSD (25% vs 12.9%, OR 1.62, 95% CI 1.14-2.30) after adjustment for general technical test results at Army induction, race, region of birth, type of enlistment, Vietnam volunteer status, Army marital status, current age, hypochondriasis, physical limitations, psychiatric limitations, postinduction alcohol and drug dependence, cigarette pack-years, education level, and current household income. The study rates as a secondary study because the *ICD-9* codes include a very broad range of conditions, including hypertension and angina.

A meta-analysis of 11 studies reporting on the association between PTSD and cardiovascular end points (either physician-diagnosed or self-reported), which included the secondary studies discussed above (but not the Kubzansky study), found that there was more angina but not more MI in war veterans with PTSD than in those without it (Gander and von Kanel 2006).

Summary and Conclusions

Clinical manifestations of cardiovascular disease take many years to develop, particularly in relatively young people like soldiers at war, so the original source of stress, in this context combat exposure and other forms of deployment stress, will have ended many years before the stress response, such as high blood pressure or MI, becomes apparent. The committee found that self-reports of many cardiovascular symptoms, such as increased heart rate and chest pains, are increased in deployed veterans, particularly those from the Gulf War, compared with their nondeployed counterparts.

Some of the studies reported an increase in hypertension related to deployment, but they are almost all based on self-reports, and others found no effect of deployment. A small increase in the prevalence of hypertension in deployed Gulf War veterans cannot be excluded, but the data cited above are inconsistent, and, because most are based on self-reports, not much reliance can be placed on them. The deployed veterans, particularly those who had unexplained symptoms after the Gulf War, probably sought more medical care, and this alone might increase the likelihood of receiving a diagnosis of hypertension. There are consistent findings that deployment to a war zone, particularly the Gulf War, is associated with an increase in self-reports of many physical symptoms, including chest pain and increased heart rate, but these symptoms do not necessarily imply any structural heart disease.

The two primary studies, one on Gulf War veterans and the other on Vietnam veterans, that used physical examinations for hypertension were both negative. Of the six secondary studies for hypertension, two were negative and four were positive.

Blood lipids, another important risk factor for CHD, do not appear to be affected by deployment, although PTSD may raise them.

Because the potential followup period after the Gulf War is still relatively short (less than 20 years) and the deployed veterans are still relatively young, it is not surprising that there has been no suggestion that Gulf War veterans are at increased risk for CHD as a result of deployment. Symptoms of chest pain are common, but they appear to be part of a nonspecific increase in general symptomatology (see "Symptom Reporting" later in this chapter) and do not themselves imply organic heart disease. Veterans of the Vietnam War are now at an age at which heart disease is prevalent, but again there is no consistent evidence that they are at increased risk as a result of their deployment. All five of the primary studies that assessed CHD in deployed and nondeployed veterans of the Gulf War and the Vietnam War showed no association; the two secondary studies were mixed.

Apart from nonspecific symptoms, the one long-term medical consequence of deployment in the Gulf War and other wars is a marked increase in the rate of PTSD. This appears to involve sensitization of the sympathetic nervous system, but the most consistent finding has been an increase in cardiovascular reactivity to simulated trauma manifested by exaggerated heart-rate and blood-pressure responses. This pattern was observed in three ambulatory studies: one found a significant increase (Muraoka et al. 1998), a second had an increase that did not quite achieve statistical significance (Beckham et al. 2004), and in the third only nighttime heart rate was increased (Haley et al. 2004). The studies that showed increased catecholamine production suggest that it may be explained by increased sympathetic nerve activity although the spectral analysis done by Haley et al. (2004) indicates that altered parasympathetic tone also contributes.

Although there may be an increase in resting heart rate, which is a risk factor for both hypertension and cardiovascular events, PTSD does not appear to lead to hypertension. The results for the association of PTSD and cardiovascular disease are mixed: one primary study and two secondary studies, all from the VES were positive, but one primary study on veterans of World War II and the Korean War found no association. The one primary study showed slight but not significant increase in total CHD in veterans with PTSD. Thus, there is suggestive, but not conclusive, evidence that PTSD increases the risk of CHD.

The committee concludes that there is inadequate/insufficient evidence of an association between deployment to a war zone and hypertension. The committee also concludes that there is inadequate/insufficient evidence of an association between deployment to a war zone and coronary heart disease.

TABLE 6-7 Cardiovascular Diseases

Study	Study Design	Population	Outcomes	Results	Adjustments	Comments
Eisen et al. 2005 NHSGWEVTF (Derived from Kang et al. 2000b)	Cross-sectional, prevalence	1061 GW-deployed veterans vs 1128 nondeployed veterans	Hypertension	Hypertension OR 0.90, 95% CI 0.60-1.33	Age, sex, race, cigarette-smoking, duty type, service branch, rank, education	Study limited by low participation rate, number of years since war
CDC 1988b VES	Retrospective cohort, prevalence, population-based, telephone interview with screening medical examination at followup	2490 Vietnam-theater veterans, 1972 Vietnam-era veterans randomly selected from 7924 theater veterans, 7364 era veterans who had entered Army in 1965-1971	Electrocardiograms, Doppler instrument for peripheral arterial system, physical examination	Hypertension OR 1.1, 95% CI 0.9-1.2; ischemia OR 1.1, 95% CI 0.7-1.7; left ventricular hypertrophy OR 1.8, 95% CI 1.0-3.3; any electrocardiographic finding OR 1.1, 95% CI 0.9-1.3; altered peripheral arterial hemodynamic finding OR 1.2, 95% CI 0.9-1.7	Age at enlistment, race, year of enlistment, enlistment status (volunteer vs draftee), score on general technical test, primary military occupational specialty	Low participation rate in control group; CI not given
Kang and Bullman 2001	Cross-sectional, mortality	621,902 GW-deployed veterans, 746,248 nondeployed veterans	Mortality and vital status determined with VA BIRLS database and SSA Master Beneficiary Record database	Cardiovascular mortality: men rate ratio 0.90, 95% CI 0.81-1.01; women rate ratio 0.96, 95% CI 0.55-1.69	Age, race, service branch, unit component, marital status	Study had good power to detect small increases in risk; limited by relying on death certificates rather than medical records
Gray et al. 1996	Retrospective cohort, hospitalization	547,076 active-duty GW veterans, 618,335 non-GW veterans	Hospital-discharge diagnoses of circulatory system disease	OR about 0.9-1.1 (exact value not given), 95% CI < 1.0 for all 3 years	Prewar hospitalization, sex, age, race, service branch, marital status, rank, length of service, salary, occupation	ORs statistically significantly below 1, but no values given; no separation of specific illnesses

TABLE 6-7 Cardiovascular Diseases

Study	Study Design	Population	Outcomes	Results	Adjustments	Comments
Gray et al. 2000	Retrospective cohort, hospitalization	652,979 GW veterans, 652,922 randomly selected non-GW-deployed veterans	Hospital-discharge diagnoses of circulatory system disease at DoD, VA, COSHPD hospital systems	Circulatory system disease: DoD PMR 0.94, 95% CI 0.91-0.98; VA PMR 0.85, 95% CI 0.76-0.93; COSHPD PMR 0.98, 95% CI 0.82-1.14	Age, sex, race (only for DoD PMR)	Able to assess only illnesses that resulted in hospitalization; possible undetected confounders
Boscarino 2005 (Derived from VES)	Cross-sectional, mortality in subset of VES	7924 Vietnam-theater veterans (836 with PTSD), 7364 Vietnam-era veterans (214 with PTSD)	Mortality determined 30 years after war, based on VA BIRLS and SSA Master Beneficiary Record databases, and National Death Index Plus	Vietnam-theater veterans with PTSD HR 1.7, 95% CI 1.0-2.7, p = 0.034; Vietnam-era veterans with PTSD HR 1.2, 95% CI 0.4-3.4, p = 0.69	Race, Army volunteer status, age at Army entry, Army discharge status, Army illicit-drug abuse, intelligence, age	Risk factors based on self-reports; PTSD status determined with nonvalidated questionnaire
Kubzanky et al. 2007 Normative Aging Study	Cohort study, prospective	1946 veterans from among 2280 community-dwelling men in Greater Boston, MA, area 21-80 years old in 1961	Mailed questionnaire containing MSCRP in 1986 or Keane PTSD scale from MMPI in 1990 used to assess PTSD, physical examination for all cardiovascular risk factors, including biochemical values	Diastolic blood pressure slight correlation (r = -0.06, p = 0.04) between lower diastolic blood pressure and score on MSCRP but not on MMPI-2; higher PTSD scores had slightly greater risk for total CHD (RR 1.21, 95% CI 0.93-1.57); nonfatal MI RR 1.30, 95% CI 0.92-1.84; angina pectoris RR 1.01, 95% CI 0.74-1.37	Age, smoking, blood pressure, serum total cholesterol, BMI, family history of CHD, education, alcohol intake	Response rate 81.2%; study participants assessed with physical examination every 3-5 years

NOTE: BIRLS = Beneficiary Identification and Records Locator Subsystem, BMI = body-mass index, CHD = coronary heart disease, CI = confidence interval, COSHPD = California Office of Statewide Health Planning and Development, DoD = Department of Defense, GW = Gulf War, HR = hazard ratio, MI= myocardial infarction, MMPI = Minnesota Multiphasic Personality Inventory, MSCRP = Mississippi Scale for Combat-Related PTSD, NHSGWEVTF = National Health Survey of Gulf War Era Veterans and Their Families, OR = odds ratio, PMR = proportional morbidity ratio, PTSD = posttraumatic stress disorder, RR = relative risk, SSA = Social Security Administration, VA = Department of Veterans Affairs, VES = Vietnam Experience Study.

RESPIRATORY SYSTEM DISEASES

The term *respiratory disease* encompasses a wide variety of conditions, of which the most prominent is chronic obstructive pulmonary disease (COPD). Asthma and emphysema are common COPDs. It is estimated that every year over 340,000 Americans die of respiratory disease and that more than 35 million Americans live with a chronic respiratory disease (American Lung Association 2007). The well-known risk factors for respiratory disease include smoking and exposure to some environmental contaminants, such as ozone. It is important to note that many factors associated with deployment, such as chemical or particulate air-pollutant exposure on the battlefield, could directly affect respiratory-disease risk.

A few studies of deployed veterans collected focused objective data on respiratory effects (for example, pulmonary-function tests, validated pulmonary outcomes, and physical examination); a larger number of studies did not have a primary focus on respiratory disease and collected more-limited information on respiratory effects and symptoms and often included a respiratory-disease assessment only as part of a larger multisymptom checklist. Although they were not the focus of this committee, a much smaller number of studies evaluated other respiratory risk factors associated with deployment, such as exposure to oil-field smoke, various chemicals, or particles.

For the purposes of this section, the committee defined a primary study according to its methodologic rigor and its use of pulmonary-function testing or a hospital record to identify respiratory effects. A secondary study used self-reported respiratory symptoms or self-reported physician-diagnosed conditions or lacked methodologic rigor. The primary studies of respiratory effects are summarized in Table 6-8.

Primary Studies

The committee identified seven primary studies and numerous secondary studies relevant to its determination of whether there is a link between deployment-related stressors and respiratory diseases. Most of the primary studies assessed veterans of the 1990-1991 Gulf War (Eisen et al. 2005; Gray et al. 1999, 2000; Ishoy et al. 1999; Karlinsky et al. 2004; Kelsall et al. 2004b); one was conducted on Vietnam veterans (CDC 1988b).

The VES was a major study of all U.S. Army Vietnam veterans conducted 15-20 years after the war (CDC 1988b). It surveyed a random sample of all 5 million Army veterans who served during the Vietnam era. The study gathered information in 1985-1986 by telephone interview from 7924 U.S. Army Vietnam veterans and 7364 non-Vietnam veterans; medical examinations were conducted for a random subset of participants (2490 Vietnam and 1972 non-Vietnam veterans). The medical evaluation included pulmonary-function testing using a wedge spirometer and chest x-ray pictures. After adjustment for age at enlistment, race, year of enlistment, and service characteristics, the prevalence of abnormal pulmonary x-ray findings was somewhat elevated (16.0% vs 14.1%, OR 1.1, 95% CI 1.0-1.4), but the frequency of adverse findings did not differ significantly between theater and era veterans for diminished forced expiratory volume in 1 second (FEV1, ≤ 80% of predicted) (10.2% vs 10.9%, OR 0.9, 95% CI 0.7-1.1), diminished forced vital capacity (FVC, ≤ 80% of predicted) (7.1% vs 6.8%, OR 1.0, 95% CI 0.8-1.3), or the FEV1/ FVC% ratio (< 70%) (6.1% vs 6.1%, OR 1.0, 95% CI 0.8-1.3).

In the first phase of VA's nationally representative study, the National Health Survey of Gulf War Era Veterans and Their Families, Kang et al. (2000b) used a stratified random-sampling method to compare 11,441 Gulf War-deployed veterans with 9476 non-Gulf War veterans from the DoD DMDC database. Deployed veterans self-reported more of all but one of the 48 symptoms evaluated for occurrence in the preceding 12 months than did the nondeployed veterans; several of them were respiratory in nature: runny nose, sore throat, coughing, shortness of breath, wheezing, tightness in the chest, sinusitis, bronchitis, and asthma. It is important to note that higher rates of exposure to respiratory irritants (such as exhaust from tent heaters and oil-well smoke) were also reported. The data were not adjusted for potential confounders.

Eisen et al. (2005), using the National Health Survey of Gulf War Era Veterans and Their Families conducted by Kang et al. (2000b), performed medical evaluations, including pulmonary-function testing, of 1061 Gulf War-deployed veterans and 1128 nondeployed veterans at VA medical centers throughout the country. The data were gathered 10 years after the Gulf War. The investigators categorized respiratory conditions as self-reported asthma, bronchitis, emphysema, or obstructive lung disease (history of disease, symptoms plus use of bronchodilators, or 15% improvement in FEV1 after bronchodilator use). After adjustment for age, sex, race, years of education, and cigarette-smoking, no significant differences were observed between deployed and nondeployed veterans in the prevalence of self-reports of asthma, bronchitis, or emphysema (5.9% vs 6.3%, OR 1.07, 95% CI 0.65-1.77) or clinical evaluation for obstructive lung disease (4.5% vs 5.9%, OR 0.91, 95% CI 0.52-1.59).

As phase III of the National Health Survey of Gulf War Era Veterans and Their Families, Karlinsky et al. (2004) conducted a cross-sectional survey of 1036 U.S. Gulf War-deployed veterans and 1103 nondeployed veterans 10 years after deployment. The goal of this phase was to assess late-onset respiratory symptoms and pulmonary-function abnormalities. The study subjects were queried about self-reported symptoms and physician-diagnosed illnesses and hospitalizations and received medical examinations in 1999-2001, including pulmonary-function tests with spirometers. The analyses did not adjust for smoking or other confounders, but slightly more deployed veterans (51%) than nondeployed veterans (44%) had a history of smoking. Deployed veterans had more self-reports of wheezing than did nondeployed veterans (OR 1.67, 95% CI 1.06-2.62), but there were no statistical differences between the two groups in cough (OR 1.12, 95% CI 0.80-1.57), physician visits for pulmonary complaints (OR 1.07, 95% CI 0.51-2.24), pulmonary hospitalizations (OR 0.91, 95% CI 0.13-6.51), asthma (OR 0.90, 95% CI 0.50-1.62), bronchitis (OR 1.08, 95% CI 0.50-2.34), or emphysema (OR 4.45, 95% CI 0.74-26.68).

Ishoy et al. (1999) evaluated respiratory effects in 1997-1998 in a population-based cohort of Danish soldiers who participated in peacekeeping operations in the Persian Gulf region in 1990-1997. The study population consisted of 686 deployed veterans and 231 age- and sex-matched nondeployed veterans. Respiratory disease was assessed by pulmonary-function testing with a Vitalograph spirometer. No differences in smoking status were observed between the groups, and no significant differences were observed between deployed and nondeployed veterans in mean FVC (100.7 ± 11.6 standard deviation [SD] vs 100.7 ± 13.1 SD), mean FEV1 (95.6 ± 11.8 SD vs 96.4 ± 13.7 SD), and peak flow (94.0 ± 19.0 SD 19.0 vs 92.8 ± 19.1 SD).

In 1994, Gray et al. (1999) surveyed U.S. Navy Seabees from 14 commands who were still on active duty for at least 3 years after the Gulf War (n = 527) and nondeployed Seabees (n = 970). The study subjects were queried about self-reported physician-diagnosed illnesses, symptoms, and exposures. They also underwent pulmonary-function testing with a spirometer and a pneumotach flow-measuring device; data were adjusted for age, height, race, and cigarette-smoking. Active-duty Gulf War Seabees were significantly more likely than nondeployed Seabees to report either cough (OR 1.8, 95% CI 1.2-2.8) or shortness of breath (OR 4.0, 95% CI 2.2-7.3). Markers of pulmonary function did not differ between the deployed and nondeployed veterans: FVC 4.96 L vs 4.99 L, respectively ($p = 0.77$), and FEV1 4.05 L vs 4.04 L, respectively ($p = 0.81$). This study is limited in that it surveyed only active-duty Seabees.

In a cross-sectional survey comparing 1456 Australian Gulf War veterans with 1588 nondeployed veterans, study subjects gave self-reports of their respiratory symptoms in the preceding 12 months and underwent spirometric pulmonary-function testing and a physical examination (Kelsall et al. 2004b). The data were gathered in 2000-2002. Deployed veterans reported significantly more respiratory symptoms (wheeze, nocturnal chest tightness, cough, and dyspnea) than did nondeployed veterans. They also reported more asthma (OR 1.4, 95% CI 1.1-1.9) and chronic bronchitis (OR 1.9, 95% CI 1.2-3.1) but were not at increased risk for airflow limitations, defined as FEV1/FCV% < 70% (OR 0.8, 95% CI 0.5-1.1) or emphysema (OR 1.0, 95% CI 0.8-1.4). Furthermore, there were no statistically significant differences between deployed and nondeployed veterans in any lung-function indexes (FEV1, FCV, or FEV1/FVC%). ORs were adjusted for age, height, smoking, weight, atopy, rank, service, education, and marital status. The study used self-reports of a physician's diagnosis or treatment for a diagnosis to determine the prevalence of asthma and bronchitis. During the medical-examination phase of the study, a physician queried each veteran about responses to the questionnaire regarding asthma and bronchitis and classified the likelihood of the diagnosis on a scale from unlikely to probable. Possible exposures to dust and oil-well fires were considered as possible contributors to the respiratory effects seen in the deployed veterans. Based on the European Community Respiratory Health Survey definition of respiratory disease, the only significant risk factor for increased asthma in deployed veterans was having an asthma attack or being awakened by shortness of breath at any time in the preceding 12 months or current use of asthma medications. For bronchitis, the only significant definition was having a doctor's first diagnosis of chronic bronchitis in 1991 or later. However, if other definitions of the diseases were used, the differences between the two groups were not significant. The study had a response rate of 80.5% for the deployed veterans and 56.8% for the nondeployed.

Gray et al. (2000) conducted a study of hospital-discharge records of three hospital systems for 1991-1994: those of DoD, VA, and California Office of Statewide Health Planning and Development. PMRs of hospital-discharge diagnoses of 652,979 Gulf War veterans and 652,922 era veterans not deployed to the gulf were compared. With adjustment for age, sex, and race, the PMRs for respiratory-disease were 1.02 (95% CI 0.99-1.04) for the DoD hospitals, 1.19 (95% CI 1.10-1.29) for the VA hospitals, and 1.06 (95% CI 0.82-1.29) for the California hospitals.

Secondary Studies

The committee identified numerous large, well-designed studies of Gulf War veterans that it considered secondary mainly because the absence of examinations for respiratory effects led to imprecision regarding evaluation of respiratory disease or lack of adequate adjustment for major confounding variables.

In addition to the study by Kang et al. (2000b) discussed above, other large, well-designed cohort studies from several countries show mixed findings regarding the presence of respiratory disease in veterans based on self-reporting via questionnaires. Proctor et al. (1998) looked at 252 U.S. Gulf War-deployed veterans—186 from the Fort Devens cohort and 66 from the New Orleans cohort—and compared them with 48 veterans deployed to Germany during the Gulf War. They did not observe any significant differences between groups in chronic lung problems, chronic respiratory symptoms, or allergies. However, a number of other studies—including Gulf War veterans from several U.S. states (Iowa Persian Gulf Study Group 1997; McCauley et al. 2002b; Spiro et al. 2006; Steele 2000), Canada (Goss Gilroy Inc. 1998), Australia (O'Toole et al. 1996b), and the United Kingdom (Hotopf et al. 2006; Simmons et al. 2004; Unwin et al. 1999)—asked veterans about respiratory symptoms and found that deployed Gulf War veterans had a higher prevalence of self-reports of a variety of respiratory symptoms (colds, asthma, emphysema, chronic bronchitis, persistent cough, and lung disease) than nondeployed controls. Because of their reliance on self-reports or questionnaires, all those studies are vulnerable to recall or reporting bias and a lack specificity regarding the outcome.

Gray et al. (2002) found that Gulf War-deployed Seabees self-reported more asthma with onset after August 1991 (2.4%) than did Seabees deployed to areas other than the gulf (1.7%) or nondeployed Seabees (1.5%); that indicated that deployed Seabees were at increased risk for asthma compared with nondeployed Seabees (OR 1.82, 95% CI 1.23-2.69). However, although adjustments were made for age, sex, active-duty or reserve status, race or ethnicity, current smoking, and current alcohol drinking, exposures to a number of toxicants were possible confounders.

Gray et al. (1996) used hospitalization records from DoD medical facilities to compare the prevalence of *ICD-9* respiratory diseases in 547,076 veterans deployed to the Gulf War compared with 618,335 nondeployed veterans. The OR for respiratory diseases decreased from slightly greater than 1 in 1991 to slightly less than 1 in 1993 (exact values not given).

Posttraumatic Stress Disorder and Respiratory Diseases

Self-reported health status was assessed in a cross-sectional survey that used a mailed questionnaire sent to 1259 female U.S. veterans who received care at the VA Puget Sound Health Care System in 1996-1998 (Dobie et al. 2004). The women were screened for PTSD with the PTSD Checklist-Civilian Version. Compared with female veterans who did not have PTSD (n = 940), those with PTSD (n = 266) had a greater prevalence of emphysema (13.8% vs 10.7%, OR 1.88, 95% CI 1.21-2.92) and asthma (24.4% vs 17.3%, OR 1.64, 95% CI 1.17-2.31%) adjusted for age. It is unclear whether the excess of respiratory symptoms could be explained by higher rates of smoking in the veterans with PTSD (39.5% vs 22.9).

Boscarino (1997), using data from the VES, found a modest but significantly higher prevalence of respiratory diseases in Vietnam veterans who had lifetime combat-related PTSD (n = 1067) than in those without PTSD (n = 332) (OR 1.54, 95% CI 1.02-2.35, p = 0.042) adjusted for a variety of demographic, social, and Army characteristics.

A study of Gulf War veterans found no statistical difference in self-reporting of pulmonary symptoms (difficulty in breathing, shortness of breath, common cold or influenza, and rapid breathing) between deployed veterans with PTSD or MDD or both (n = 20) and deployed veterans with neither psychiatric condition (n = 178) or veterans who were deployed to Germany during the Gulf War (n = 48) (Wolfe et al. 1999).

Summary and Conclusions

The committee placed the greatest weight on studies that included a medical evaluation, identified specific respiratory diagnoses, and adjusted for potential confounding variables.

Although an association between deployment and respiratory effects was noted in some studies that assessed respiratory effects on the basis of self-reports of symptoms, studies that used more objective markers of respiratory disease (such as pulmonary-function tests and respiratory examinations) did not document a consistent relationship between deployment and respiratory disease.

None of the primary studies considered for respiratory effects (one study in Vietnam veterans and six in Gulf War veterans) found a higher risk of chronic respiratory effects in deployed than in nondeployed veterans on the basis of objective measures of pulmonary function and disease. However, deployed veterans reported more symptoms of respiratory effects, such as cough and shortness of breath, in one Gulf War study and of asthma and chronic bronchitis in a second Gulf War study than did the nondeployed veterans. In both studies, on examination, pulmonary function was not compromised in the deployed groups. Of the 12 secondary studies that relied on self-reports of respiratory effects, 11 found that deployed Gulf War veterans reported more symptoms of respiratory effects. The one secondary study that assessed hospitalizations of Gulf War veterans for respiratory disease found no increase in risk.

Results regarding the relationship between PTSD and respiratory effects are mixed. No primary studies were identified; in the secondary studies, although modest increases in respiratory symptoms were reported in Vietnam veterans and in female veterans with PTSD, no such increase was seen in a small study of Gulf War veterans.

Respiratory conditions are common in veterans regardless of deployment status. The population burden of asthma and COPD in all U.S. adults is high, but COPD takes many years to develop and is uncommon in people under the age of 50 years. The prevalence of respiratory disease is even higher in adults with a history of cigarette-smoking. Thus, with additional followup of the veterans, future studies might show an effect of war-related stress. Many studies fail to make clear whether there is a direct relationship between deployment stress and increased pulmonary complaints as opposed to some other mediating or moderating factor. Veterans of the Gulf War were exposed to numerous air pollutants, including smoke from oil-well fires, pesticides, exhaust from tent heaters, and possibly chemical-warfare agents. Veterans of other conflicts may have similar exposures to toxicants and to other agents, such as Agent Orange in the case of Vietnam veterans. Many of the studies considered by the committee identified other possible exposures of veterans, particular those who were deployed to the Gulf War, but were unable to eliminate possible confounding when assessing risks. The association between increased Gulf War deployment and cigarette-smoking is unknown. Cigarette-smoking was not controlled in the analyses in a number of the studies so it is unclear to what degree smoking may account for any increase in respiratory symptoms, complaints, or disease.

The few studies that collected more-objective data on respiratory outcomes—such as data on pulmonary-function testing, data from physical examinations, and data on verified pulmonary events from medical-record review or physician questionnaires—did not find strong indications of increased risk among veterans with combat deployment. The vast majority of available studies of veterans with respiratory diseases were not specifically designed to focus on these outcomes as primary variables but derived information from a larger nonspecific self-administered symptom checklist.

The committee concludes that there is inadequate/insufficient evidence to determine whether an association exists between deployment to a war zone and chronic respiratory effects.

TABLE 6-8 Respiratory System Diseases

Study	Study Design	Population	Outcomes	Results	Adjustments	Comments
CDC 1988 VES	Retrospective cohort, prevalence, population-based, telephone interview with screening medical examination at followup	2490 Vietnam-theater veterans, 1972 Vietnam-era veterans randomly selected from 7924 theater veterans and 7364 era veterans who entered Army in 1965-1971	Chest x-ray findings, pulmonary-function tests	Chest x-ray OR 1.1, 95% CI 1.0-1.4; FEV1 ≤ 80% of predicted OR 0.9, 95% CI 0.7-1.1; FVC ≤ 80% of predicted OR 1.0, 95% CI 0.8-1.3; FEV1/ FVC < 70% OR 1.0, 95% CI 0.8-1.3	Age at enlistment, race, year of enlistment, enlistment status (volunteer vs draftee), score on general technical test, primary military occupational specialty	Low participation rate in control group
Eisen et al. 2005 NHSGWEVTF (Derived from Kang et al. 2000b)	Cross-sectional, prevalence	1061 GW-deployed veterans, 1128 nondeployed veterans	Self-reported asthma, bronchitis, or emphysema; obstructive lung disease (history of disease or symptoms and use of bronchodilators or 15% improvement in FEV1 after bronchodilator use)	Asthma, bronchitis, or emphysema OR 1.07, 95% CI 0.65-1.77; obstructive lung disease OR 0.91, 95% CI 0.52-1.59	Age, sex, race, cigarette-smoking, duty type, service branch, rank	Study limited by low participation rate and number of years since war
Karlinsky et al. 2004 NHSGWEVTF (Derived from Kang et al. 2000b)	Cross-sectional	1036 GW-deployed, 1103 nondeployed, assessed 10 years after war	Pulmonary-function tests with spirometer, self-reports of respiratory symptoms or use of medication	Cough OR 1.12, 95% CI 0.80-1.57; wheezing OR 1.67, 95% CI 1.06-2.62; physician visits for pulmonary complaints OR 1.07, 95% CI 0.51-2.24; pulmonary hospitalization: OR 0.91, 95% CI 0.13-6.51; asthma OR 0.90, 95% CI 0.50-1.62; bronchitis OR 1.08, 95% CI 0.50-2.34; emphysema OR 4.45, 95% CI 0.74-26.68	Age, height, smoking status, weight, education, service characteristics	No adjustment for smoking although smoking history reported

TABLE 6-8 Respiratory System Diseases

Study	Study Design	Population	Outcomes	Results	Adjustments	Comments
Ishoy et al. 1999	Cross-sectional	686 Danish peacekeepers deployed to gulf in 1990-1997, 231 age- and sex-matched armed forces nondeployed controls	Health examination by physician, including lung function and self-report questionnaire	No significant differences in lung-function values for FVC, FEV1, peak flow between groups		Participation rate 83.6% deployed, 57.8% nondeployed
Gray et al. 1999	Cross-sectional, medical evaluation	527 GW veterans, 970 nondeployed from 14 U.S. Navy Seabees commands	Pulmonary-function testing with spirometer with Fleisch-type pneumotach flow-measuring device	Cough OR 1.8, 95% CI 1.2-2.8; shortness of breath OR 4.0, 95% CI 2.2-7.3; FVC 4.96 L deployed, 4.99 L nondeployed, p = 0.77; FEV1 4.05 L deployed, 4.04 L nondeployed, p = 0.81	Age, height, race, smoking status	Only active-duty Seabees surveyed
Kelsall et al. 2004b	Cross-sectional	1456 deployed Australian GW veterans, 1588 nondeployed veterans	Self reports of symptoms, pulmonary-function testing with spirometer	Self-reported asthma OR 1.4, 95% CI 1.1-1.9; bronchitis OR 1.9, 95% CI 1.2-3.1; air flow limitation OR 0.8, 95% CI 0.5-1.1; emphysema OR 1.0, 95% CI 0.8-1.4; lung-function indexes all ORs -0.04-0.7	Age, height, smoking, weight, atopy, education, marital status, service, rank	Although physician reviewed and classified likelihood of accuracy of self-report of diagnosis, no physical examinations conducted except for lung function
Gray et al. 2000	Retrospective cohort, hospitalization	652,979 GW veterans, 652,922 randomly selected nondeployed veterans	Hospital-discharge diagnoses of respiratory disease in DoD, VA, COSHPD hospital systems	DoD PMR 1.02, 95% CI 0.99-1.04; VA PMR 1.19, 95% CI 1.10-1.29; CA PMR 1.06, 95% CI 0.82-1.29	Age, sex, race	Able to assess only illnesses that resulted in hospitalization; possible undetected confounders

NOTE: CDC = Centers for Disease Control and Prevention, CI = confidence interval, COSHPD = California Office of Statewide Health Planning and Development, DoD = Department of Defense, FEV1 = forced expiratory volume in 1 second, FVC = forced vital capacity, GW = Gulf War, OR = odds ratio, NHSGWEVTF = National Health Survey of Gulf War Era Veterans and Their Families, PMR = proportional morbidity ratio, VA = Department of Veterans Affairs, VES = Vietnam Experience Study.

DIGESTIVE SYSTEM DISORDERS

Soon after the Gulf War, veterans reported gastrointestinal (GI) symptoms more frequently than most other symptoms (Kang et al. 2000b). That is understandable because there is a common and scientifically recognized association between acute and chronic stress and GI dysfunction (Creed et al. 2006; Drossman and Chang 2003). This dysfunction can lead to changes in intestinal movements (motility) that affect gastric emptying rates and intestinal transit time which in turn cause nausea, vomiting, bloating, diarrhea, and constipation. Psychological distress can also affect sensitivity of the visceral nerves, thus producing abdominal discomfort and pain (Drossman 2002, 2006a,b; Kellow et al. 2006a,b) (see Chapter 4 for more discussion on GI dysfunction in response to stress).

The functional GI disorders or syndromes, such as irritable bowel syndrome (IBS) and functional dyspepsia, are characterized by recurrent or prolonged clusters of symptoms that range in severity from occasional mild episodes to more persistent and disabling episodes with impaired health-related quality of life. So named because they are disturbances of GI functioning rather than diseases, these disorders are understood in a biopsychosocial construct (Drossman 1998); that is, genetic or early environmental predisposing factors, including family enablement of illness behaviors (Levy et al. 2000) and a history of early trauma or abuse (Drossman et al. 1995), coupled with acute or chronic exposure to stress or acute GI infection (Spiller and Campbell 2006) can precipitate or exacerbate the disorders. The disorders are then sustained or perpetuated in the presence of psychologic comorbidities, including PTSD, anxiety, depression, maladaptive coping style, and impaired social networks (Creed et al. 2006; Drossman et al. 2002; Levy et al. 2006).

Of particular relevance here is the growing evidence of development of postinfectious IBS. In some cases, functional GI disorders are triggered by pathogens, which usually cause acute gastroenteritis, and the symptoms are then sustained by stressful conditions (Drossman 1999; Dunlop et al. 2003; McKeown et al. 2006; Spiller and Campbell 2006). From a biologic perspective, the functional GI syndromes are characterized by dysregulation of neural pathways between the brain and gut (that is, the brain-gut axis) that produces persistent motility and sensory disturbances (visceral hypersensitivity), dysregulation of the hypothalamic-pituitary-adrenal (HPA) axis (see Chapter 4), alteration in corticolimbic pain modulation, and inflammation of the bowel mucosa associated with altered bacterial flora (Drossman 2006a,b; Drossman et al. 2002). Diagnosis of a functional GI disorder is based on identification of specific bowel symptoms that fulfill the Rome Criteria[1] and a minimal period of symptoms, usually 6 months (Drossman 2006a,b). The diagnostic criteria have rarely been included in the assessment of Gulf War veterans, so the veterans' diagnoses have been presumptive, that is, based on sufficient clusters of symptoms that are consistent with the Rome criteria for diagnosis. However, diagnostic criteria were used in a few supportive studies of selected cohorts of Gulf War veterans that yielded relevant physiologic data (Dunphy et al. 2003).

---

[1]The Rome Criteria, developed by the Rome Foundation, are symptom-based diagnostic criteria for functional GI disorders, including functional gastroduodenal disorders, functional bowel disorders, and the group of disorders formerly referred to as functional biliary disorders. IBS is defined by Rome III criteria as abdominal discomfort or pain of at least 3 months' duration in which two of the following three are present: pain that is improved by defecation, association of the onset of pain with a change in the frequency of the stool, and association of the onset of pain with a change in the consistency (looser or harder) of the stool (http://www.romecriteria.org).

GI diseases, sometimes called organic or structural, such as peptic ulcer or inflammatory bowel disease (that is, ulcerative colitis or Crohn's disease), are characterized by morphologic abnormalities seen on x-ray pictures, endoscopically, or through laboratory tests. For example, in inflammatory bowel disease, intestinal inflammation may lead to ulcerations, strictures, and bowel injury. Acute stress can produce symptoms and even activate symptoms in people with existing disease (see Chapter 4), but the relationship of chronic stress to the onset of disease is difficult to study because onset may take years.

For the purposes of this section, the committee defined primary studies according to their methodologic rigor (see Chapter 2) and outcome assessment, requiring sufficiently valid symptom clusters consistent with a functional GI diagnosis or, in the case of structural diseases, physical examination. Although the committee identified several papers that assessed the development of GI effects in veterans with PTSD, none met the criteria for a primary study, so they are discussed only as secondary studies. The primary studies and several secondary studies are summarized in Table 6-9.

Primary Studies

To determine the link between deployment-related stressors and GI diseases and disorders, the committee identified three primary studies (Eisen et al. 2005; Gray et al. 2002; Sostek et al. 1996) of deployment and GI effects and several secondary studies. During the Gulf War, U.S. Navy Seabees were responsible for building airports, supply points, and roads. Gray et al. (2002) surveyed nearly 12,000 active-duty, deployed and nondeployed Seabees in 14 commands who were still on active duty at least 3 years after the Gulf War. The subjects gave self-reports of physician-diagnosed illnesses, symptoms, and exposures. IBS was one of the physician-diagnosed illnesses listed on the survey. Active-duty Gulf War Seabees were much more likely than nondeployed Seabees to report having a diagnosis of peptic ulcer disease (OR 3.11, 95% CI 1.67-5.78), any new GI disease diagnosed after September 1990 (OR 2.10, 95% CI 1.39-3.17), or IBS (2.48% vs 0.81%, OR 3.57, 95% CI 2.22-5.73). IBS was one of a cluster of four physician-diagnosed conditions—PTSD, CFS, and multiple chemical sensitivity were the other three—found to be more prevalent among Gulf War-deployed Seabees, and the four conditions were highly associated with one another. Among the deployed Seabees, receiving a diagnosis of one of the four also was associated with reporting 13-18 other symptoms, whereas deployed Seabees who did not report any of the four had fewer (average, six) other symptoms. The clustering of the symptoms and conditions is consistent with emerging data that indicate that multiple symptom reporting is associated with psychologic trauma, which may disrupt central mechanisms for filtering incoming visceral and somatic neural signals (Drossman et al. 1996; Mayer 2006; Whitehead et al. 2002). Because the focus of the study was to cluster symptoms and conditions that might shed light on a unique Gulf War illness, the analysis undertook no further evaluation of GI conditions in isolation. It was not possible to discern how a diagnosis of IBS was made. Another limitation is that the study included only active-duty veterans and thus was not representative of all Gulf War veterans.

A study by Sostek et al. (1996) focused on evaluating the prevalence and spectrum of GI complaints in a group of 57 Gulf War-deployed veterans and 44 veteran controls from the same National Guard who were not deployed to the gulf. A 68-item survey asked the veterans to rate the frequency of their GI symptoms and other symptoms before, during, and after the war. There were no differences between the groups in demographics and no differences in prewar smoking, alcohol or medication consumption, or psychologic problems. The reporting of medical, including GI, symptoms was low (0-9%) and not different between groups. During the war, Gulf War veterans reported markedly higher rates of GI symptoms (abdominal pain, 63%; gas, 60%; nausea and vomiting, 39%; diarrhea, 67%; and blood in the stool, 23%) than the nondeployed veterans, and about 80% remained symptomatic after the war. The high reported proportion with blood in the stool suggests that the symptoms may have been related in part to intestinal infections. Postwar comparisons showed significant differences between deployed veterans and controls in abdominal pain (70% vs 9%, p = 0.001), relief of pain with bowel movements (47% vs 16%, p = 0.05), postprandial pain (46% vs 14%, p = 0.05), pain associated with increased or watery bowel movements (44% vs 5%, p = 0.001), loose stools (74% vs 18%, p = 0.001), mucus in the stools (19% vs 0%, p = 0.05), and incomplete rectal evacuation (60% vs 7%, p = 0.001). The frequency of blood in the stool was low and not significantly different between groups. In addition, deployed veterans reported significantly higher frequencies of all 10 non-GI symptoms, including headache, fatigue, and joint pains. A strength of the study is that it asked specific GI questions that were more than sufficient to meet the Rome criteria for IBS, functional dyspepsia, and possibly other functional GI disorders (Drossman 2006; Longstreth et al. 2006a,b). Furthermore, the temporal association of symptom development in deployed veterans, possibly enabled by exposure to infectious bacteria, and the retention of symptoms to a significantly higher degree than the controls after the war, strongly supports an association of GI-symptom development with war-zone exposure. The study may be limited by the relatively small sample compared with samples in larger epidemiologic studies, although type I error given these findings is unlikely. Considering the study design, there is also a possibility of retrospective recall bias.

Ten years after the Gulf War, in the National Health Survey of Gulf War Era Veterans and Their Families, a nationally representative population-based study, VA conducted medical evaluations that included dyspepsia to determine the prevalence of common diseases in deployed veterans (Eisen et al. 2005). In 1999-2001, 1061 deployed and 1128 nondeployed veterans were evaluated at several VA centers. The veterans had been randomly selected from 11,441 deployed and 9476 nondeployed veterans who had participated in a 1995 VA survey (Kang et al. 2000b) that used a self-report questionnaire. Dyspepsia was diagnosed through in-person interviews according to two criteria: a history or symptoms of dyspepsia (frequent heartburn and recurrent abdominal pain) and use of antacids, histamine-2 receptor blockers, or other medications to treat dyspepsia. The prevalence of dyspepsia was 9.1% and 6.0% in deployed and nondeployed veterans, respectively (OR 1.87, 95% CI 1.16-2.99); the prevalence of gastritis was 5.9% and 4.2%, respectively (OR 1.57, 95% CI 0.88-2.78). A study limitation is that dyspepsia was diagnosed crudely as recurrent abdominal pain or frequent heartburn, which is more commonly associated with gastroesophageal reflux disease. Furthermore, IBS, a more common functional GI disorder, was not evaluated. Finally, despite three recruitment waves, the participation rate in the 2005 study was low: only 53% of Gulf War veterans and 39% of nondeployed veterans invited to participate were examined during the second phase of the study. To determine nonparticipation bias, the authors gathered previously collected findings from participants and nonparticipants from the DMDC and sociodemographic and self-reported health findings from the earlier VA study (Kang et al. 2000b). Both deployed and nondeployed participants were more likely than nonparticipants to report heartburn or indigestion; although this could limit the generalizability of findings, the authors adjusted for the disparity in their analysis of population prevalence.

Secondary Studies

Most large-scale Gulf War cohort studies conducted in several countries found a postwar excess of self-reported GI symptoms in deployed vs nondeployed military personnel (Kelsall et al. 2004a; Proctor et al. 1998; Simmons et al. 2004; Unwin et al. 1999). Some specifically reported increased rates of "bowel disorder, including diarrhea, constipation, or bleeding" (Kelsall et al. 2004a). Those studies are limited by being based largely on self-reports. Furthermore, most did not address functional GI disorders, such as IBS, through questionnaires or medical evaluations. A final limitation of many studies is that the outcome being measured was too broad, such as the *ICD* category Diseases of the Digestive System.

In the 1995 prevalence survey of Gulf War veterans by Kang et al. (2000b) discussed above, gastritis and frequent diarrhea were among the top five medical conditions self-reported by deployed (25.2% and 21.2%, respectively) vs non-deployed veterans (11% and 5.9%, respectively) during the preceding 12 months. Enteritis and colitis were reported less frequently but were also more prevalent in deployed than in nondeployed veterans (6.6% vs 2.8% and 4.6% vs 2.2%, respectively). When asked about individual symptoms on the same questionnaire, veterans often reported GI symptoms at high rates. Of more than 50 symptoms, heartburn and indigestion were among the 10 most frequently reported; they also were among the top 10 symptoms reported as severe. Gulf War veterans reported many other symptoms, and that is consistent with the possibility that the stress of war is associated physiologically with the setting of low central nervous system (CNS) thresholds for symptom experience and reporting (see Chapter 4). Because these are self-report data, it is likely that the reports of gastritis, enteritis, and colitis represent functional GI symptoms rather than organic diseases. Nevertheless, the findings support a greater prevalence of those GI and other symptoms in deployed veterans than in nondeployed controls.

Eisen et al. (1991) assessed data from the Vietnam Era Twin Registry to determine whether service in the Vietnam theater increased the risk of physical health problems. Twin pairs (n = 2260) that were discordant for currently having, ever having, or having been hospitalized for stomach conditions were surveyed for self-reports of a variety of physical health problems. Deployed twins were at slightly greater risk for ever having a stomach condition, such as dyspepsia (OR 1.4, 95% CI 1.0-1.9), or having been hospitalized for a stomach condition (OR 2.6, 95% CI 1.4-4.9) than the nondeployed twins. Being hospitalized for a stomach condition was also associated with combat exposure although the relationship was not linear.

Some studies that did not assess war-zone deployment but did assess surrogate traumatic exposures in other populations lend support to the primary data. One prospective cohort study of IBS patients in a gastroenterology practice in Romania (Dumitrascu and Baban 1991) had several evaluation times beginning with the death of Nikolai Ceausescu in December 1990. Sixty IBS patients were tracked with regard to their bowel symptoms after a political uprising in Romania in December 1989 and in January, March, and June 1990. The trauma was related not only to the political upheaval but to exposure to television images of street fighting when previously all television programs had been censored. Painful GI episodes were reported by 80% of the patients at the onset of the uprising but only 33% of them reported painful episodes 6 months later. The value of this study is in the certainty of the IBS diagnosis and in its prospective design.

A case-control study of patients hospitalized in Israel for non-GI complaints (Stermer et al. 1991) looked at the prevalence of GI symptoms in 239 Eastern European Holocaust survivors and 384 Eastern Europeans not exposed to the Nazis. The study used a checklist of 13 GI symptoms—including abdominal pain, irregular bowels, diarrhea, constipation, distention, nausea, and vomiting—that were consistent with criteria for IBS, dyspepsia, aerophagia, and other functional symptoms; the results showed that all the symptoms were significantly more common in the Holocaust survivors ($p < 0.0001$-0.02). The study concluded that functional GI symptoms were more severe and more protracted (often for 15-40 years) among those more heavily exposed to trauma.

A study involving victims of a severe flash flood and mudslides in Puerto Rico, in which almost 200 people were killed, reported more new-onset GI symptoms than in unexposed controls (Escobar et al. 1992). Over 1550 people had been interviewed in 1984, one year before the disaster as part of an epidemiologic study; 375 of them were reinterviewed in 1987, a little more than a year after the disaster. This prospective study reported incident symptoms.

Finally, physiologic studies have yielded strong evidence of an association of acute or chronic stress with altered GI functioning and symptoms. One study of 12 Gulf War veterans, who reported the development of chronic abdominal pain and diarrhea during their time in gulf, showed that those veterans had greater pain intensity, pain unpleasantness, visceral sensitivity, and anxiety in relation to rectal distention and cutaneous hand stimulation than had deployed veterans without reports of chronic abdominal pain or civilians (Dunphy et al. 2003). Other studies in civilians with IBS have shown altered autonomic activity and lower pain thresholds in response to acute physical and psychologic stress (Murray et al. 2004) and a greater association of altered GI motility and GI symptoms with corticotropin-releasing hormone, a stress hormone, compared with controls without IBS (Fukudo et al. 1998). A full review of this subject can be found in Kellow et al. (2006a,b).

Studies of associations of war-zone deployment with structural GI diseases, such as peptic ulcer or inflammatory bowel disease, have been reported in some epidemiologic studies. However, none provides sufficient evidence to document a diagnosis. Furthermore, several studies have attributed such diagnoses as gastritis and colitis to functional GI symptoms in the absence of sufficient documentation that the criteria for the diseases have been met.

Posttraumatic Stress Disorder and Gastrointestinal Effects

An association between functional GI disorders and PTSD appears to be caused by more than chance; however, the committee was unable to identify any studies on PTSD and functional GI disorders that met its criteria for primary studies, mainly because PTSD was assessed only by screening and not by an actual diagnosis. The studies discussed below are all secondary studies.

As many as 36% of patients with IBS have been found to have PTSD and other psychiatric comorbidities (Irwin et al. 1996). Several studies have dealt with the question of whether deployment-related PTSD is associated with GI symptoms. Studying OIF veterans a year after their return, Hoge et al. (2007) found that veterans who had PTSD (16.6% of them on the basis of the PTSD Symptom Checklist) were about 2-3 times more likely than veterans without PTSD to report being frequently bothered by stomach pain (OR 3.86, 95% CI 2.80-5.33); constipation, loose bowels, or diarrhea (OR 3.02, 95% CI 2.28-4.00); and nausea, gas, or indigestion (OR 3.44, 95% CI 2.65-4.48).

Gulf War veterans who screened positive for PTSD reported a higher prevalence of GI symptoms and conditions than those without PTSD although the symptoms were not specified (Barrett et al. 2002a). Using data from the Normative Aging Study of older male World War II and Korean War veterans, Schnurr et al. (2000) found that veterans who screened positive for PTSD ($n > 590$) were more likely also to have new-onset lower GI-tract symptoms (hazard rate

1.23, 95% CI 1.04-1.45) according to physical examinations conducted periodically since the 1960s. PTSD was assessed with the Mississippi Scale for Combat-Related TPSD. In the final multivariate model, lower GI disorders increased by 23% for every 10-point increment in PTSD symptom scores. A study of Vietnam veterans from the VES found GI disturbances of a nonspecific nature to be more common in those with a diagnosis of combat-related PTSD (n = 332) than in those without PTSD (n = 1067) (OR 1.47, 95% CI 1.02-2.10) (Boscarino 1997). Finally, Dobie et al. (2004), in a study of female veterans who had received treatment at the VA Puget Sound Health Care System, found that women who screened positive for current PTSD (n = 266) were more likely than those who screened negative (n = 940) to report IBS (37% vs 18%, OR 2.82, 95% CI 2.06-3.85).

Overall, most of the secondary studies are limited by self-reporting and cross-sectional design, which enables them to assess only comorbidity. Furthermore, the reported GI symptoms are among many other somatic symptoms reported at high frequency, and this raises the likelihood that PTSD may be like other stress-related conditions in being associated with a general tendency to set lower sensation thresholds and thus to lead to multiple symptom reporting. A limitation of studies that aimed to link PTSD with GI illness is that they used screening criteria, rather than in-person psychiatric evaluation, to assess PTSD.

Summary and Conclusions

GI symptoms and functional GI disorders have been associated with war-zone deployment in two large-scale and well-designed primary studies of veteran populations and one smaller primary study that used adequate criteria to identify functional GI disorders in Gulf War veterans. The nationally representative study of Gulf War veterans, which relied on medical evaluations, found a relationship between deployment and symptoms of dyspepsia (Eisen et al. 2005); Gulf War veterans also reported a higher prevalence of colitis, enteritis, heartburn, and indigestion. A large questionnaire survey of U.S. Navy Seabees deployed during the Gulf War found more self-reporting of physician-diagnosed IBS compared with nondeployed Seabees (Gray et al. 2002). And a study of Gulf War veterans found that the prevalence of GI symptoms consistent with functional GI disorders that developed during war-zone exposure was higher than the prevalence before deployment and persisted after deployment. The prevalence of those GI symptoms with non-GI symptoms was significantly greater in deployed than in nondeployed veterans (Sostek et al. 1996).

Results of six secondary studies are consistent with those of the primary studies in showing higher reporting frequencies of GI symptoms in deployed veterans than in control populations. Vietnam theater veterans reported higher rates of hospitalizations for stomach conditions than era veterans (Eisen et al. 1991). Large cohort studies of Gulf War and Vietnam veterans found excess reporting of GI symptoms (Boscarino 1997; Kelsall et al. 2004a; Proctor et al. 1998; Simmons et al. 2004; Sostek et al. 1996; Unwin et al. 1999). Like the primary Gulf War study by Sostek et al., the Boscarino study (Boscarino 1997) of the Vietnam War provided the appropriate timeline between exposure and onset of GI disturbances. Symptoms were reported to begin during deployment and to persist for years thereafter (Schnurr et al. 2000). There is also some evidence that the development of these syndromes were enabled by exposure to GI infections during the stress of deployment (Sostek et al. 1996; Spiller and Campbell 2006).

Three civilian populations exposed to war or severe trauma found a greater prevalence of GI symptoms or disorders in those with greater trauma exposure (Dumitrascu and Baban 1991; Escobar et al. 1992; Stermer et al. 1991).

PTSD was associated with increased GI symptoms in several studies of veterans. In the largest military study, which had the longest followup period (nearly 20 years), combat-related PTSD was associated with more frequent later development of GI diseases in Vietnam-theater veterans than in Vietnam-era veterans (Boscarino 1997). Other studies corroborated the relationship between GI disturbances and combat or PTSD (a surrogate for trauma exposure) in veterans of the Vietnam War (Eisen et al. 1991), OIF (Hoge et al. 2007), and of World War II and the Korean War (Schnurr et al. 2000).

The committee notes that a substantial number of physiologic studies support associations of acute and chronic stress with lowered pain-sensation threshold and with visceral hypersensitivity, increased motility, altered brain circuitry involving pain regulation, and altered HPA-axis reactivity (Chang 2006; Dunphy et al. 2003; Kellow et al. 2006a,b; Murray et al. 2004). It is possible that combat stress leads to central amplification of visceral and somatic symptoms via a variety of CNS-peripheral mechanisms, such as the HPA axis, pain-modulating circuits, and autonomic function (see Chapter 4).

There are some limitations in this body of evidence, mostly related to methods of effect assessment. One is that the self-reporting of GI symptoms in most cases did not fulfill the criteria for diagnosing a functional GI disorder. None of the studies used contemporary criteria to assess functional GI disorders although in some cases the diagnoses can be inferred. There was also a lack of adequate medical diagnostic testing to identify a GI structural disease.

Nevertheless, taken together, the overall pattern of symptoms found in many primary and secondary studies confirms an association of deployment-related stress and functional GI symptoms, including abdominal pain, diarrhea, nausea, and vomiting. Changes in GI functioning mark the acute stress response, and this is well supported in the physiologic literature. Furthermore, the findings suggest the development of deployment-related IBS, functional dyspepsia, and some other functional GI syndromes. The relationship provides a strong biologic rationale, as explained in Chapter 4, for the epidemiologic relationship found here between severe trauma exposure and long-term GI illness in veterans.

The methods of the veteran studies are insufficient to determine a clear association between acute or chronic stress and the onset of a structural disorder (Drossman and Ringel 2004). Furthermore, the diagnosis of these diseases should be validated by medical records because physicians not infrequently place an organic label on a patient's symptoms (for example, gastritis or peptic ulcer) without performing diagnostic studies, and this will confound the diagnosis in a survey, particularly if the data are based on the subjects' recollections of physicians' diagnoses.

Thus, the association of deployment-related stress with GI symptoms is accepted, the association with functional GI disorders is supported but not complete, and an association with structural GI diseases cannot be determined.

> **The committee concludes that there is limited but suggestive evidence of an association between deployment to a war zone and gastrointestinal symptoms consistent with functional gastrointestinal disorders, such as irritable bowel syndrome and functional dyspepsia. The committee also concludes that there is inadequate/insufficient evidence to determine whether an association exists between deployment to a war zone and the development of structural gastrointestinal diseases.**

TABLE 6-9 Digestive System Disorders

Study	Study Design	Population	Outcomes	Results	Adjustments	Comments
Gray et al. 2002	Retrospective, case-control	U.S. Navy Seabees: 3831 GW-deployed veterans, 4933 veterans deployed elsewhere, 3104 nondeployed veterans	Self-reported physician diagnoses, self-reported symptoms from mailed questionnaire	Deployed vs nondeployed: peptic ulcer disease OR 3.11, 95% CI 1.67-5.78; IBS OR 3.57, 95% CI 2.22-5.73; new GI disease OR 2.10, 95% CI 1.39-3.17; clustering of CFS, PTSD, MCS, IBS: Seabees who had one had 13-18 other symptoms, Seabees without any averaged 6 other symptoms	Age, sex, active-duty or reserve status, race or ethnicity, current smoking, current alcohol drinking	Study limited by recall bias, IBS not analyzed exclusively, response rate 70%, large sample
Sosteck et al. 1996	Cross-sectional, prevalence	57 male GW-deployed veterans, 44 nondeployed veterans of National Guard unit	Questionnaire about GI and non-GI symptoms with recall before, during, after GW period	Prevalence of GI symptoms: abdominal pain 70% vs 9%; diarrhea 74% vs 18%; incomplete rectal evacuation 60% vs 7%; gas 74% vs 23%; decreased appetite 42% vs 7% (all $p < 0.001$)		Response rate 74%; limitations include small sample and self-report questionnaire for recall before, during, after GW
Eisen et al. 2005 NHSGWEVTF (Derived from Kang et al. 2000b)	Cross-sectional, prevalence	1061 GW-deployed veterans vs 1128 non-GW-deployed veterans	Physician evaluation, questionnaire for dyspepsia; GI symptoms and medical conditions reported from earlier survey	Dyspepsia OR 1.87, 95% CI 1.16-2.99; gastritis OR 1.57, 95% CI 0.88-2.78	Age, sex, race, cigarette-smoking, duty type, service branch, rank	Study limited by low participation rate, number of years since war; weak diagnostic criteria

TABLE 6-9 Digestive System Disorders

Study	Study Design	Population	Outcomes	Results	Adjustments	Comments
Kang et al. 2000b NHSGWEVTF	Cohort, prevalence, conducted in 1995	11,441 GW-deployed veterans vs 9476 nondeployed veterans	Self-reports of 48 medical conditions during preceding 12 months; self-reports of exposure of veterans in health registry; medical-record review of subset of 4200 veterans for clinic records, hospital records	Estimated prevalence: heartburn 37% vs 25%; diarrhea 31% vs 15%; abdominal pain 23% vs 12%; nausea 19% vs 11%; constipation 13% vs 7%; trouble swallowing 12% vs 5%; colitis 4.6% vs 2.2%; vomiting 10% vs 6%; gastritis 25.2% vs 11.7%; enteritis 6.6% vs 2.8%; frequent diarrhea 21.2% vs 5.9% (all significant at $p \leq 0.05$)		Mailed questionnaires followed by telephone interviews
Eisen et al. 1991 VET Registry	Case-control, mail or telephone survey	2260 male monozygotic twins from twin registry who were on active duty during Vietnam war	Mail or telephone interviews of whether veteran had at time of interview, had since service, or had been hospitalized for 13 categories of health problems; index of combat exposure	Twins who served in Vietnam and been hospitalized for stomach conditions OR 2.6, 95% CI 1.4-4.9	PTSD; did not alter results	Response rate 75%; potential for reporting bias; self-reports; comparing monozygotic twins naturally adjusts for genetic susceptibilities
Dumitrascu and Baban 1991	Cohort study done at 4 times	60 civilians with IBS from medical clinic in Cluj, Romania	In-person interview on bowel symptoms after Romanian uprising in December 1989 and in January, March, June 1990	Painful IBS episodes high in January 1990, decreased in March, June 1990 (80%, 38%, 33%, respectively), but diarrheal episodes did not change (13%, 12%, 10%, respectively)		
Stermer et al. 1991	Case-control	239 holocaust survivors vs 384 Eastern Europeans not exposed to Nazis; all born before 1941, hospitalized in Israel in 1985-1986 for non-GI complaints	In-person interviews on medical history with emphasis on GI symptoms	Compared prevalence of GI symptoms: abdominal pain, irregular bowels, diarrhea, constipation, distention, heartburn, flatulence, anorexia, nausea, vomiting, mucus, tenesmus, aerophagia; all significant ($p < 0.001$-0.0001)		

TABLE 6-9 Digestive System Disorders

Study	Study Design	Population	Outcomes	Results	Adjustments	Comments
Boscarino 1997 (Derived from VES)	Nested case-control study in retrospective cohort study conducted 17 years after war	332 PTSD-positive Army Vietnam War veterans with high-combat exposure, 1067 PTSD-negative controls mostly with low-combat exposure	Lifetime PTSD evaluation by in-person interview with DIS; postservice self-reported physician-diagnosed digestive system diseases at in-person interviews; Combat Exposure Index	Digestive diseases OR 1.47, 95% CI 1.02-2.10	Preservice, in-service, postservice factors, including intelligence, race, region of birth, enlistment status, volunteer status, Army marital status, Army medical profile, hypochondriasis	Large sample, generalizability to Army Vietnam veterans; in-person diagnoses of PTSD; lack of specificity as to particular disease; no verification of health reporting against medical records
Dobie et al. 2004	Cross-sectional	266 female veterans with PTSD, 940 veterans without PTSD; women had all received care at one VA medical center in 1996-1998	Mailed questionnaire for health history, SF-36, PCL-C (screening instrument)	IBS OR 2.8, 95% CI 2.1-3.9	Age; no adjustment for other confounders	Response rate 65%; self-administered questionnaire; without criteria, IBS symptom reporting may be part of generalized somatic reporting tendency

NOTE: CFS = chronic fatigue syndrome, CI = confidence interval, DIS = Diagnostic Interview Schedule, GI = gastrointestinal, GW = Gulf War, IBS = irritable bowel syndrome, MCS = multiple chemical sensitivity, NHSGWEVTF = National Health Survey of Gulf War Era Veterans and Their Families, OR = odds ratio; PCL-C = PTSD Checklist-Civilian, PMR = proportional morbidity ratio, PTSD = posttraumatic stress disorder, SF-36 = Short form 36, VA = Department of Veterans Affairs, VES = Vietnam Experience Study, VET Registry = Vietnam Era Twin Registry.

SKIN DISORDERS

Rashes were among the most frequently reported health problem soon after the Gulf War (Murphy et al. 1999). *Rash* usually refers to dermatitis, an umbrella term covering several subtypes, including atopic dermatitis, contact dermatitis, seborrheic dermatitis, and psoriasis. In both the Gulf War and the Vietnam War, troops were exposed to several toxicants that could cause allergic skin reactions, including pesticides; Agent Orange has been associated with the chloracne seen in some Vietnam veterans.

For the purposes of this section on deployment-related stress and dermatologic effects, the committee defined a primary study according to methodologic rigor (Chapter 2) and use of a dermatologic examination. In a secondary study, the determination of a dermatologic effect was based on veterans' self-reports of symptoms or self-reported physician-diagnosed conditions. This section excludes one skin condition, chloracne, because its cause in veterans was herbicide exposure peculiar to the Vietnam War (IOM 2007). Primary studies are summarized in Table 6-10.

Primary Studies

To determine the link between deployment-related stressors and dermatologic diseases, the committee identified four primary studies (CDC 1988b; Eisen et al. 2005; Higgins et al. 2002; Ishoy et al. 1999) and numerous secondary studies. In the large, nationally representative study of U.S. Gulf War veterans, Eisen et al. (2005) performed medical evaluations of more than 2,000 veterans. The study was performed 10 years after the Gulf War and used data derived from the 1995 VA National Health Survey of Gulf War Era Veterans and Their Families (Kang et al. 2000b). The investigators searched for dermatologic conditions by dividing them into two categories: group 1 consisted of freckles, seborrheic keratoses, moles, cherry hemangiomas, skin tags, and scars; group 2 consisted of dermatologic diagnoses not included in group 1. Diagnoses were made by a board-certified dermatologist, who evaluated group 2 conditions through teledermatology by using at least two digital photographs and results of a standardized history and physical examination. The prevalence of group 1 diagnoses did not differ between deployed and nondeployed veterans (OR 0.87, 95% CI 0.68-1.12). After adjustment for age, sex, race, years of education, cigarette-smoking, duty type, service branch, and rank, the prevalence of a diagnosis of one or more group 2 skin conditions was 34.6% in deployed veterans and 26.8% in nondeployed veterans (OR 1.38, 95% CI 1.06-1.80). Two skin conditions in group 2 were diagnosed more frequently ($p = 0.02$) in deployed than in nondeployed veterans: verruca vulgaris (warts) (1.6% vs 0.6%, OR 4.02, 95% CI 1.28-12.6) and atopic dermatitis (1.2% vs 0.3%, OR 8.1, 95% CI 2.4-27.7). Atopic dermatitis (a form of eczema) is an inflammatory condition manifested on the skin by dry, eczematous skin and papules. It tends to run in families (with allergic rhinitis and other allergies), and its course is often chronically relapsing (Leung 2000). Atopic dermatitis is not to be confused with contact dermatitis, a delayed hypersensitivity response to a specific agent that directly or indirectly injures the skin.

Researchers in the UK conducted in-person dermatologic evaluations of UK Gulf War-deployed veterans (111 disabled and 98 nondisabled) and 133 disabled veterans not deployed to the Gulf War (Higgins et al. 2002). The cross-sectional study was conducted in 1999-2000; participants were randomly selected from three representative cohorts that had served in the gulf or in Bosnia or had been on active duty but not deployed to either location. Disability was defined as reduced physical functioning according to the SF-36. All participants were examined by a dermatologist who was blinded as to deployment and health status. The prevalence of any skin condition was 47.7% in disabled Gulf War veterans, 36.7% in nondisabled Gulf War veterans, and 42.8% in disabled non-Gulf War veterans. The investigators found no differences among groups in any dermatologic conditions other than seborrheic dermatitis (8.1% in deployed vs 2.3% in nondeployed), which was more common in Gulf War veterans than in the two comparison groups. The prevalence of seborrheic dermatitis in the general UK population is estimated to be about 3%. The excess in deployed veterans was irrespective of disability status.

Ishoy et al. (1999) reported on Danish peacekeepers deployed to the gulf during 1990-1997. The 686 deployed veterans and 231 nondeployed age-, sex-, and profession-matched veterans each received a medical examination and were interviewed for a full medical history by a physician. Veterans indicated whether any condition had its onset before or after deployment to the gulf. The examinations found that the prevalence of the following conditions with onset during or after deployment or August 1990 was higher in deployed veterans than in nondeployed veterans: eczema (15.0% vs 3.0%, $p < 0.001$), retarded wound healing (6.0% vs 1.7%, $p < 0.01$), other skin problems (17.1% vs 5.2%, $p < 0.001$), hair loss or hair disease (4.2% vs 0.9%, $p < 0.01$), and sweaty, clammy, or damp hands (7.9% vs 3.9%, $p < 0.05$). The study limitations included performance of only multiple univariate observations and a lack of information on possible confounders, although such lifestyle factors as smoking, alcohol use, and physical activity were reported.

The VES was a major study of all U.S. Army veterans conducted 17 years after the Vietnam War (CDC 1988b). It surveyed a random sample of the 5 million Army veterans who served during the Vietnam era: 2490 Vietnam-theater veterans and 1972 era veterans were interviewed and examined in 1985-1986. During the medical-examination phase of the study, a significantly higher prevalence of skin conditions as a global category (excluding chloracne) was found in theater veterans than in era veterans (33.0% vs 21.8%, OR 1.7, 95% CI excludes 1.0, $p < 0.05$). Upon dermatologic examination, none of the selected dermatologic conditions were found to be more prevalent in theater veterans than in era veterans; ORs for hyperpigmentation, hirsutism, folliculitis, tinea, any skin infection, and postinflammatory scars were all 0.9-1.2 (95% CIs 0.8-1.7).

Secondary Studies

The committee identified numerous large well-designed studies of Gulf War veterans that it considered secondary studies primarily because they lacked a dermatologic examination or were imprecise regarding specific dermatologic disorders. Most secondary studies found higher prevalence of dermatologic conditions in deployed vs nondeployed veterans. In the first phase of the VA National Health Survey of Gulf War Era Veterans and Their Families, Kang et al. (2000b) used a stratified random-sampling method to compare 11,441 Gulf War-deployed veterans with 9,476 nondeployed veterans on the basis of the DMDC. The study found that dermatologic conditions were in the top five self-reported medical conditions diagnosed by physicians in the preceding 12 months. The skin conditions listed were eczema or psoriasis (7.7% vs 4.4%, rate difference 3.34, 95% CI 3.26-3.42), other dermatitis (25.1% vs 12.0%, rate difference 13.16, 95% CI 13.04-13.28), and diseases of the hair or scalp or hair loss (16.9% vs 7.2, rate difference 9.65, 95% CI 9.55-9.75). A sample of participants were later evaluated by clinical examination in the Eisen et al. study (2005), which was the study's final phase.

Other large cohort studies conducted in several countries reported similar findings in Gulf War veterans based on self-reports via questionnaires. The population-based survey of UK Gulf War-deployed veterans found the prevalence of dermatitis to be 21%, a rate higher than that in two control groups: one dispatched to Bosnia (OR 1.6, 95% CI 1.3-2.0) and the other era controls (OR 1.6, 95% CI 1.4-1.9) (Unwin et al. 1999). Simmons et al. (2004) found that male UK Gulf War veterans reported more skin allergies with onset after 1991 than their nondeployed counterparts (OR 3.3, 95% CI 3.0-3.7). Proctor et al. (1998) compared the prevalence of dermatologic conditions—such as rashes, eczema, and skin allergies—in 252 U.S. Gulf War-deployed veterans. The estimated prevalence was 15.5% for the 186 veterans from the Fort Devens cohort, 11.7% for the 66 veterans from the New Orleans cohort, and 1.9% for the 48 veterans deployed to Germany during the Gulf War. A higher prevalence of skin conditions was also reported in Australian population-based studies (Kelsall et al. 2004a). Moderate to severe rash and skin irritation was reported at a higher rate in 1456 deployed veterans than in 1588 nondeployed veterans (OR 2.0, 95% CI 1.6-2.5). On the basis of a diagnosis by a physician after 1991 (deemed by the investigators to be a probable diagnosis), deployed veterans reported more dermatitis (OR 1.8, 95% CI 1.3-2.6) and skin diseases other than dermatitis, skin cancer, eczema, or psoriasis (OR 1.3, 95% CI 1.1-1.7) compared with nondeployed veterans. In light of their reliance on self-reports or questionnaires, all those studies are susceptible to recall or reporting bias. They also lack specificity regarding specific skin effects.

Eisen et al. (1991) performed a co-twin study in 1987 to determine the health effects of the Vietnam War. One member of each of 2260 male monozygotic twin pairs reported having a health problem and the other did not; it was then determined how many of the affected twins and unaffected twins had served in Vietnam. The study established the validity of self-reported health responses against medical records for a subset of the twins. It also searched for relationships between health problems and levels of combat exposure. The investigators constructed a combat exposure index by using responses to a separate questionnaire. Twins with persistent skin conditions (such as severe acne and rashes) that were present at any time since service were more likely to have served in Vietnam than were unaffected twins (OR 2.1, 95% CI 1.5-3.0). The prevalence of skin problems (either currently or ever) was significantly associated with increasing levels of combat exposure. At the highest level of combat exposure, skin problems were 3 times more likely than at the lowest combat level. The study is limited in that skin problems included "severe acne," which may have included chloracne associated with Agent Orange, although the VES showed its prevalence to be lower (1.9% in theater veterans) than that of other skin conditions (33% in theater veterans) upon examination (CDC 1988b).

A study of Australian veterans deployed to the Vietnam War (a simple random sample of Army veterans, n = 641) found that combat exposure, as determined by Army records and a self-reported combat exposure scale, was related to self-reported chronic "rash" in an increasing linear relationship ($p = 0.041$) (O'Toole et al. 1996b). There was nearly a linear dose-response relationship for eczema, but it did not reach significance ($p = 0.062$). The study did not have dermatologic examinations, but trained interviewers did ask questions about chronic health conditions in person through the standardized Australian Bureau of Statistics Health Interview Survey 1989-1990.

Posttraumatic Stress Disorder and Skin Disorders

Gulf War veterans with PTSD display higher rates of dermatologic symptoms or conditions, according to two studies, one of Gulf War veterans and one of Vietnam veterans. The studies were questionnaire-based, used self-reports of symptoms or physician-diagnosed conditions, and used veterans without PTSD as the comparison population. The assessment of PTSD, which was similar in the two studies, was based on a screening questionnaire, the PTSD Checklist, with standard cutoffs. In a nested case-control study drawn from the population-based study of Iowa veterans of the Gulf War, Barrett et al. (2002a) found the prevalence of current dermatologic conditions and dermatologic symptoms to be higher in 53 veterans with current PTSD (over 90%) than in 3629 veterans without PTSD (about 25%). The study was conducted by telephone interview 5 years after the Gulf War. This nested case-control component of the larger cohort study conducted by the Iowa Persian Gulf Study Group (1997) is limited by lack of specification in the analysis of which particular dermatologic symptoms or conditions might be more prevalent.

The Veterans Health Study of 2425 consecutive male ambulatory-care patients seen at four VA medical centers screened veterans for PTSD with the PTSD Checklist. Patients who screened positive (n = 456) reported higher rates of dermatitis than those without PTSD (OR 2.37, 95% CI 1.88-3.0) (Spiro et al. 2006). The study is limited, however, by its lack of a control population, lack of reporting of veterans' previous deployment status, and absence of identification as to whether PTSD was related to a deployment-related trauma.

Another case-control study was nested within the VES. It sought to determine whether combat-related PTSD was associated with development of a wide variety of medical disorders (Boscarino 1997). Case subjects were PTSD-positive Vietnam veterans with high combat exposure, and controls were PTSD-negative veterans with low combat exposure. Lifetime PTSD status was determined with in-person interviews that used the DIS, and combat exposure was determined with the Laufer Combat Exposure Scale. Medical disorders were ascertained during the in-person interviews by asking veterans to respond affirmatively or negatively to a list of specific medical conditions as to whether they had been diagnosed by a physician and whether the condition occurred before or after discharge. The conditions were later collapsed into general medical categories to minimize the likelihood of reporting bias. The study found no excess of dermatologic diseases occurring after discharge in veterans with PTSD vs those without PTSD (OR 1.09, 95% CI 0.59-1.04) after adjustment for general technical test results, race, region of birth, type of enlistment, Vietnam volunteer status, marital status, age, hypochondriasis, physical limitations in the military record, and psychiatric limitations in the military record. Key advantages of the study are its focus on combat-related PTSD, its ascertainment of PTSD with the DIS, a well-validated structured psychiatric interview based on *DSM* criteria, and use of a combat exposure scale. Another study strength is its adjustment for a host of preservice and postservice behavioral risk factors and physical or psychiatric limitations reported in the military record at the time of service. The major study limitation is the lack of specificity regarding particular dermatologic diseases.

In a later case-control analysis of the VES, Boscarino (2004) tested the hypothesis that combat-related PTSD increases the risk of autoimmune disease after discharge. The prevalence of 20 autoimmune diseases was examined in 124 Vietnam-theater veterans with comorbid PTSD and 54 veterans with current but noncomorbid PTSD (less severe PTSD according to the author). Psoriasis was the one of nine autoimmune diseases with dermatologic manifestations. After multivariate analysis—adjusted for age, education, race, intelligence, geographic region, Army volunteer status, number of times married, smoking, and history of psychiatric disorder—psoriasis was found to be nearly 5 times more prevalent in veterans with comorbid PTSD than in veterans without PTSD (OR 4.7, 95% CI 1.9-11.7).

Finally, older male World War II and Korean War veterans participating in the Normative Aging Study who screened positive for lifetime PTSD (n > 580) using the Mississippi Scale for Combat-Related PTSD were more likely to have new onset of dermatologic disorders (hazard rate 1.18, 95% CI 1.05-1.34) according to physical examinations conducted periodically beginning in the 1960s, than veterans without PTSD (Schnurr et al. 2000). Dermatologic diseases (*ICD* 690-698) included eczema, dermatitis, and psoriasis. Dermatologic disorders increased by 18% for every 10-point increment in PTSD symptom scores.

Summary and Conclusions

The committee placed the greatest weight on studies that included medical evaluation and identification of specific dermatologic diagnoses. All four primary studies showed a higher prevalence of some skin diseases or conditions in deployed than in nondeployed veterans. A nationally representative study of Gulf War veterans found a relationship between deployment and atopic dermatitis and verruca vulgaris (warts), but not other skin conditions (Eisen et al. 2005). A UK study of Gulf War veterans found a relationship between deployment and seborrheic dermatitis (Higgins et al. 2002). Each of those dermatologic associations is supported by a single primary study, although Ishoy et al. (1999) also found an increased prevalence of eczema in deployed Gulf War veterans. The VES showed no increase in selected skin conditions not related to exposure to Agent Orange in Vietnam-theater veterans (CDC 1988b).

Secondary studies are largely consistent with the primary studies but lack specificity regarding dermatologic outcomes. Many report higher prevalences of self-reported symptoms or physician-diagnosed dermatologic conditions in deployed than in nondeployed veterans. Some secondary studies are somewhat more specific in reporting a greater prevalence of eczema or psoriasis (Kang et al. 2000b) or eczema alone (Wolfe et al. 1998).

Dermatologic conditions are highly common in veterans regardless of deployment status. Verruca vulgaris is known to be caused by a virus, and seborrheic dermatitis is thought to be caused by a combination of sebaceous gland secretions, microfloral metabolism, and individual susceptibility (Ro and Dawson 2005). Therefore, the higher prevalence of those two conditions in deployed than in nondeployed veterans are more likely related to environmental conditions in the Gulf War or may simply be due to chance.

The other two conditions—atopic dermatitis and psoriasis—have more plausible relationships with deployment stressors. Both are mediated by the immune system, which has strong interrelationships with the stress response. In the case of psoriasis, the epidemiologic evidence comes directly from one of the primary studies implicating combat-related PTSD of high severity in the onset of psoriasis (Boscarino 2004). Case subjects not only had a higher prevalence of other autoimmune diseases but displayed five biologic markers of autoimmune and other inflammatory diseases. Other controlled studies of psoriasis patients found that introduction of psychologic stressors is associated with biologic alterations in the stress response (Buske-Kirschbaum et al. 2007).

In the case of atopic dermatitis, a large body of research over the last decade suggests immune dysregulation in its pathophysiology and psychologic stress as a key trigger in its maintenance or exacerbation (Leung and Soter 2001). Controlled clinical trials found that patients with atopic dermatitis show attenuated activity of the HPA axis and overreactivity of the sympathetic adrenomedullary system in response to psychologic stressors (Buske-Kirschbaum et al. 2002). Those findings are consistent with the findings from veteran studies. Skin conditions (as a broad category) were directly linked to deployment stressors via a combat exposure index in two secondary studies (Eisen et al. 1991; O'Toole et al. 1996b). In addition, the rate of incident skin conditions—including dermatitis, psoriasis, and eczema—had a dose-response relationship with PTSD symptom levels in a secondary study of Korean War and World War II veterans (Schnurr et al. 2000).

In summary, there is a high frequency of self-reports of various types of rash and other skin conditions among deployed vs nondeployed veterans, and, in general, these reports are confirmed by dermatologic examination, particularly for eczema. Overall, very few studies have rigorously assessed the prevalence of skin conditions in Vietnam War and Gulf War veterans and results are mixed with increases for some skin conditions but not for others. Most are weak in design and limited by self-selection and possible reporting bias. (Skin cancer was discussed earlier in the section "Cancer.")

The committee concludes that there is limited but suggestive evidence of an association between deployment to a war zone and skin disorders.

TABLE 6-10 Skin Disorders

Reference	Study Design	Population	Outcomes	Results	Adjustments	Limitations/Comments
Eisen et al. 2005 NHSGWEVTF (Derived from Kang et al. 2000b)	Population-based, cross-sectional, prevalence, medical evaluation	1061 GW-deployed vs 1128 nondeployed	Full-body skin examination by physician; dermatologist used teledermatology for group 2 diagnoses	Atopic dermatitis OR 8.1, 95% CI 2.4-27.7; verruca vulgaris OR 4.02, 95% CI 1.28-12.6; any group 2 diagnosis OR 1.38, 95% CI 1.06-1.80; any group 1 diagnosis OR 0.87, 95% CI 1.06-1.80	Age, sex, race, years of education, smoking, duty type, service branch, rank	Low participation rates 53% deployed, 39% nondeployed; study conducted 10 years after war
Higgins et al. 2002	Prospective case-comparison, cross-sectional prevalence	111 UK disabled GW veterans, 98 nondisabled GW veterans, 133 disabled non-GW veterans; samples derived from larger cohort study of UK veterans of GW, Bosnia peacekeepers, active-duty but nondeployed veterans	Skin examination by dermatologist blind to service history, health status	Any skin condition 47.7% vs 36.7% vs 42.8%; seborrheic dermatitis 8.1% deployed vs 2.3% nondeployed (disabled and nondisabled)	Age, sex, rank, smoking, alcohol	Skin disorders are common in veterans; finding could have been by chance; study conducted 9-10 years after war
Ishoy et al. 1999	Cross-sectional, prevalence	686 Danish peacekeepers deployed to gulf in 1990-1997 vs 231 age- and sex-matched armed forces nondeployed controls	Health examination by physician, self-report questionnaire	Prevalence of skin conditions with onset after gulf: eczema 15.0% vs 3.0%, $p < 0.001$; retarded wound healing 6.0% vs 1.7%, $p < 0.01$; other forms of skin problems 17.1% vs 5.2%, $p < 0.001$; hair loss or hair disease		Participation rate 83.6% deployed, 57.7% nondeployed; lack of information on adjustment for confounders in multivariate analysis

TABLE 6-10 Skin Disorders

Reference	Study Design	Population	Outcomes	Results	Adjustments	Limitations/Comments
				4.2% vs 0.9%, $p < 0.01$; sweaty, clammy, or damp hands 7.9% vs 3.9%, $p < 0.05$		
CDC 1988b VES	Retrospective cohort, prevalence, population-based, telephone interview with screening medical examination at followup	2490 Vietnam-theater veterans, 1972 Vietnam-era veterans randomly selected from 7924 theater veterans, 7364 era veterans who had entered Army in 1965-1971	Dermatologic examinations, laboratory testing at medical examination	Other skin conditions OR 1.7, 95% CI excludes 1.0, $p < 0.05$; hyperpigmentation OR 1.2, 95% CI 0.9-1.7; folliculitis OR 0.9, 95% CI 0.8-1.1; tinea OR 1.0, 95% CI 0.8-1.1; any skin infection OR 1.0, 95% CI 0.8-1.1; postinflammatory scars OR 1.0, 95% CI 0.9-1.2	Age at enlistment, race, year of enlistment, enlistment status (volunteer vs draftee), score on general technical test, primary military occupational specialty	Low participation rate in control group; conducted 17 years after war

NOTE: CI = confidence interval, GW = Gulf War, NHSGWEVTF = National Health Survey of Gulf War Era Veterans and Their Families, OR = odds ratio, VES = Vietnam Experience Study.

FIBROMYALGIA AND CHRONIC WIDESPREAD PAIN

Fibromyalgia, also called fibrositis, is a chronic and variable rheumatic condition characterized by widespread muscle and skeletal tenderness and fatigue. Diagnosis is based on two criteria of the American College of Rheumatology (ACR): a history of widespread pain lasting at least 3 months and the presence of 11 or more of 18 designated tender points on the body. Other nonspecific symptoms of fibromyalgia are sleep disturbance, morning stiffness, and cognitive impairment. The ACR has developed a definition of chronic widespread pain (CWP) as part of the diagnostic criteria for fibromyalgia: CWP is pain reported in the axial skeleton and two contralateral quadrants that persists for 3 months or longer, that is both right and left sides of the body and both above and below the waist. One of the predesignated pain sites is considered a true tender point only if the person feels pain on application of 4 kg of pressure to the site. There are no laboratory tests to diagnose fibromyalgia or CWP, and their etiology is unknown. It has been noted that fibromyalgia cannot be diagnosed without a physical examination (Buskila 2000) and it has been suggested that CWP and fibromyalgia are points on a continuum of chronic pain disorders (Kuzma and Black 2006). Chronic pain, as distinct from CWP, is discussed in the final section of this chapter, "Symptom Reporting."

Fibromyalgia has a prevalence in the general population of about 2.0%—3.4% in women and 0.5% in men—and its prevalence increases with age (Johnson 1989). As many as 4 million Americans, mostly women, may have fibromyalgia (American Pain Foundation 2007). CWP has been estimated to occur in 5% of patients seen in general internal-medicine practice and up to 20% of rheumatology-clinic patients (Wolfe 1989). In the United Kingdom, 10-11% of the general population reported having symptoms consistent with the ACR definition of CWP (Papageorgiou et al. 2002).

Primary studies of fibromyalgia include a diagnosis based on symptom reporting and physical examination, preferably using ACR criteria. Primary studies of CWP also needed to include a diagnosis based on ACR criteria. Self-reports, even those using pain manikins (a drawing of a person on which areas of pain can be identified), were not considered to be sufficient for a primary study of either condition. The primary studies for fibromyalgia and CWP are summarized in Table 6-11.

Primary Studies

The committee identified three primary studies: two of fibromyalgia (Eisen et al. 2005; Smith et al. 2000) and one of CWP (Ang et al. 2006). In 1999-2001, Eisen et al. (2005) reported on the prevalence of 12 medical conditions in 1061 Gulf War-deployed veterans and 1128 nondeployed veterans who were randomly selected from a national cohort of 11,441 deployed and 9476 nondeployed veterans in all service branches. The veterans were part of the National Health Survey of Gulf War Era Veterans and Their Families, whose first phase was a mail and telephone interview conducted in 1995 (Kang et al. 2000b). Researchers were blinded to deployment status, and combat exposure was not assessed. On the basis of self-reports using the SF-36, the prevalence of fibromyalgia in deployed and nondeployed veterans was 0.6% and 0.8%, respectively, for a nonsignificant OR of 1.21 (95% CI 0.36-4.10). However, when fibromyalgia was diagnosed by physical examination following the ACR criteria (Wolfe et al. 1990), the prevalence was 2% in deployed veterans and 1.2% in nondeployed for a significant

OR of 2.32 (95% CI 1.02-5.27, $p = 0.04$) adjusted for age, sex, race, cigarette-smoking, duty type, service branch, and rank. Deployed veterans were slightly younger, less educated, less likely to be married, and of lower income, but the analysis adjusted for most of those factors. Strengths of the study include the population-based sampling strategy, blinding of evaluating physicians, and use of validated diagnostic criteria based on physical examination. Limitations include the potential for substantial selection bias due to modest participation rates—53% of deployed veterans and 39% of nondeployed veterans—and lack of information on potential exposures.

Using a different approach, Smith et al. (2000) examined all hospital records in DoD medical facilities from 1991 to 1997 to assess whether 551,841 Gulf War-deployed and 1,478,704 nondeployed active-duty military personnel were at increased risk for hospitalization with a diagnosis of fibromyalgia. During the 6-year period, 239 Gulf War veterans and 621 nondeployed veterans were hospitalized for fibromyalgia. Cox proportional-hazards models showed a slightly higher hospitalization rate for fibromyalgia among the deployed than among the nondeployed veterans (RR 1.23, 95% CI 1.05-1.43). The risk of hospitalization was 3 times greater for female veterans than for male veterans, twice as likely if the person had been hospitalized for any cause before the war, and more than twice as likely for Army veterans than veterans in other service branches. The authors attributed the increase to the DoD Comprehensive Clinical Evaluation Program (CCEP)—which began in June 1994 and ended in mid-1995—during which many veterans were admitted to the hospital only for purposes of evaluation. Before the inception of the CCEP, there was no difference in hospitalization for fibromyalgia between deployed and nondeployed veterans (RR 0.92, 95% CI 0.74-1.13); after CCEP in 1994, there was almost twice the rate of hospitalization for fibromyalgia (RR 1.76, 95% CI 1.39-2.22). CCEP participants were 26 times more likely to be hospitalized for fibromyalgia than were nonparticipants, and adding a CCEP covariate to the analysis resulted in a reduction in the risk for deployed veterans (RR 0.56, 95% CI 0.41-0.78). The Smith et al. study has the advantage of being a large population-based sample and having good statistical power for detection of an effect. Its major limitations are the inclusion of only active-duty personnel, changes in hospitalization rates for fibromyalgia in association with the practices of the CCEP, use of hospitalization data only from DoD medical facilities, lack of assessment of combat exposure or deployment stress, and the fact that fibromyalgia is rarely severe enough to warrant hospitalization.

The committee identified only one primary paper that looked specifically at CWP in deployed and nondeployed Gulf War veterans. A random sample of a population-based cohort of regular military and National Guard and reserve veterans (Iowa Persian Gulf Study Group 1997), 1896 deployed and 1799 nondeployed, who listed Iowa as their home state at the time of enlistment were surveyed in 1995-1996. Veterans were identified through the DMDC. The study was conducted through structured telephone interviews to determine the prevalence of CWP on the basis of responses to the SF-36. Gulf War veterans reported significantly more bodily pain than did nondeployed veterans ($p < 0.01$). In a followup study of a subset of this cohort 5 years after the baseline survey, Ang et al. (2006) conducted in-person followup examinations of 370 Gulf War veterans who had not met the case definition of CWP at baseline. The goal of the followup study was to identify predictors of delayed-onset CWP. Of the 370 veterans, 69 (18.6%) had met the classification criteria for CWP at the followup evaluation: 51 in the deployed group and 18 in the nondeployed group. According to a logistic multiple-regression model, CWP was significantly associated with perceived life stress (based on responses to the

Brief Life Stress Questionnaire) at the time of the Gulf War, whether military-related or not (OR 1.4, 95% CI 1.0-2.0), and with perceived life stress in the 6 months after returning home (OR 1.3, 95% CI 1.0-1.8). CWP also correlated with combat exposure during deployment (OR 1.5, 95% CI 1.1-2.0) although not specifically with deployment to the gulf itself (OR 1.1, 95% CI 0.6-2.0). Symptoms of alcohol use at the 5-year baseline survey were protective for CWP at 10 years (OR 0.2, 95% CI 0.1-0.6, p = 0.0039). The authors used the Expanded Combat Exposure Scale in the baseline survey and reported that for every 5-point increase in combat exposure score, there was a 50% increase in the likelihood that a veteran would develop CWP. Although the study had the advantage of using an in-person evaluation for the medical diagnosis of CWP and had a relatively large population of deployed and nondeployed veterans, there was a possibility of recall bias for life and deployment stressors reported 5 years after the conflict, and only veterans from Iowa were evaluated. Furthermore, only veterans who did not meet the CWP criteria at baseline were considered for the followup evaluation; veterans who may have developed CWP during the first 5 years after the conflict were not included in the followup examination.

Secondary Studies

Several studies have looked at self-reports of fibromyalgia, symptoms of fibromyalgia, or CWP in Gulf War veterans. The Iowa Persian Gulf Study Group (1997) surveyed 1896 Gulf War-deployed and 1799 nondeployed veterans who listed Iowa as their home state at the time of enlistment to determine whether there was a unique Gulf War illness. In telephone interviews, veterans were asked about symptoms of fibromyalgia on the basis of questions keyed to the symptom criteria of Wolfe et al. (1990), which included the presence of widespread pain for at least 3 months. Symptoms of fibromyalgia were present in 18.2% of 985 deployed regular military veterans and 23.8% of 911 deployed National Guard or reserve veterans compared with 9.2% of 968 nondeployed regular military veterans and 13.2% of 831 nondeployed National Guard or reserve veterans. The authors found a statistically significant Cochran-Mantel-Haenszel rate difference of 9.3 (95% CI 7.3-11.2) after adjustment for age, sex, race, branch of military, and rank. Although the study used a large population-based sample, the determination of fibromyalgia was based solely on self-reported symptoms, not a physical examination. Participants were asked about a number of military exposures during deployment, including chemical and psychologic stressors, although combat was not specifically mentioned. The study had a high response rate: interviews were completed with 78% of the eligible deployed veterans and 73% of the eligible nondeployed veterans.

In a similar study conducted by Steele (2000), 1545 deployed and 435 nondeployed Gulf War veterans who were residents of Kansas in 1998 were asked about their health status in telephone interviews. Specifically, they were asked whether they had ever received a physician's diagnosis of or treatment for fibromyalgia and, if so, when it had developed. Of the deployed and nondeployed veterans, 2% (n = 24) and less than 0.5% (n = 2), respectively, reported having a diagnosis of fibromyalgia with new onset between 1990 and 1998 (OR 3.69, 95% CI 0.86-15.84 adjusted for sex, age, income, and education level). Although the study included a population-based sample, its goal was to ascertain the prevalence of symptoms that might be indicative of Gulf War illness and the circumstances that increased their prevalence. No physical examinations were conducted to confirm a diagnosis of fibromyalgia or to link it to specific exposures.

A 1997 mail survey of the entire cohort of Canadian Gulf War-deployed veterans and a comparison group of nondeployed veterans—group-matched to cases on sex, age, and regular or reserve status—found that the Gulf War veterans were more likely (16%) to report symptoms of fibromyalgia than nondeployed veterans (about 10%) (Goss Gilroy Inc. 1998). Veterans were also asked about exposure to psychologic stressors, physical trauma, ionizing radiation, and other CNS agents. After adjustment for income, service branch, rank, and age, an OR of 1.81 (95% CI 1.55-2.13) was derived from the prevalence of fibromyalgia in deployed and nondeployed veterans. However, among deployed veterans, exposure to psychologic stressors and physical trauma also increased the likelihood of symptoms of fibromyalgia (OR 1.86, 95% CI 1.47-2.37 and OR 1.64, 95% CI 1.28-2.11, respectively), as did reported exposure to CNS agents and radiation and having lower rank and income. In both deployed and nondeployed veterans, the prevalence of fibromyalgia symptoms did not vary according to whether the veteran had other theater experience in the preceding 12 years. The main study limitation was diagnosis of fibromyalgia based on symptoms or self-reported diagnosis without physical examination.

Using data from the Iowa Persian Gulf Study Group (1997), Forman-Hoffman et al. (2007) analyzed information from the structured telephone interview conducted with 1896 deployed regular military, National Guard, and reserves and 1799 nondeployed veterans in 1995-1996. They looked for self-reports of symptoms of CWP according to the following criteria: the veteran reported having fibromyalgia or fibrositis in the previous 12 months or reported overall body pain that occurred almost every day for at least 3 months during the previous 12 months and had body pain in the 24 hours before the interview. The deployed veterans reported significantly more symptoms of CWP than did nondeployed veterans (OR 2.03, 95% CI 1.60-2.58), whether in the regular military or in the National Guard or reserves; the OR was adjusted for age, sex, race, rank, branch of service, military status, smoking, and current income. Veterans who met the researchers' definition of CWP also had more impairment, such as bed days and VA disability and compensation, and they were more likely to be unemployed, to report their health status as fair or poor, and to have greater use of health care than those without CWP.

Stimpson et al. (2006) surveyed UK veterans who had served only in the Gulf War (n = 2959), only in Bosnia (n = 2052), or both in the Gulf War and in Bosnia (n = 570) and a comparison era group of veterans who had not been deployed to either the Gulf War or Bosnia (n = 2614) for self-reports of CWP. A mailed questionnaire containing a pain manikin to ascertain the pattern and intensity of pain was sent to 12,592 male and female veterans in 1997; the response rate was 60-70%. Veterans were selected for each deployment group on the basis of stratified random sampling of all UK Gulf War veterans. Data from the shaded manikins were used to determine whether the pain pattern met the ACR definition of CWP. The prevalence of reporting of CWP in the Gulf War-deployed group (16.8%) and the Gulf War- and Bosnia-deployed group (15.8%), but not in the Bosnia only-deployed group (7.6%), was statistically significantly higher ($p < 0.0001$) than that in the era group (8.5%) even when adjusted for socioeconomic and demographic factors. The pattern of pain was similar in all the groups; the most common sites of pain were the back and knees. Veterans who reported pain in one limb were also 30 times more likely to report pain in the symmetrically opposite limb rather than a second limb on the same side of the body; the authors found this suggestive of "systemic pain" rather than pain from an injury. Although the sample was large, the study is limited by a lack of physical examination and a lack of indication as to whether the veterans had sustained injuries during deployment or were using pain medication at the time of the survey.

A similar study by Cherry et al. (2001a,b) 6-8 years after the Gulf War also used a pain manikin to identify whether and where veterans had experienced pain for at least 24 hours in the preceding month. Among the 9588 male and female UK Gulf War veterans in all service branches, 12.2% reported widespread pain on a manikin compared with 6.5% of 4790 nondeployed veterans; widespread pain was considered to be present if the manikin showed axial skeletal and contralateral body pain. CWP was not associated with exposure to combat although it was associated with other deployment exposures, specifically to insect repellent, medical attention, and side effects of nerve-agent prophylaxis. The study had response rates of 93% of the active-duty military and 80% of those who had left the military.

Posttraumatic Stress Disorder, Fibromyalgia, and Chronic Widespread Pain

As noted earlier, PTSD is highly comorbid with other health problems, particularly chronic pain and psychiatric disorders. Some studies have assessed whether PTSD is comorbid with fibromyalgia and CWP. Two studies that looked at the comorbidity of PTSD and fibromyalgia were identified.

Amital et al. (2006) found that 49% of 55 male Israeli veterans suffering from combat-related current PTSD met the ACR criteria for fibromyalgia, whereas only 5% of 20 veterans with MDD had fibromyalgia; none of 49 healthy control veterans had fibromyalgia. The PTSD veterans also had more tenderness points (assessed by a rheumatologist) than the MDD veterans (mean, 8.85 vs 2.85). Patients who had both PTSD and fibromyalgia also had more severe PTSD symptoms, primarily re-experiencing symptoms, and scored significantly higher on the CAPS than did veterans without fibromyalgia (97.6 ± 13.2 vs 88.2 ± 14.0). The traumatic event that preceded PTSD had occurred during military service 22-36 years before the study.

Fibromyalgia and PTSD are more prevalent in women than in men. Dobie et al. (2004) sent a mail survey to 1206 female Gulf War veterans who received care at VA medical centers in 1996-1998. The presence of PTSD was determined with the PTSD Checklist-Civilian Version, and fibromyalgia was self-reported. Of the 1206 women, 266 (22%) screened positive for current PTSD; these 266 were more likely to screen positive for fibromyalgia (19.2% of the 266) than were the 940 women without PTSD (8.0%) for an age-adjusted OR of 3.00 (95% CI 1.98-4.45). This cross-sectional survey has several limitations, including lack of identification of the trauma associated with the PTSD, use of a treatment-seeking population, lack of diagnostic examinations for either PTSD or fibromyalgia, and reporting bias.

The committee identified only one study that looked at CWP in veterans with PTSD. Ang et al. (2006) found that CWP was associated with symptoms of PTSD in Gulf War veterans (OR 4.5, 95% CI 0.6-32.3, $p = 0.1383$) more than in nondeployed veterans. Because the veterans were screened for current PTSD with the PTSD Checklist-Military Version, this is a secondary study.

Summary and Conclusions

The diagnosis of fibromyalgia is based on meeting the ACR criteria in a physical examination for tender points and the presence of CWP. The committee identified only two primary studies that diagnosed fibromyalgia on the basis of the ACR criteria and included both Gulf War-deployed and nondeployed veterans: Eisen et al. (2005) and Smith et al. (2000). The committee was unable to locate any studies of fibromyalgia in Vietnam veterans or veterans of other U.S. conflicts. The Eisen et al. (2005) study found that Gulf War-deployed veterans' risk of fibromyalgia was more than twice that of nondeployed veterans. Smith et al. (2000) found no association between Gulf War deployment and hospitalization for fibromyalgia, but it should be noted that fibromyalgia is rarely severe enough to warrant hospitalization, so this finding can not be used to contradict that of Eisen et al. (2005).

Steele (2000) also found fibromyalgia in about 2% in Gulf War-deployed forces but had no nondeployed comparison group. Both the Iowa study and the Canadian study found significantly increased fibromyalgia symptoms in deployed Gulf War veterans than in nondeployed veterans, but the findings from these studies are limited because of the self-reporting of the diagnosis of fibromyalgia.

Two studies looked at the presence of fibromyalgia in veterans with PTSD. Amital et al. (2006) found that almost half the Israeli veterans with combat-related PTSD also had fibromyalgia, but the sample was small. Similar but less dramatic results were seen by Dobie et al. (2004), who found that female Gulf War veterans with PTSD were three times as likely to have fibromyalgia as those without PTSD.

The committee reviewed one primary study and three secondary studies on deployment-related stress and CWP. Although each of the studies found a higher prevalence of CWP in deployed than nondeployed veterans, all had considerable limitations. In Ang et al. (2006), the prevalence of CWP was found to increase both with increased combat exposure and with increased perception of life stress at the time of deployment; the study is limited in that only veterans with no pain 5 years after the conflict were evaluated 10 years after the conflict. The Stimpson et al. study (2006) also found an increase in CWP associated with deployment to a war zone. The other two secondary studies also showed more CWP in deployed than in nondeployed veterans. The committee reviewed one study of PTSD and CWP, which found a strong association between the two disorders (Ang et al. 2006).

Several studies have reviewed the presence of chronic pain in veterans but the definition of chronic pain varied with the study (Hyams et al. 1996; Kuzma and Black 2006; Thomas et al. 2006). Kuzma and Black (2006) noted that many studies of Gulf War veterans reported increased pain symptoms that could be clustered into CWP, but the terminology used in the studies was not consistent and included joint pain and general aches and pain; these pain clusters may or may not have met the ACR criteria for CWP.

The committee concludes that there is limited but suggestive evidence of an association between deployment to a war zone and both fibromyalgia and chronic widespread pain.

TABLE 6-11 Fibromyalgia and Chronic Widespread Pain

Study	Study Design	Population	Outcomes	Results	Adjustments	Comments
Eisen et al. 2005 NHSGWEVTF (Derived from Kang et al. 2000b)	Population-based, cross-sectional, prevalence, medical evaluation	1061 GW-deployed veterans, 1128 nondeployed veterans	Symptoms and physical examination for fibromyalgia with ACR criteria	OR 2.32, 95% CI 1.02-5.27	Age, sex, race, years of education, cigarette-smoking, duty type, service branch, rank	Uses gold standard for diagnosis of fibromyalgia; participation rates 53% deployed, 39% nondeployed
Smith et al. 2000	Postwar hospitalization	551,841 GW-deployed, 1,478,704 nondeployed	Hospitalization records in 1991-1997 for fibromyalgia	RR 1.23, 95% CI 1.05-1.43; however, survival curves indicate excess due to hospitalization for purposes of evaluation during CCEP; before CCEP RR 0.92, 95% CI 0.74-1.13	Sex, age, branch of service	No increase after accounting for CCEP effect; limited to active duty; most cases of fibromyalgia not severe enough to warrant hospitalization
Ang et al. 2006	Cohort of veterans from IPGWSG	370 veterans who were free of CWP at 5 years were examined 10 years after war: 267 GW-deployed, 103 nondeployed	Structured telephone interview about 5 years after GW; in-person followup medical examination 10 years after war of 370 veterans who did not report chronic widespread pain 5 years after war	Neither deployment to nor time in gulf significantly correlated with CWP: OR 1.1, 95% CI 0.6-2.0 and OR 1.0, 95% CI 0.7-13, respectively; combat exposure correlated: OR 1.5, 95% CI 1.1-2.0; perception of stress due to military experience at time of GW correlated more significantly with CWP: OR 1.6, 95% CI 1.1-2.3, p = 0.0084	Controls matched for age, sex, branch of service	Potential for recall bias; only veterans who were free of CWP at 5 years were assessed 10 years after war

NOTE: ACR = American College of Rheumatology, CCEP = Comprehensive Clinical Evaluation Program, CI = confidence interval, CWP = chronic widespread pain, GW = Gulf War, IPGWSG = Iowa Persian Gulf War Study Group, NHSGWEVTF = National Health Survey of Gulf War Era Veterans and Their Families, OR = odds ratio, RR = relative risk.

REPRODUCTIVE EFFECTS

Several studies of deployed veterans have indicated that veterans express concerns about the effects of deployment on child-bearing—both their ability to conceive children and the health of those children. This section reviews studies on three subjects related to reproductive health: birth defects and miscarriage, fertility, and sexual function.

To determine the association between deployment-related stress and adverse reproductive effects, the committee identified six primary studies and nine secondary studies. Primary studies obtained information from both deployed and nondeployed veterans and assessed relevant outcomes with methods beyond self-reporting, such as review of hospital or public-health records. Secondary studies obtained information relevant to the effects in question but had methodologic limitations, such as reliance on self-reports of symptoms or effects, or the examination of small or potentially biased samples of veterans. The primary studies of reproductive effects are summarized in Table 6-12.

Birth Defects and Miscarriage

Primary Studies

The committee identified five citations of four studies that examined the prevalence of birth defects or miscarriage in veterans. One study was on veterans of the Vietnam War and four of the citations were to three studies of offspring of Gulf War veterans.

The VES was a cross-sectional retrospective cohort study of all U.S. Army veterans conducted 17 years after the Vietnam War (CDC 1988b). It surveyed a random sample of the 5 million Army veterans who served during the Vietnam era. In the 1985-1986 phase 1 telephone survey, 7924 theater veterans and 7364 era veterans were asked about various reproductive outcomes in their offspring: live births, pregnancies that ended early (including miscarriages, induced abortions, and tubal pregnancies), stillbirths, major health problems in the first five years of life, low birth weight, leukemia or other cancer, birth defects, infant and child mortality, and cerebrospinal malformations (CDC 1988c). In a substudy, hospital birth records of the children of a random subsample of 1237 theater veterans and 1045 era veterans, selected without regard to phone interview results, were sought. Records were obtained for 1791 children of theater veterans and 1575 children of era veterans.

During the interview phase, Vietnam-theater veterans reported more pregnancies that ended in miscarriage (OR 1.3, 95% CI 1.2-1.4) and more birth defects in their children (OR 1.3, 95% CI 1.2-1.4) than did era veterans, but there was no significant difference between the veteran groups in the other reproductive outcomes examined—pregnancies ending in induced abortions, tubal pregnancies, stillbirths, and infant mortality (CDC 1988c). However, in the birth-defects substudy, the rates for all birth defects as documented by hospital birth records were similar for theater veterans and era veterans (72.6 and 71.1 per 1000 total births, respectively) for an OR of 1.0 (95% CI 0.8-1.4), adjusted for veteran's age at the time of the child's birth, race, year of entry into Army, enlistment status, general technical test score, primary military occupational specialty, years between entry and birth, maternal age, and gravidity. Cerebrospinal malformations, including anencephaly, spina bifida, and hydrocephalus, were observed in 26 children of theater veterans (expected number 18.3-32.4, based on rates from the nationwide Birth Defects Monitoring Program) and in 12 children of era veterans (expected number 17.0-30.3). Limitations of the study include the lack of data on mothers' risk factors and possible exposures of the fathers in Vietnam, possible recall bias, and lack of verification of many of the reproductive effects reported by the veterans.

Cowan et al. (1997) examined routinely collected data on all live births in 135 military hospitals in 1991-1993 to compare the frequency of birth defects in children of active-duty Gulf War veterans and nondeployed active-duty veterans. Information on 33,998 infants born to Gulf War-deployed veterans (30,151 men and 3847 women) and 41,463 born to nondeployed veterans (32,638 men and 8825 women) was reviewed. The risk of any birth defect was 7.45% for deployed veterans and 7.59% for nondeployed veterans (RR 0.98, 95% CI 0.93-1.03). There was no significant association between service in the Gulf War and the risk of any birth defect for male veterans (OR 0.97, 95% CI 0.91-1.03) or female veterans (OR 1.07, 95% CI 0.94-1.22) after adjustment for mother's age at delivery, race or ethnicity, and marital status of parent at the time of the Gulf War. The unadjusted risk of having an infant with severe birth defects was 1.03 (95% CI 0.92-1.15) for male active-duty veterans, 0.92 (95% CI 0.71-1.20) for female active-duty veterans, and 1.00 (95% CI 0.90-1.10) for men and women combined; the authors note that when the adjusted ORs were calculated, no associations were seen but did not provide the data. A limitation of the study is that it examined data only from live births to active-duty personnel in military hospitals.

After conducting a pilot study (Araneta et al. 2000) in Hawaii on birth-defects in the offspring of Gulf War veterans, Araneta et al. (2003) conducted an expanded study examining hospital records of births in 1989-1993 to military personnel in Arizona, Hawaii, Iowa, and selected counties of Arkansas, California, and Georgia. Data from the DMDC on people in military service in February 1991 were linked to data from state and county birth-defects surveillance programs to identify infants born to military personnel who served during the Gulf War. The researchers identified 11,961 infants born to Gulf War veterans (including 450 female veterans) and 33,052 infants born to Gulf War-era veterans (including 3966 female veterans). In infants conceived before and during the Gulf War, there was no significant difference in birth defects between those born to Gulf War veterans and those born to era veterans. In infants conceived after the war, the rate of hypospadias was significantly higher in male infants born to Gulf War mothers than to era mothers (RR 6.3, 95% CI 1.5-26.3, $p = 0.015$). The prevalence of congenital tricuspid valve insufficiency was higher in infants born to Gulf War male veterans than to era male veterans (RR 2.7, 95% CI 1.1-6.6, $p = 0.039$), as was the prevalence of aortic valve stenosis (RR 6.0, 95% CI 1.2-31.0, $p = 0.026$). A significant limitation on the interpretation of these findings is that comparisons were made for 26 birth-defect categories without correction for multiple comparisons; this raises the possibility that the statistical significance of the associations observed is due to chance (Ryan et al. 2004).

In a case-control study performed by Werler et al. (2005), birth records of infants born with the malformation hemifacial microsomia were examined to determine whether there was an association between Gulf War service of the parents and the birth defect. Hemifacial microsomia was identified in 232 cases from craniofacial clinics in 26 cities and matched to 832 controls by pediatrician and child's age. Mothers of case subjects and controls were interviewed by telephone in 1996-2002 to identify pregnancy exposures, including military service, particularly in the Gulf War, of the mother or father 5-11 years before the child's birth. Of the cases, four mothers and 30 fathers had served in the military, as had 10 control mothers and 100 control fathers; of those, four case parents (all in the Army) and 23 control parents (including nine in the Army) had served in the Gulf War. The risk associated with Army service overall was significant

(OR 2.4, 95% CI 1.4-4.2), but the risk associated with having served in the Gulf War was not (OR 0.8, 95% CI 0.3-2.3).

Secondary Studies

Four secondary studies, one of Vietnam veterans and three of Gulf War veterans, were identified that assessed birth defects or miscarriages.

Kang et al. (2000a) compared the self-reported pregnancy outcome of 3392 female Vietnam-theater veterans and 3038 female veterans not deployed to Vietnam. A structured health questionnaire was administered by telephone interview in 1992, and hospital records were obtained to verify reports of moderate to severe birth defects in 13 children. Although there were no significant differences between groups in rates of miscarriage or stillbirth, low birth weight, preterm delivery, or infant death, reports of "moderate to severe" birth defects were significantly higher in female Vietnam veterans (OR 1.46, 95% CI 1.06-2.02), after adjustment for demographic and military characteristics and a number of factors associated with pregnancy.

Researchers obtained information on a cohort of 52,811 Gulf War veterans from the United Kingdom and a randomly selected comparison group of 52,924 nondeployed veterans regarding adverse reproductive outcomes (Doyle et al. 2004; Maconochie et al. 2003). Data were collected with a validated mailed questionnaire in 1998-2001, and 25,084 Gulf War veterans and 19,003 nondeployed veterans responded. There were 27,959 pregnancies reported by male veterans and 861 by female veterans. Miscarriages were reported more frequently by male Gulf War-deployed veterans than nondeployed veterans (OR 1.4, 95% CI 1.3-1.5). Malformations in infants were also more frequently reported among male Gulf War veterans than among nondeployed veterans (OR 1.5, 95% CI 1.3-1.7). No association between Gulf War service and miscarriage was found among women; when restricted to cases that had been clinically confirmed, the maternal results were too few to analyze for malformations and stillbirths.

Kelsall et al. (2007) obtained information on reproductive function from 1424 Australian Gulf War-deployed veterans and 1548 nondeployed veterans with a mail questionnaire in 2000-2002. There was no increased risk in veterans of miscarriage, stillbirth, or terminations. Children of male Gulf War veterans born after the Gulf War were not at greater risk of being born prematurely, having a low birth weight, or having a birth defect or chromosomal abnormality (OR 1.0, 95% CI 0.6-1.6).

A mail survey with telephone followup of 10,000 married U.S. veterans deployed to the Gulf War and 10,000 married U.S. veterans not deployed to the Gulf War was conducted in 1996-1997 (Wells et al. 2006). The response rate in both groups was 51%. Among the subset of 2233 female deployed and nondeployed veterans and 2159 male deployed and nondeployed veterans who had reported one or more pregnancies, no significant differences were found between deployed men and women and nondeployed men and women in reported pregnancies, birth weight, ectopic pregnancies, stillbirths, or miscarriages.

Fertility Difficulties

Primary Studies

The VES examined fertility (CDC 1988b) in theater and era veterans. During the 1985-1986 physical-examination phase, fertility difficulties were reported in 21.0% and 14.5% of the 2490 Vietnam-theater and 1972 Vietnam-era veterans, respectively, for an OR of 1.5 ($p < 0.05$). Because of concerns about fertility, the 705 veterans without vasectomies who had physical examinations in the last 5 months of the study were asked to participate in a study of semen characteristics; 571 (81%) participated. The characteristics examined were sperm concentration, percentage of motile cells, and percentage of morphologically normal cells. A significant difference was seen between theater and era veterans only in sperm concentration (OR 2.3, 95% CI 1.2-4.3). Theater and era veterans were similar in terms of proportion who had not fathered any children (31% and 25%, respectively) as well as the average number of children fathered after primary tour of duty (1.4 and 1.5, respectively).

The sperm of that VES subsample of 705 veterans was reanalyzed in another study that used a more sensitive measure of semen abnormalities (DeStefano et al. 1989). The results confirmed those of the original analysis, showing no difference in sperm characteristics except that more theater veterans than era veterans had low sperm concentration (≤ 20 million cells/mL) for an OR of 2.7 (95% CI 1.3-5.7) adjusted for year of entry into the service, age at entry, enlistment status, enlistment general technical score, military occupational specialty, race, smoking status, illicit drug use, alcohol consumption, abstinence from sexual activity, time between sample collection and analysis, and videotaping magnification (used to measure sperm motility).

Secondary Studies

The study of Kelsall et al. (2007) described above also provided self-reported information on the fertility of male Australian veterans of the Gulf War. Compared with nondeployed veterans, the deployed veterans reported more fertility difficulties after the war (OR 1.4, 95% CI 1.0-1.8) although they were more successful at later fathering children (OR 1.8, 95% CI 1.3-2.6). The groups reported similar rates of pregnancies and live births.

The UK Gulf War veteran study included an examination of infertility based on self-reported inability to achieve conception (type I infertility) and to achieve a live birth (type II infertility) (Maconochie et al. 2004). Reported infertility was significantly higher among male Gulf War veterans than among nondeployed veterans (type I infertility OR 1.41, 95% CI 1.05-1.89; type II OR 1.50, 95% CI 1.18-1.89). In addition, among men not reporting infertility, time to conception was longer among Gulf War fathers than nondeployed fathers (OR 1.18, 95% CI 1.04-1.34). The studies had several limitations including low response rates that made response and recall biases possible.

Sexual Dysfunction

In a primary study, researchers conducted a clinical examination of 661 Danish peacekeepers who served in the gulf in 1990-1997 and 215 Danish military personnel who were not deployed to the gulf; all had previously completed a health interview that included questions about sexual problems (Ishoy et al. 2001). Veterans were asked whether they experienced any sexual problems (decreased libido or nonorganic erectile dysfunction) that they attributed to service in the gulf. Self-reported sexual problems were higher among Gulf War veterans (12%) than among controls (3.7%) for an age-adjusted OR of 2.9 (95% CI 1.4-6.0, $p = 0.003$). A clinical evaluation for serum concentrations of reproductive hormones—including luteinizing hormone, follicle-stimulating hormone, serum hormone-binding globulin, and testosterone—found no significant differences between the deployed and nondeployed veterans. The deployed veterans were more likely to report sexual problems if they had seen killed or wounded people ($p = 0.002$), watched a friend or colleague being threatened or shot at ($p = 0.02$), or been threatened with arms themselves ($p = 0.04$) than if they had not had these experiences. Deployed veterans with sexual dysfunction also reported more perceived psychologic stress during deployment than veterans without sexual dysfunction.

Simmons et al. (2004) used a mail questionnaire to survey all UK Gulf War veterans and demographically similar veterans who had served at the same time but were not deployed to the gulf. Of the 42,818 male veterans who responded, 24,379 had been deployed and 18,439 had not. Sexual dysfunction or a lack of sexual drive was reported by 0.8% and 0.2% of the deployed and nondeployed veterans, respectively, for an OR of 4.6 (95% CI 3.2-6.6, $p < 0.001$) adjusted for age and service status at the time of the survey, service and rank at the time of the war, alcohol consumption, and smoking.

Posttraumatic Stress Disorder and Reproductive Effects

One study examined the association between PTSD and sexual dysfunction in combat veterans. Cosgrove et al. (2002) administered the International Index of Erectile Function to 44 combat veterans undergoing treatment for PTSD at a VA clinic and 46 age-comparable combat veterans without PTSD. Of the veterans with and without PTSD, 85% and 22% had erectile dysfunction, respectively. Severity of PTSD was associated with severity of erectile dysfunction; however, more than half the PTSD veterans were using psychotropic medications compared with only 17% of non-PTSD veterans.

Summary and Conclusions

There is some evidence that deployed veterans of the Vietnam War and the Gulf War report more difficulties with reproductive function, such as increased rates of miscarriage and birth defects, than do nondeployed veterans, based on four primary studies. Several studies have examined the frequency of birth defects, as ascertained from hospital records or registries, in the children of deployed and nondeployed veterans; in general, the studies have not detected a higher rate of birth defects in the children of deployed veterans. The one study in Vietnam veterans and the three studies in Gulf War veterans found no increases in birth defects in children born to deployed fathers (or mothers for the Gulf War) compared to nondeployed fathers (or mothers), although the Vietnam veterans reported more miscarriages and birth defects. One study of Gulf War veterans found an increase in the risk for male children of deployed female veterans having hypospadia and infants of male Gulf War veterans were at increased risk of congenital tricuspid valve insufficiency and aortic valve stenosis. The studies did not examine the relationship between exposure to deployment-related stressors and such self-reported problems. Furthermore, virtually none of the studies has examined the potential influence of deployment-related stress.

One primary study in male Vietnam veterans did find theater veterans had lower sperm counts than did era veterans; there were no primary studies of fertility difficulties in Gulf War veterans. The two secondary studies found that Australian and UK Gulf War veterans reported more fertility difficulties than their nondeployed counterparts. One secondary study examined sexual dysfunction in deployed Danish peacekeepers and found it to be linked it to deployment-related stressors (Ishoy et al. 2001) and a second study found sexual dysfunction was also reported by UK Gulf War veterans.

The committee concludes that there is inadequate/insufficient evidence to determine whether an association exists between deployment to a war zone and reproductive effects.

TABLE 6-12 Reproductive Effects

Reference	Study Design	Population	Outcomes	Results	Adjustments	Comments
CDC 1988c VES	Retrospective cohort, prevalence, population-based, telephone interview with medical examination at followup	3366 birth records of veterans' children: 1791 of Vietnam veterans, 1575 of era veterans	Reproductive outcomes and child health measured through telephone interview and hospital birth records: pregnancies that ended early, including miscarriages, induced abortions, tubal pregnancies, DOB, sex of child, status (live birth or stillbirth), major health problems, low birth weight, leukemia or other cancer, birth defects and CSMs, infant and child mortality	Fathering pregnancy that ended in miscarriage OR 1.3, 95% CI 1.2-1.4); other reproductive outcomes no difference; birth defects OR 1.0, 95% CI 0.8-1.4; based on hospital birth records	Age of veteran at birth of child (or adverse pregnancy outcome), race, year of entry into Army, enlistment status, general technical aptitude test score, primary military occupational specialty, time between enlistment and birth of child, maternal age, gravidity	Lack of data on mothers of children studied concerning potentially important exposures: tobacco, alcohol, drug use, exposure of father Recall bias of veteran regarding adverse reproductive outcomes, such as miscarriages
Cowan et al. 1997	Cohort, routinely collected data on all live births in military hospitals 1991-1993	33,998 infants born to GW-deployed veterans, 41,463 to nondeployed veterans	Occurrence of birth defects recorded in medical file	Any birth defect: men OR 0.97, 95% CI 0.91-1.03; women OR 1.07, 95% CI 0.94-1.22 Severe birth defects (men and women) OR 1.00, 95% CI 0.90-1.10	Mother's age, ethnicity, marital status	Obtained information only on live births in military hospitals and only on children of active-duty personnel; no data from later monitoring; information was only on live births, not, for example, miscarriages

TABLE 6-12 Reproductive Effects

Reference	Study Design	Population	Outcomes	Results	Adjustments	Comments
Araneta et al. 2003	Cohort, prevalence	684,645 GW-deployed veterans, 1,587,102 nondeployed veterans; 11961 infants from deployed parents, 33,052 from nondeployed parents	Military records of veterans linked to birth certificates in Arizona, Hawaii, Iowa, and selected counties in Arkansas, California, and Georgia that had active case ascertainment of birth defects	Male veterans: congenital tricuspid valve insufficiency RR 2.7, 95% CI 1.1-6.6, $p = 0.039$; aortic valve stenosis RR 6.0, 95% CI 1.2-31.0, $p = 0.026$ Female veterans: hypospadias RR 6.3, 95% CI 1.5-26.3, $p = 0.015$		Significant limitation is that comparisons were made for 26 birth-defect categories without correction for multiple comparisons, so observed associations may be due to chance; no information on possible deployment exposures
CDC 1988b VES	Retrospective cohort, prevalence, population-based, telephone interview with screening medical examination at followup	2490 Vietnam-theater veterans, 1972 Vietnam-era veterans randomly selected from 7924 theater veterans and 7364 era veterans who entered Army in 1965-1971; of 705 veterans without vasectomy who were eligible for sperm substudy, 571 (81%) participated	Telephone interview followed by medical examination, including semen analysis	Fertility difficulties OR 1.5, $p < 0.05$; sperm concentration OR 2.3, 95% CI 1.2-4.3; no other characteristics significantly different	Age at enlistment, race, year of enlistment, enlistment status (volunteer vs draftee), score on general technical test, primary military occupational specialty	Low participation rate in control group, CI not given, conducted 17 years after war, participation bias in semen substudy by men who perceived negative reproductive outcomes
Werler et al. 2005	Case-control	232 cases of hemifacial microsomia identified in craniofacial clinics in 26 cities, 832 controls matched by age and pediatrician	Mothers interviewed in 1996-2002 about pregnancy events and exposures, including GW deployment of either parent 5-11 years before child was born	Risk of hemifacial microsomia based on parental GW service OR 0.8, 95% CI 0.3-2.3	Family income, race, BMI in pregnancy	Small sample; possible confounding by lifestyle factors

TABLE 6-12 Reproductive Effects

Reference	Study Design	Population	Outcomes	Results	Adjustments	Comments
DeStefano et al. 1989 (Derived from VES)	Cross-sectional, prevalence, population based, telephone interview followed by screening medical examination	2490 Vietnam-theater veterans, 1972 Vietnam-era veterans randomly selected from 7924 theater veterans and 7364 era veterans who entered Army in 1965-1971; of 705 veterans without vasectomy who were eligible for semen-analysis substudy, 571 (81%) participated	Computer-assisted semen-analysis system for more sensitive analysis than CDC 1988b	Sperm concentration (≤20 million cells/mL) OR 2.7, 95% CI 1.3-5.7	Six covariates as above plus race, age at entry into Army, year of entry, type of enlistment, general technical test score, military occupational specialty	Semen analysis performed only on subsample of men
Ishoy et al. 2001	Cross-sectional, prevalence	661 Danish peacekeepers deployed to Gulf in 1990-1997, 215 Danish nondeployed military controls	Clinical examination, including hormone measurements; interview	Sexual problems OR 2.9, 95% CI 1.4-6.0, $p = 0.003$; no difference in concentrations of reproductive hormones	Age	Deployed veterans reported more sexual problems if they had seen killed or wounded people ($p = 0.002$), watched friend or colleague be threatened or shot at ($p = 0.02$), or been threatened with arms themselves ($p = 0.04$), or perceived psychologic stress during deployment

NOTE: BMI = body-mass index, CDC = Centers for Disease Control and Prevention, CI = confidence interval, CSM = cerebrospinal malformation, DOB = date of birth, GW = Gulf War, OR = odds ratio, RR = relative risk, VES = Vietnam Experience Study.

SUICIDE AND ACCIDENTAL DEATH

Suicide occurs when a person takes his or her own life. By definition, suicide is fatal and it affects not only those who die from or attempt suicide, but families and communities as well. In the United States, it is the 11th leading cause of death in the general population. Over 32,000 people die from suicide in the United States each year (CDC 2007b). Men are 4 times more likely than women to die from suicide, although women are more likely to attempt suicide. Accidental death is considered to be death resulting solely through violent, external, and accidental means.

Primary studies provided the basis of the committee's findings on the relationship between deployment-related stress and suicide. Primary studies had to meet the criteria established in Chapter 2. Primary studies were considered to be studies in which exposure was determined by deployment status or studies that used a diagnosis of PTSD as a marker of war-related trauma. Primary studies also included those in which the cause of death was confirmed through at least one supplemental source, for example, through linkage of death-certificate data to the National Death Index or by a qualified nosologist or medical-review team that was blinded to subjects' deployment status. Secondary studies typically had methodologic limitations, such as assessment of suicidal behaviors solely on the basis of self-report data. Most of the secondary studies did not confirm causes of death through a supplemental source. Understanding of the relationship between deployment-related stress and suicide or accidental death is hampered by the use of different case definitions for suicide or accidental death among cohorts of veterans. Suicide is an outcome that is rare even in the highly vulnerable population being considered here, so studies with low statistical power would have limited ability to establish an association between it and deployment-related stress. Primary studies are summarized in Table 6-13.

Primary Studies

The committee identified seven primary articles (Boehmer et al. 2004; Bullman and Kang 1996; CDC 1987; Kang and Bullman 1996, 2001; Kaplan et al. 2007; Thomas et al. 1991) and one government report (MHAT 2006a) relevant to determining whether there is a relationship between deployment-related stress and suicide or accidental death.

The VES is a major comprehensive study of the health of Vietnam veterans, an initial historical cohort of 9324 Vietnam-theater veterans who were compared with 8989 Vietnam-era veterans who served in the military during the Vietnam War but were deployed in Korea, Germany, or the United States. To be included in the study, veterans had to be male U.S. Army veterans who initially entered military service from 1965 to 1971, served a single term of enlistment, and were discharged alive in enlisted pay grades E-1 through E-5; participants were randomly selected from military personnel files of veterans discharged after 1971.

The first component of the VES to be completed was an assessment of mortality (CDC 1987). Nearly complete ascertainment of vital status of both veteran cohorts was obtained with multiple methods. In addition to determination of cause of death through inspection of all death certificates by persons blinded to the veterans' Vietnam status, a medical review board, also blinded to Vietnam status, independently coded the underlying causes of all 426 deaths by using data from additional sources, including physicians, hospital records, autopsy records, and coroner and law-enforcement files. In the first followup period, which began at discharge from active duty (1965) and ended at death or on December 31, 1983, whichever came first, the total death rate of theater veterans was 17% higher than that of era veterans, and theater veterans had a 25% higher mortality due to external causes. The excess mortality during the early followup period (considered to be the first 5 years) was due largely to external causes (rate ratio 1.25, 95% CI 1.00-1.55), including motor-vehicle accident (rate ratio 1.93, 95% CI 1.16-3.22), suicide (rate ratio 1.72, 95% CI 0.76-3.88), homicide (rate ratio 1.52, 95% CI 0.59-3.91), and accidental poisoning (rate ratio 1.69, 95% CI 0.49-5.77); the death rate ratio for all causes of death was 1.45 (95% CI 1.08-1.96) for the first 5 years after discharge and 1.01 (95% CI 0.79-1.28) after 6 or more years. Death from motor-vehicle crashes was almost 2 times more likely in theater veterans than in era veterans during the early followup period. Alcohol use did not appear to account for the excess risk of a fatal motor-vehicle crash. A similar increase in risk was found for suicide during the early followup period; adjustment for covariates increased the risk ratio for suicide in the early followup period from 1.7 (95% CI 0.76-3.88) to 2.59 (95% CI 1.09-6.17) based on death certificates analyses and to 2.56 (95% CI 1.11-5.87) based on medical review panel assessment. Thereafter, the ratio for suicide declined until it was no more than 1.0. The rate ratios for homicide and other accidents also were below 1.0 in the later followup period and the rate ratio for motor vehicle accidents was 1.16 (95% CI 0.72-1.87).

Boehmer et al. (2004) studied postservice mortality in a 30-year followup of Vietnam veterans by obtaining data on vital status and underlying causes of death on 18,313 male U.S. Army veterans in the VES cohort, thus extending followup an additional 17 years. Vital status was retrospectively ascertained from the end of the original study (1984) through 2000 by using three national databases: the VA BIRLS, the Social Security Administration's Death Master File, and the National Death Index Plus. Potential matches from each data source were reviewed manually, and underlying cause-of-death codes were obtained from the National Death Index Plus. If data on cause of death were not available from the National Death Index Plus, official copies of death certificates were obtained, and an experienced nosologist at National Center for Health Statistics (NCHS) coded the cause of death. NCHS converted *ICD-9* and *ICD-10* causes of death to the NCHS list of 113 selected causes of death, which were then categorized for external causes to allow comparisons with the original study.

Crude death rates were calculated separately for Vietnam-theater and Vietnam-era veterans by using person-years at risk, beginning with the day of discharge from service and ending with the date of death or December 31, 2000, whichever came first. Cox proportional-hazards models were used to approximate the adjusted relative risks for all-causes mortality; for each model, potential confounding and effect modification were assessed. Standardized mortality ratios were used to compare veteran death rates with those in the U.S. male population; they were adjusted for age, race, and calendar year but were limited to deaths through 1998 because U.S. rates had not yet incorporated *ICD-10* codes when the analysis was conducted. There were 1138 new deaths during the additional followup period, five of which occurred during the previous study but had not been identified then. At 5 years since discharge, the only significant external cause of death was accidental poisoning (rate ratio 2.58, 95% CI 1.09-6.14). Mortality due to motor-vehicle accidents or suicide was not significantly higher in theater veterans than in era veterans more than 5 years after discharge from the service (rate ratio 1.02, 95% CI 0.73-1.43 and rate ratio 0.93, 95% CI 0.64-1.34, respectively). However, there continued to be an excess of drug-related deaths among Vietnam veterans during the entire followup period, and there was some overlap between the definitions of unintentional poisoning and drug-related death. The authors noted that even though theater veterans were more likely than era veterans to die from drug-related causes, the contribution to the overall number of deaths was small. The strengths of the study lie in the relatively long followup time after the Vietnam War and, as in the other primary studies reviewed above, the use of multiple databases.

In a retrospective cohort study, Thomas et al. (1991) examined excess mortality in 4582 female veterans who served in Vietnam during the period July 1965-March 1973, and 5324 female veterans who never served in Vietnam. The investigators reported a nonsignificant excess mortality due to external causes, including suicide, in female theater veterans compared with era veterans (RR 1.33, 95% CI 0.80-2.23). There was a significant excess of motor-vehicle accidents (RR 3.19, 95% CI 1.03-9.86). There was no increase in risk of suicide in this cohort of female theater veterans (RR 0.96, 95% CI 0.39-2.39).

Some caution is advisable in using these findings to support a relationship between deployment-related stress and accidental death in that many women deployed to Vietnam were nurses and generally did not witness combat although they were exposed to dead bodies and other traumatic events. However, the investigators estimated cause-specific mortality in the female theater veterans relative to the female era veterans by using a proportional-hazards multivariate model that adjusted for rank (officer or enlisted), military occupation (nursing or other), duration of military service, age at entry into followup, and race. With regard to the nonsignificant finding when suicide alone was used as the outcome, the small number of female veterans who served in Vietnam may not provide sufficient statistical power to detect an association between serving in Vietnam and suicide. Although the study cohort of female Vietnam veterans had sufficient power (95%) to detect an increase in relative risk of death from all causes of 1.3 or greater, the investigators noted that the study had insufficient statistical power to detect moderate increases in deaths from rare causes. Taking the power calculations into consideration may explain why when suicide, accidental death, and nonintentional poisoning are included together as an external cause of death there is sufficient power to detect an increased risk of death in female theater veterans from external causes, especially accidental death, but not suicide.

Bullman and Kang (1996) sought to determine whether there was an association between Vietnam veterans' exposure to trauma, as indicated by being wounded in combat, and risk of suicide. Subjects were identified from a computerized database, the Casualty Information System, which covered casualties sustained by U.S. Army military and civilian personnel and their dependents worldwide from 1961 to 1981. Of about 70,000 veterans who received nonlethal wounds in 1969-1973, 34,534 were selected randomly for inclusion in the study. Cause-specific mortality in all wounded veterans was compared with that in the U.S. population after adjustment for age, race, and calendar year. In study subjects, there was a slight decrease in overall mortality (standardized mortality ratio 0.97, 95% CI 0.93-1.02). However, study subjects had a statistically significant increase in risk of death from all motor-vehicle accidents (standardized mortality ratio 1.23, 95% CI 1.10-1.37), and all accidents (standardized mortality ratio 1.18, 95% CI 1.09-1.29).

The rate of suicide was slightly, but not significantly, higher in wounded veterans than in U.S. men (standardized mortality ratio 1.12, 95% CI 0.96-1.30). The relative risk of suicide for veterans wounded two or more times compared to those wounded once was 1.50 (95% CI 1.01-2.24). There was a statistically significant increase in risk of suicide in veterans who were wounded more than once and hospitalized for a wound (rate ratio 1.82, 95% CI 1.12-2.96) compared with those wounded once and not hospitalized. In addition, there was a significant trend of increasing risk of suicide with increasing occurrences of combat trauma ($\chi^2 = 5.3$, $p <$

0.05). When study subjects were stratified by hospitalization status and number of times wounded and compared with U.S. men, those who received at least one wound that required hospitalization had a higher risk of suicide than those not hospitalized (standardized mortality ratio 1.22, 95% CI 1.00-1.46), and those wounded more than once had a higher risk of suicide than those wounded only once (standardized mortality ratio 1.58, 95% CI 1.06-2.26). Vietnam veterans who were wounded only once and never required hospitalization had the lowest risk of suicide (standardized mortality ratio 0.96, 95% CI 0.72-1.24), and those who were wounded more than once and required hospitalization for at least one wound had the highest risk of suicide (standardized mortality ratio 1.73, 95% CI 1.10-2.60). Strengths of the study included a 95% statistical power to detect a 1.2-fold increase in relative risk of motor-vehicle accidents and a 1.28-fold increase in relative risk of suicide in comparison with the U.S. general population using an alpha level of 0.05 and a two-sided test. Furthermore, although most studies of exposure to combat trauma rely on interview data to ascertain exposure, this study was able to minimize that source of potential bias by using military records (that is, military reports of casualties) to determine exposure. However, this study, like many, was unable to include data on potentially predisposing psychologic and behavioral characteristics that might be important risk factors for suicide after military service.

Kang and Bullman (1996) obtained death certificates of Gulf War veterans, of a control group that was mobilized and deployed elsewhere, and of a control group of veterans who were not deployed at all. Death certificates were provided through VA regional offices, as identified from combined data sources, which included the BIRLS database and the files from Social Security Administration. A qualified nosologist used the *ICD-9* to code all causes of death and was blinded to subjects' deployment status. Of 695,516 Gulf War veterans, 1765 had died, and death certificates were located for 1654 (93.7%). Of 746,291 controls deployed elsewhere or not deployed, 1729 had died, and death certificates were located for 1615 (93.4%). Gulf War veterans had a significantly higher mortality than veterans deployed elsewhere or never deployed during the period (adjusted mortality rate ratio 1.09, 95% CI 1.01-1.16). Accidental death accounted for the largest part of the difference (rate ratio 1.25, 95% CI 1.13-1.39), but the suicide rate in Gulf War veterans was not higher (rate ratio 0.94, 95% CI 0.79-1.12); rate ratios were adjusted for age, race, sex, branch of service, and type of unit. In general, the contrast between mortality for all causes in female veterans who served in the Gulf War and the general U.S. population was greater (standardized mortality ratio 0.56, 95% CI 0.44-0.71); however, the excess risk of suicide in female veterans approached significance in comparison with women in the general U.S. population (standardized mortality ratio 1.81, 95% CI 0.90-3.24).

Kang and Bullman (2001) extended their 1996 study for an additional 4 years and evaluated changing patterns of mortality in U.S. veterans of the Gulf War for almost 7 years of followup. They compared cause-specific mortality in 621,902 Gulf War veterans who arrived in the Persian Gulf before March 1, 1991, with nondeployed veterans. That excluded people who arrived in the Persian Gulf after hostilities had ended and therefore were not likely to have received the exposures of interest, which included the psychologic stresses of combat. A stratified random sample of all military personnel who served during the war but were not deployed to the Persian Gulf made up the control group of 746,248 veterans. Vital status was determined by using multiple databases, including those of the VA BIRLS and Social Security Administration. Death certificates were requested from VA regional offices. For death certificates that could not be located in that manner, the National Death Index was used to capture causes of death. As in their previous study of Vietnam veterans, the investigators used a qualified nosologist who coded causes of death according to the *ICD-9* without knowledge of the subjects' deployment status.

Kang and Bullman (2001) reported four analyses. The first yielded unadjusted rate ratios calculated from crude death rates. The second used Cox proportional-hazards models to account for possible confounding and effect modification by selected covariates related to veterans' risk of dying (or hazard) from specific causes from the time they entered the cohort. Adjusted rate ratios derived from the models were used to approximate relative risk. The third analysis compared cause-specific mortality in Gulf War veterans and nondeployed veterans with expected numbers of deaths in the overall U.S. population. Finally, changes in relative mortality in Gulf War veterans and nondeployed veterans during four 20-month followup periods were examined with a chi-squared test for trend. For each of followup periods beginning in January 1993 and extending to December 1997, an adjusted rate ratio was derived from the Cox proportional-hazards model after adjustment for age, race, marital status, branch of service, and type of unit. In the analyses, there was no excess all-cause-specific mortality and no excess mortality from all external causes combined, but there was an excess risk of death from motor-vehicle accidents in Gulf War veterans compared with nondeployed veterans that decreased steadily from the first followup (rate ratio 1.32, 95% CI 1.13-1.53) to the last followup (rate ratio 1.00, 95% CI 0.82-1.22). The chi-squared value ($\chi^2 = 7.53$) indicated that there was a significant decreasing trend ($p = 0.0061$) in the risk of motor-vehicle accidental death with time since the Gulf War in contrast with a steadily increasing trend in disease-related causes of death in Gulf War veterans compared with nondeployed veterans; deaths from disease was about the same for deployed and nondeployed veterans by the end of the last followup period. The authors concluded that 7 years after the Gulf War, mortality in both Gulf War and nondeployed veterans was half that in their civilian counterparts.

A report from the Mental Health Advisory Team-III (MHAT-III) (MHAT 2006a) issued by the Office of the Surgeon General, U.S. Army Medical Command, is included as a primary source because it used a direct measure of deployment exposure in Iraq. The MHAT-III found that in 2005 the confirmed OIF suicide rate for soliders deployed in Iraq was 19.9 per 100,000 troops. That was compared with a suicide rate in the entire Army of 12.3 per 100,000 in the same year and an average suicide rate of 11.6 per 100,000 in 1995-2005 in the Army.

Secondary Studies

Eight publications were identified as secondary studies (Adams et al. 1998; Boscarino 2005; Kaplan et al. 2007; Kramer et al. 1994; Macfarlane et al. 2000, 2005; Price et al. 2004; Writer et al. 1996). Two publications by Macfarlane et al. (2000, 2005) identified veterans from the UK who served in the Gulf War and veterans who were not deployed to the region. Data on the deployed and era cohorts were obtained from the National Health Service but not confirmed with a supplemental source. The initial study (2000) by the investigators found that the deployed cohort had higher mortality from external causes than the era cohort. However, the difference was nonsignificant and was due primarily to accidents. The second study (2005) by the investigators found no differences in external causes of death between Gulf War and era veterans at followup in June 2004. The study was considered secondary because it did not confirm cause of death.

Writer et al. (1996) used the same retrospective cohort data as Kang and Bullman (1996). Cause-specific mortality from August 1990 though July 1991 was compared for Gulf War-deployed veterans and active-duty troops deployed elsewhere. All active-duty military deaths were reported on a Report of Casualty Form collected routinely and unrelated to the study. Cause of death was reviewed on every casualty report, and the investigators changed the casualty code on the form if it was found to be clearly incorrect. When possible, the cause of death of those who served in the Persian Gulf was verified through a registry of autopsies maintained by the Office of the Armed Forces Medical Examiner; however, no central repository of autopsy data was available to determine the accuracy of deaths of service members deployed elsewhere. The investigators reported that although death rates from unintentional injury were significantly higher in those deployed to the gulf region than in those deployed elsewhere (69.1 vs 41.2 per 100,000 person-years), suicide rates were significantly lower in those deployed to the gulf (3.78 vs 10.82 per 100,000 person-years). The standardized mortality ratios were 0.34 (95% CI 0.16-0.63) for suicides and 1.54 (95% CI 1.32-1.77) for unintentional deaths. This study was considered secondary because no supplemental source was used to determine causes of death in the control group.

Adams et al. (1998) used the Southeast Asia Combat Area Casualties Database to assess the risk of suicide in U.S. ground troops during their tours of duty in Vietnam between 1957 and 1973. They found a higher risk of suicide in men serving in the Army than in other branches of the military (OR 7.86, 95% CI 1.64-5.31). The study was included as a secondary study because no confirmatory sources were used to check the accuracy of the cause of death and only deaths during deployment in country were considered.

Kaplan et al. (2007) examined suicide rates in a nationally representative sample of male community residents in the United States who had completed National Health Interview Surveys in 1986-1994. Vital status and causes of death were determined for survey respondents from 1986 through 1997. Data were collected with face-to-face household interviews; response rates were 94-98%. The outcome variable in the study was death by suicide. The relative risk of suicide was estimated with the Cox proportional-hazards model and adjusted for demographics and socioeconomic, health, and functional status. Time to death was measured from the month of the interview to the month of suicide. Analyses that adjusted for self-reports of demographic characteristics, socioeconomic factors, and health status found that respondents who reported having ever served on active duty in the armed forces had twice the risk of suicide of those who reported being nonveterans (hazard ratio 2.04, 95% CI 1.10-3.80). The committee emphasizes that a major limitation of this study that the investigators did not include a measure of deployment, which is the exposure of interest for this report.

Several studies of suicide in veterans that confined their samples to VA populations (Fontana and Rosenheck 1995b; Lambert and Fowler 1997; Thompson et al. 2002) could not avoid the inherent bias of a self-selected population that elects to receive health care from VA, and so were not considered in this review.

PTSD and Suicide or Accidental Death

Boscarino (2005) and Kramer et al. (1994) found that the risk of suicide or suicidal behavior was higher in Vietnam veterans with PTSD than in those without it. Boscarino (2005) used data from the VES to examine causes of death in 15,288 Vietnam Army veterans 30 years after the war and 15 years after the phase I telephone surveys and personal interviews. When the DIS was used, 10.6% of the theater veterans and 2.9% of the era veterans were found to have PTSD. Vital status and cause-specific mortality were determined with the VA BIRLS, the Social Security Administration Death Master File, and the National Death Index Plus. Veterans with PTSD were more likely than those without PTSD to have died since the 1985-1986 survey

(11.8% vs 4.9%, $p < 0.001$). The hazard ratio for death from external causes in theater veterans with PTSD compared with those without PTSD was 2.3 (95% CI 1.4-3.9). External causes of death were motor-vehicle collision, accidental poisoning, suicide, homicide, and injury of undetermined intent. The hazard ratio was adjusted for race, Army volunteer status, Army entry age, Army discharge status, Army illicit drug use, age at interview, and intelligence.

Price et al. (2004) used data from phase III of the VES survey, conducted in 1996-1997, to assess the effect of PTSD on the risk of nonfatal suicidality (suicidal thinking or behavior) from 1972 to 1996 in 637 male Vietnam-theater veterans. Comparing veterans with PTSD to those without PTSD, the hazard ratio was 1.51 (risk limits 0.65-3.48); during that time, nine of 943 veterans in the cohort database died from suicide, and 15.7% of the 641 veterans interviewed in 1996-1997 reported suicidality. MDD was also significantly associated with nonfatal suicidality over the 25 years (hazard ratio 3.21, risk limits 1.93-5.34), as was drug dependence (hazard ratio 2.06, risk limit 1.31-3.24) but not alcohol dependence (hazard ratio 1.18, risk limit 0.84-1.68). Both PTSD and drug dependence prolonged the duration of suicidality; although the influence of PTSD remaining high during the 25 years, the influence of drug dependence on suicidality decreased with time.

Kramer et al. (1994) assessed the impact of PTSD on suicidality in 131 Vietnam veterans who lived in the community, 64 veterans in a clinical outreach program, and 37 veterans who were psychotherapy patients. PTSD and suicidality were assessed with the Schedule for Affective Disorders and Schizophrenia-Lifetime Version. Suicidal thoughts were more highly correlated with lifetime and current PTSD ($p < 0.001$) than were suicidal behaviors.

Summary and Conclusions

The results of the studies based on cohorts from the Vietnam War and the 1991 Gulf War demonstrate consensus and divergence with regard to the strength of an association between deployment and suicide or accidental death. The conclusions on suicide and accidental death are presented separately.

One study from the Vietnam era provides evidence of a dose-response relationship between the degree of traumatic injury suffered during deployment and suicide. Considering that study with two other primary studies, one in the early followup period after the Vietnam War and the other a study of female Vietnam veterans, the committee concluded that there is sufficient evidence that, at least for some period after deployment, Vietnam veterans were at increased risk of dying from suicide compared with nondeployed veterans. That conclusion is supported in part by the recent report of a higher suicide rate in deployed OIF troops in 2005 than in the Army in that year. The risk may also be increased for some veteran groups, namely, those suffering from PTSD, depression, or substance abuse, and those with specific war-related traumas. The association was not strongly supported by studies conducted in those deployed to the Gulf War, but the brevity of that war and the limited involvement of troops in the region may have kept the statistical power of those studies too low to detect an association between a rare effect—suicide—and deployment.

The committee concluded that there is also sufficient evidence for an association between deployment and accidental death, again, especially potent during the early years postexposure. These conclusions are based on evidence from both the Vietnam War and the Gulf War and from primary and secondary studies.

The studies considered in this section have limitations. In the United States, the coding of mortality data changed substantially in 1999 from *ICD-9* to *ICD-10*, and the number of deaths and death rates due to suicide and accidental death before 1999 may not be readily comparable with data from 1999 on (Anderson et al. 2001; Hoyert et al. 2001). In 2003, the National Center for Health Statistics (NCHS) revised the *ICD-10* Injury Mortality Matrix to finalize groupings of external cause-of-injury classifications; this affected groupings related to both suicide and motor-vehicle accidental deaths. The best way to address discrepancies in how clinicians and researchers define suicidal behaviors is still being debated. Thus, underlying all the studies considered in this section is an inevitable limitation related to a potential for bias due to the inconsistency of case definition of suicide and accidental death among studies of veterans that were conducted over decades. Further limitations may be related to the presence of unknown bias due to misclassification of accidental deaths, some of which may be suicides, and to potential underreporting. However, those potential sources of bias are likely to occur equally among veterans and nonveterans, so it was critical to assess the inclusion of an appropriate control or reference group in the studies evaluated here.

> **The committee concludes that there is sufficient evidence of an association between deployment to a war zone and suicide in the early years after deployment. The committee also concludes that there is sufficient evidence of an association between deployment to a war zone and accidental death in the early years after deployment.**

TABLE 6-13 Suicide and Accidental Death

Reference	Study Design	Population	Outcomes	Results	Adjustments	Comments
CDC 1987 VES	Retrospective cohort, mortality, prevalence	9324 Vietnam-theater veterans, 8989 Vietnam-era veterans who entered Army in 1965-1971	Follow-up began at date of discharge, ended at death or December 31, 1983, whichever came first; mortality data from death certificates coded by *ICD-9* and blind to Vietnam status; review panel of two physicians reviewed cause of death, using medical and legal records for each of 426 deaths; all causes of death were coded by *ICD-9* and blind to Vietnam status	Mortality 17% higher in theater than era; all deaths ≤ 5 years rate ratio 1.45, 95% CI 1.08-1.96, > 5 years rate ratio 1.01, 95% CI 0.79-1.28; all external causes rate ratio 1.25, 95% CI 1.00-1.55; death from motor-vehicle accidents ≤ 5 years rate ratio 1.93, 95% CI 1.16-3.22), > 5 years rate ratio 1.16, 0.72-1.87; suicide ≤ 5 years rate ratio 1.72, 95% CI 0.76-3.88 (adjusted for covariates based on death certificates risk ratio 2.59, 95% CI 1.09-6.17 or medical review panel risk ratio 2.56, 95% CI 1.11-5.87), > 5 years rate ratio 0.64, 95% CI 0.32-1.30; homicide ≤ 5 years rate ratio 1.52, 95% CI 0.59-3.91, > 5 years rate ratio 0.78, 95% CI 0.39-1.55; accidental poisoning (mostly drugs) ≤ 5 years rate ratio 1.69, 95% CI 0.49-5.77	Unadjusted	
Boehmer et al. 2004 (Derived from VES)	Cohort, mortality 30 years after war	9324 Vietnam-theater veterans, 8989 Vietnam-era veterans	Vital-status and cause-of-death followup using VA BIRLS, SSA, and NDI Plus databases; mortality data from death certificates; causes of death coded by *ICD-9* and *ICD-10* and blind to deployment status	All external causes ≤ 5 years rate ratio 1.62, 95% CI 1.16-2.26, > 5 years rate ratio 1.08, 95% CI 0.89-1.29; motor-vehicle accidents ≤ 5 years rate ratio 1.93, 95% CI 1.16-3.22, > 5 years rate ratio 1.02, 95% CI 0.73-1.43; suicide ≤ 5 years rate ratio 1.72, 95% CI 0.76-3.88, > 5 years rate ratio 0.93, 95% CI 0.64-1.34; accidental poisoning (mostly drugs) ≤ 5 years rate ratio 1.69, 95% CI 0.50-5.77, > 5 years rate ratio 2.58, 95% CI 1.09-6.14; homicide ≤ 5 years rate ratio 1.52, 95% CI 0.59-3.91, > 5 years rate ratio 0.80, 95% CI 0.50-1.26; undetermined intent > 5 years rate ratio 3.19, 95% CI 0.88-11.58	Crude death rate per 100,000 person-years	Used multiple sources for vital-status ascertainment; death certificates may not be accurate as to cause of death, particularly suicide; long followup after Vietnam war; large number of deaths

TABLE 6-13 Suicide and Accidental Death

Reference	Study Design	Population	Outcomes	Results	Adjustments	Comments
Thomas et al. 1991	Retrospective cohort, mortality	4582 female Vietnam-theater veterans, 5324 female Vietnam-era veterans; theater veterans served in Vietnam in 1965-1973	Mortality data from death certificates coded by *ICD-9* and blind to Vietnam status	Cause-specific mortality rates; all causes of death combined rate ratio 0.93, 95% CI 0.74-1.16; external causes rate ratio 1.33, 95% CI 0.80-2.23; motor-vehicle accidents rate ratio 3.19, 95% CI 1.03-9.86; suicide rate ratio 0.96, 95% CI 0.39-2.39	Rank, military occupation, duration of military service, age at entry into followup, race	Small cohort of women, short followup period, small number of deaths
Bullman and Kang 1996	Retrospective cohort, average length of followup 21 years	34,534 wounded Vietnam-theater veterans selected randomly from sample of 70,000 wounded veterans included in Casualty Information System database in 1969-1973	Followup from date of wounding until death or December 31, 1991, whichever was earlier; cause of death was based on data from each veteran's death certificate coded by *ICD-9*; Casualty Information System data used to measure date of wounding, severity of wound, number of times wounded	Suicide among veterans who were wounded once and not hospitalized rate ratio 1.00; wounded once and hospitalized rate ratio 1.19, 95% CI 0.85-1.66; wounded two or more times and not hospitalized rate ratio 1.24, 95% CI 0.53-2.88; wounded two or more times and hospitalized for wound rate ratio 1.82, 95% CI 1.12-2.96; compared with U.S. population, wounded veterans had slightly higher risk of death from suicide standardized mortality ratio 1.12, 95% CI 0.96-1.30		1990 data showing military population in general had lower suicide risk than U.S. population (standardized mortality ratio = 0.69, 95% CI 0.56-0.82); risk is almost twice that for peace time, supporting association between exposure to combat trauma and increased risk of suicide
Kang and Bullman 1996	Retrospective cohort, postwar mortality, 2.4-year followup	695,516 GW-deployed veterans, 746,291 nondeployed veterans, including 49,919 female GW veterans, 84,517 female active-duty controls	Vital-status followup using VA and SSA databases; mortality data from death certificates; causes of death coded by *ICD-9* and blind to deployment status	Mortality in men: all causes rate ratio 1.09, 95% CI 1.01-1.18; external causes rate ratio 1.17, 95% CI 1.07-1.29; all accidents rate ratio 1.26, 95% CI 1.11-1.42; motor-vehicle accidents rate ratio 1.27, 95% CI 1.09-1.48; suicide rate ratio 0.88, 95% CI 0.72-1.08 Mortality in women: all causes rate ratio 1.32, 95% CI 0.95-1.83; external causes rate ratio 1.78, 95% CI	Crude death rate per 10,000 person-years; Cox proportional-hazards model adjusted for age, race, sex, service branch, type of unit	Interview data, small sample—alcohol-related accident group may have differed from suicides in undetected ways (unrecognized confounders)

TABLE 6-13 Suicide and Accidental Death

Reference	Study Design	Population	Outcomes	Results	Adjustments	Comments
				1.16-2.73; all accidents rate ratio 1.83, 95% CI 1.02-3.28; motor-vehicle accidents rate ratio 1.81, 95% CI 0.96-3.41; suicide rate ratio 1.47, 95% CI 0.63-3.43		
Kang and Bullman 2001 (Followup to Kang and Bullman 1996)	Retrospective cohort; initial study was 2.4 years; this study was nearly 7 years	621,902 GW-deployed veterans, 746,248 nondeployed veterans (stratified random sample of all military personnel, including active-duty, reserves, National Guard units who served during conflict but not deployed in Persian Gulf)	Vital status followup using VA and SSA databases; mortality data from death certificates; causes of death coded by *ICD-9* and blind to deployment status	Mortality in men: all causes rate ratio 0.95, 95% CI 0.92-0.99; external causes rate ratio 1.04, 95% CI 0.99-1.10; all accidents rate ratio 1.15, 95% CI 1.07-1.23; motor-vehicle accidents rate ratio 1.19, 95% CI 1.09-1.30; suicide rate ratio 0.92, 95% CI 0.83-1.02 Mortality in women: all causes rate ratio 1.16, 95% CI 0.97-1.38; external causes rate ratio 1.39, 95% CI 1.08-1.80; all accidents rate ratio 1.36, 95% CI 0.95-1.96; motor-vehicle accidents rate ratio 1.63, 95% CI 1.09-2.45; suicide rate ratio 1.29, 95% CI 0.78-2.31	Crude death rate per 10,000 person-years; Cox proportional-hazards model adjusted for age, race, sex, service branch, type of unit	Interview data, small sample—alcohol-related accident group may have differed from suicides in undetected ways (unrecognized confounders)
MHAT 2006a	Survey of OIF troops during deployment in Iraq	1320 U.S. Army soldiers (79% active-duty, 8% reserve, 13% National Guard), 447 Marines	MHAT Soldier and Marine Well-Being Survey of anonymous troops; observations by authors; focus-group interviews; behavioral-health surveys, primary care, unit ministry-care surveys	Suicide rate in Iraq (per 100,000) 18.8 (2003), 9.6 (2004), 19.9 (2005), 16.1 (2006), $p < 0.01$; U.S. Army 10-year average suicide rate 11.6 per 100,000 year	Report states suicide rates were adjusted, but no details given	Report is prepared periodically as requested by Army; it is not a formal, methodologically rigorous survey, but is included because it contains recent data on troops surveyed in Iraq

NOTE: BIRLS = Beneficiary Identification Record Locator Subsystem Death File, BMI = body-mass index, CI = confidence interval, GW = Gulf War, *ICD-9* = *International Statistical Classification of Diseases*, 9th edition, MHAT = Mental Health Advisory Team, NDI = National Death Index, OIF = Operation Iraqi Freedom, OR = odds ratio, SSA = Social Security Administration, VA = Department of Veterans Affairs, VES = Vietnam Experience Study.

SYMPTOM REPORTING

Numerous studies, many of them discussed earlier in this chapter, indicate that war-zone-deployed veterans, both men and women and regardless of the conflict in which they served, consistently report more symptoms, more adverse health effects, and poorer health status than do veterans who served in the military at the same time but were not deployed or were deployed but not to a war zone (CDC 1988b; Cherry et al. 2001a; Eisen et al. 2005; Goss Gilroy Inc. 1998; Gray et al. 1999, 2002; Hotopf et al. 2003b; Iowa Persian Gulf Study Group 1997; Ishoy et al. 1999; Kang et al. 2000b; Kelsall et al. 2004a; Kulka et al. 1990; O'Toole et al. 1996b; Ozakinci et al. 2006; Pierce 1997; Proctor et al. 1998; Simmons et al. 2004; Steele 2000; Unwin et al. 1999; Wolfe et al. 1999). In particular, Gulf War veterans reported markedly more symptoms compared to their nondeployed counterparts, whether the veterans were from the United States, the UK, Canada, Australia, or Denmark. Increased symptoms have also been reported in Vietnam veterans from the United States and Australia (CDC 1988b; O'Toole et al. 1996b).

This section considers three aspects of this excess symptom reporting by deployed veterans from the Vietnam War, the Gulf War, and OEF and OIF that do not readily fit with the health outcomes already discussed: general symptoms that do not appear to be indicative of a specific illness or disorder, symptoms that appear to cluster into the *ICD* category of unexplained illness, and chronic pain of unknown origin. The committee has included the primary studies for general symptoms and unexplained illness in Table 6-14.

General Symptoms and Signs

Gulf War-deployed veterans reported many symptoms at rates 2-3 times higher than those seen in nondeployed veterans in several large studies from five countries: the United States (Kang et al. 2000b; Gray et al. 2002), the United Kingdom (Cherry et al. 2001a; Simmons et al. 2004; Unwin et al. 1999), Denmark (Ishoy et al. 1999), Canada (Goss Gilroy Inc. 1998), and Australia (Kelsall et al. 2004a). Similar results have been seen in veterans of the Vietnam War (CDC 1988b; Kulka et al. 1990) and World War II (Villa et al. 2002). Furthermore, the symptoms and reports of poor health persist, often for many years after the war (Ozakinci et al. 2006).

Among the symptoms most commonly reported by Gulf War and Vietnam veterans are fatigue, headaches, irritability or feeling anxious, poor memory, joint stiffness or pain, sleep difficulties (including problems in falling asleep or staying asleep and unrefreshing sleep, such as waking up feeling tired), and poor concentration. Several of the symptoms—such as sleep problems, abdominal pain, and chest pain—and neurologic problems have been discussed by the committee in previous sections on sleep disturbances, neurocognitive effects, cardiovascular diseases, and digestive system diseases.

CDC undertook the VES to assess the health status of Vietnam-theater and Vietnam-era veterans who served in the U.S. Army during 1965-1971; the study was completed in 1988, about 15-20 years after the war (CDC 1988b). A nationally representative random sample of 7924 theater veterans and 7364 era veterans completed a phase 1 telephone interview; in phase 2, a subsample of 2490 of the theater veterans and 1972 of the era veterans also completed physical- and psychologic-health screening examinations in 1985-1986. In phase 1, 19.6% of the 7924 theater veterans reported their health as fair or poor compared with 11.1% of 7364 era veterans (OR 1.8, 95% CI excludes 1.0, $p < 0.05$); similar results were found on examination (OR 1.9, 95% CI excludes 1.0). On examination, 10.2% of theater veterans and 6.2% of era veterans had somatic symptoms, which included nervousness, fatigue, gastrointestinal tract ailments, dizziness, and headaches for a significant OR of 1.7 (95% CI excludes 1.0); symptoms of peripheral neuropathy (numbness, tingling, burning sensation, or weakness of arms or legs) were found in 3.5% of the theater veterans and 1.9% of the era veterans (OR 1.5, 95% CI 1.0-2.2). The OR was adjusted for age at enlistment, race, year of enlistment, enlistment status, score on a general technical test, and primary military occupational specialty. The study had the advantage of including a physical examination and a large study population; the response rate was 75% for theater veterans and 63% for era veterans.

Ishoy et al. (1999) assessed the health status of 686 Danish peacekeepers deployed to the Persian Gulf during 1991-1996 and compared them with 231 nondeployed military personnel. All study participants underwent a health examination in 1997-1998. The deployed veterans had significantly ($p < 0.001$) more repeated headaches (19.2% vs 6.5%), balance disturbances or dizziness (13.65 vs 3.9%), concentration or memory difficulties (31.2% vs 8.2%), abnormal fatigue (26.4% vs 10.8%), sleep problems (19.8% vs 6.9%), and feeling nervous, irritable, or agitated (21.0% vs 9.1%) with onset during or after deployment than the nondeployed controls.

Some surveys have asked veterans about more than 95 symptoms and found that for all symptoms—ranging from the less severe, such as loss of appetite, to the more severe, such as chest infections and abscesses—deployed veterans report having more symptoms and being more troubled by the symptoms than nondeployed veterans (Cherry et al. 2001a). In a telephone survey conducted in 2000-2002, 674 World War II veterans, 983 Korean War veterans, 1420 Vietnam War veterans, and 137 Gulf War veterans living in southern California and Nevada were asked about their health and activities of daily living (Villa et al. 2002). World War II and Korean veterans reported the best mental health, but World War II veterans were also more likely to report their health status as poor and to have more impairment in activities of daily living than the other veteran groups even when socioeconomic status, disease prevalence, and mental-health status were held constant. Vietnam veterans, however, were more likely than Korean War or Gulf War veterans to report difficulty in performing activities of daily living.

In a comprehensive review, Barrett et al. (2002b) examined symptom prevalence in various Gulf War veteran populations. They concluded that reports of symptoms were higher in Gulf War veterans than in controls but the pattern of symptoms being reported was neither abnormal for, nor peculiar to, a veteran population.

The primary precipitating event for increased reporting of adverse health effects after deployment is combat experience. Combat stressors were discussed in Chapter 3. McFarlane (1997) reported on World War II veterans who were followed until the age of 65 years for PTSD. They found that men who had experienced heavy combat had died earlier, and this finding was independent of PTSD. Of the men who experienced heavy combat, 56% were dead or chronically ill by the age of 65 years compared with only 39% of the men who had not experienced heavy combat (Lee et al. 1995). Increasing combat exposure results in an increase in the reporting of stress-related symptoms (Sutker et al. 1993b; Wolfe et al. 1998).

Kulka et al. (1990) found that male Vietnam veterans who had experienced high war-zone stress were twice as likely to report their physical health as poor as were veterans who experienced low war-zone stress (25% vs 13%). In a study of Australian Vietnam veterans; however, O'Toole et al. (1996b) did not find a significant increase in symptoms, signs, and ill-defined conditions with increasing combat exposure ($p = 0.029$). The impact of combat on PTSD and other psychiatric disorders is discussed in Chapter 5.

PTSD and General Symptom Reporting

PTSD is associated with increased reports of poor physical health in veterans and civilian populations, regardless of how physical health is determined, that is, through physical examination or self-reports (Baker et al. 1997; Barrett et al. 2002a; Beckham et al. 1998; Schnurr and Jankowski 1999; Sloan et al. 2005). That has been seen in studies of male and female Vietnam veterans (Beckham et al. 1998; Boscarino 1997; Kulka et al. 1990; Taft et al. 1999; Zatzick et al. 1997a,b), Gulf War veterans (Baker et al. 1997), and World War II and Korean War veterans in the VA Normative Aging Study (Schnurr and Spiro 1999). Several researchers have attempted to identify links between war-zone exposures and physical health of veterans (Friedman et al. 1995; Taft et al. 1999; Wolfe et al. 1994). In each case, PTSD was the major mediator between war-zone exposure and poor physical health; the presence of PTSD was a better predictor of poor health than was being in a war zone. People with PTSD also tend to engage in poor behavioral practices, such as increased alcohol consumption and smoking, which in turn put them at risk for other health problems (Friedman et al. 1995).

Asmundson et al. (2002) studied the effects of PTSD on health in 1187 Canadian men deployed to war zones for UN peacekeeping missions and compared them with the health of 669 Canadians who had served in the military but had never been deployed. According to the PTSD Checklist-Military Version, 11% of the deployed and 3% of the nondeployed troops met the screening criteria for current PTSD. Those with PTSD had more self-reported poor health than those without PTSD regardless of deployment status. PTSD symptoms also contributed to depression, which in turn, resulted in even more poor health. PTSD was also predictive of alcohol use, however, the latter, unlike depression, was not associated with poorer health beyond that associated with symptoms of PTSD alone.

In a study of 107 Harvard graduates who fought in World War II discussed above (Lee et al. 1995), symptoms of PTSD in both 1946 and 1988 were correlated significantly ($p < 0.001$) with combat exposure and with the number of physical symptoms experienced by the veterans during their combat exposure; however, the PTSD symptoms were not associated with any premorbid vulnerabilities, such as low socioeconomic status or childhood emotional problems. Combat exposure was also a predictor of later poor health: 59% of those with both heavy combat and PTSD were chronically ill or dead by the age of 65 years, compared with only 39% of those without heavy combat experience.

World War II veterans (70-74 years old) who had participated in secret military tests of mustard gas during the war were assessed for current PTSD in 1996 using the PTSD Checklist (Schnurr et al. 2000). Veterans with PTSD had significantly higher rates of the following self-reported illnesses than veterans without PTSD: coronary heart disease, pulmonary disease, dermatologic conditions, ophthalmologic diseases, GI disorders, sexual dysfunction, and urologic disorders. Veterans with PTSD also had greater pain and fatigue, greater impairment in physical and psychosocial functioning, and were more likely to have lifetime disability, including lifetime VA psychiatric disability. Health care use was also significantly higher for veterans with PTSD.

The VA Normative Aging Study, begun in 1963, consists of 2280 men, 95% of whom are World War II or Korean War veterans. At study entry, 84% of the veterans reported combat exposure; in 1990, using the Combat Exposure Scale, 79% reported combat exposure. In 1990,

Schnurr et al. (2000) screened 605 of the veterans (98% white and 85% World War II veterans) for PTSD symptoms with the Mississippi Scale for Combat-Related PTSD. They found that 1% of the study participants had a score on the scale that indicated symptoms of PTSD. More combat exposure was correlated with more PTSD symptoms, and both combat and PTSD symptoms were correlated with increased self-reports of poor physical and mental health (Schnurr and Spiro 1999). When PTSD symptoms were associated with various physician-diagnosed health outcomes, a 10-point increase in PTSD symptom scores was found to increase the risk of having an arterial disorder by 27%, a lower GI disorder by 23%, a dermatologic disorder by 18%, and a musculoskeletal disorder by 9%. Increases in arterial, pulmonary, and upper GI disorders, but decreases in onset of other heart disorders, were associated with increased combat exposure. No association was found between PTSD and cancer, genitourinary disorders, or endocrine disorders (Boscarino 1997; Schnurr et al. 2000). The ambulatory care veterans from the VA Veterans Health Study who screened positive for PTSD were found to have significantly more chronic lower back pain than veterans without PTSD (OR 2.85, 95% CI 2.25-3.63, $p \leq 0.05$) adjusted for age and for depression (Spiro et al. 2005).

Women with PTSD have a greater risk of poor health status than do women without PTSD. Using NVVRS data, Zatzick et al. (1997b) found that female veterans with PTSD reported poorer health status and well-being, had more days in bed, were more likely not to be working currently, and had more limitations in physical functioning than female veterans without PTSD. In a mailed survey of female veterans who attended a VA medical facility, those who screened positive for PTSD (n = 266) using the PTSD Checklist-Civilian Version were significantly more likely than those without PTSD (n = 940) to also screen positively for a drinking problem (OR 1.68, 95% CI 1.22-2.30), a drug problem (OR 3.56, 95% CI 2.36-5.37), being a victim of domestic violence (OR 2.58, 95% CI 1.92-3.46), and various psychiatric disorders, including panic disorder and major depression. Female veterans who screened positive for PTSD were also more likely to have several self-reported medical problems, including fibromyalgia, stroke, irritable bowel syndrome, chronic pelvic pain, premenstrual syndrome, and polycystic ovary disease (all ORs > 2.0, 95% CIs > 1.0) (Dobie et al. 2004).

Unexplained Illness

Unexplained illnesses have been described primarily in the Gulf War veteran literature. As discussed above, veterans who were deployed to the Persian Gulf region report more symptoms than their nondeployed counterparts. The numerous symptoms or clusters of symptoms have been referred to by a variety of terms, such as Gulf War syndrome, chronic multisymptom illness, and "unexplained" illness. They are "unexplained" not in the sense that they are of unknown etiology (which is true of many medical conditions) but rather in the sense that they do not fit into established medical diagnostic categories (IOM 2006). The *ICD* includes a category "unknown and unspecified causes of morbidity," R69, that might be appropriate for this health effect. Several studies for unexplained illness that met the committee's criteria for primary studies because they did not rely on self-reports are included in Table 6-14.

The committee identified eight studies of unexplained illness in Gulf War veterans beginning with a study by Fukuda et al. (1998) that established the CDC case definition for chronic multisymptom illness. In response to a request from DoD, VA, and the Commonwealth of Pennsylvania, Fukuda et al. (1998) assessed the health status of Air Force veterans who had been deployed to the Gulf War. Their focus was to assess the prevalence and causes of an unexplained illness in members of one Air National Guard unit. They administered a 35-item symptom inventory that included symptom severity (mild, moderate, or severe) and duration (less than 6 months or 6 months or longer) and randomly divided the 3255 participants who had answered all symptom questions into subsamples of 1631 and 1624. They used factor analysis to organize symptoms into a case definition for the CDC. The case definition consisted of having one or more chronic symptoms (present for 6 months or longer) in each of at least two of three categories: fatigue, mood-cognition (symptoms of feeling depressed, difficulty in remembering or concentrating, feeling moody, feeling anxious, trouble in finding words, and difficulty in sleeping), and musculoskeletal (symptoms of joint pain, joint stiffness, and muscle pain). A case was classified as severe if each reported symptom that was used to meet the case definition was rated as severe.

Of the survey participants, those deployed to the Gulf War experienced a higher prevalence of chronic symptoms than nondeployed veterans (33 of 35 symptoms with more than 6-month duration were reported to be more prevalent). According to the case definition, 39% of Gulf War-deployed veterans and 14% of nondeployed veterans had mild to moderate cases, and 6% and 0.7%, respectively, had severe cases. On the basis of a total of 158 clinical examinations performed in one Air National Guard unit, there were no abnormal physical or laboratory findings that differentiated those who met the case definition from those who did not meet the case definition. Case subjects, however, reported significantly lower functioning and well-being. Because such a large fraction (14%) of nondeployed veterans met the definition of mild to moderate cases, the investigators concluded that the case definition could not specifically characterize Gulf War veterans who had unexplained illnesses (Fukuda et al. 1998).

The study has several limitations, including the fact that its coverage of only current Air Force personnel several years after the Gulf War makes it difficult to generalize its results to other branches of service and to those who might have left the service because of illness. The use of self-reported symptoms introduced the possibility of reporting bias, and the low participation rates in two of the four units (62% and 35%) introduced the possibility of selection bias. Nonetheless, symptom reporting and prevalence were similar among the four units. A particular strength of the study was its use of a symptom inventory rather than asking veterans about specific diagnoses, such as CFS, multiple chemical sensitivity, depression, and various neurologic abnormalities. Its use of a more intensive examination of Gulf War veterans from one unit—including an additional clinical questionnaire, a variety of laboratory tests, and interviewer-administered modules on major depression, somatization disorder, and panic disorder—provided important additional data even though participation rates were low (62%).

A nested case-control secondary study of the Fukuda et al. (1998) cohort (n = 1002) sought to identify self-reported exposures associated with cases of chronic mutisymptom illness (Nisenbaum et al. 2000). Having an injury requiring medical attention was associated with having a severe case of chronic mutisymptom illness. Symptom clustering in the Fort Devens cohort was studied in 1997 with CDC's case definition of chronic mutisymptom illness (Wolfe et al. 2002). The case definition was applied to findings from use of the 52-item health checklist. About 60% of respondents met the CDC case definition. That group was divided between "mild to moderate" and "severe" cases. Both Nisenbaum et al. (2000) and Wolfe et al. (2002) found that many Gulf War exposures—including exposure to pyridostigmine bromide, anthrax vaccination, tent-heater exhaust, oil-fire smoke, and chemical odors—and psychologic distress such as fear of a chemical attack, were associated with meeting the case definition of chronic mutisymptom illness.

In a primary study, Blanchard et al. (2006) sought to determine the prevalence of unexplained illnesses in Gulf War veterans 10 years after the Gulf War. The study applied CDC's definition of chronic multisymptom illness (Fukuda et al. 1998). Data were collected from 1035 deployed veterans and 1116 nondeployed veterans. Participants were asked about symptoms in face-to-face interviews, and those who reported at least one symptom in each of three clusters—fatigability, mood and cognition, and musculoskeletal—were considered to meet the case definition. Cases were classified as severe if at least one symptom in each cluster was rated as severe. The investigators found that overall 29% of deployed participants and 16% of nondeployed participants met the criteria for chronic mutisymptom illness (OR 2.16, 95% CI 1.61-2.90); deployed veterans were more likely than nondeployed veterans to have severe chronic mutisymptom illness (OR 4.65, 95% CI 2.27-9.52), and among deployed veterans it was associated with a higher score on the Combat Exposure Scale ($p < 0.001$). Both deployed and nondeployed veterans who met the case definition had lower mean scores on the SF-36 for physical and mental health, more nonroutine clinic visits, more prescriptions, and were more likely to be using psychotropic medications, than deployed or nondeployed veterans without chronic mutisymptom illness. Veterans with chronic mutisymptom illness were also more likely than veterans without it to also have fibromyalgia, CFS, symptomatic arthralgia, dyspepsia, metabolic syndrome, PTSD, anxiety disorders, major depression, nicotine dependence, alcohol dependence (deployed veterans only), and more than one psychiatric diagnosis during the year preceding the examination. The study was limited by low participation rates and the self-reporting of symptoms, but it provided evidence that the cluster of symptoms used to define chronic mutisymptom illness persisted in Gulf War veterans 10 years after the war.

Ozakinci et al. (2006), in a secondary study, also investigated widespread symptomatic illness in Gulf War veterans. Participants were identified from the VA Gulf War Health Registry, contacted twice (in 1995 and 2000), and asked to respond to symptom survey questionnaires. Statistical analyses were conducted to assess changes in symptoms over time. No significant changes were found in the cohort in symptom number or severity. Thus, Gulf War Health Registry veterans 10 years after deployment continued to experience significant symptoms. Limitations of the study include the problem of generalizability to all Gulf War veterans—the study included only veterans in a registry, and there was no nondeployed comparison group—and the possibility of reporting bias because of the self-reporting nature of the questionnaire.

Self-reports of health status in Australian Vietnam veterans 20-25 years after the war, and the impact of combat exposure, were investigated. O'Toole et al. (1996b) used the Australian Bureau of Statistics Health Interview Survey questionnaire to interview in-person a random sample of Army veterans posted to Vietnam during 1964-1972 and compared the veterans with the general Australian population. A 21-item combat exposure index was also used to measure the relationship between combat and physical health. Combat exposure was related to recent but not chronic symptoms, signs, and ill-defined conditions. Comparison of Australian Vietnam Veterans with the Australian population for prevalence of self-reported symptoms, signs, and ill-defined conditions, adjusted for response bias, yielded an RR of 2.77 (99% CI 1.88-3.66).

In the first of three primary hospitalization studies, Gray et al. (1996) used a retrospective cohort and data from DoD hospitals for the period 1991-1993. The study examined hospitalizations of 547,076 Army, Navy, Marine Corps, and Air Force Gulf War veterans and 618,335 nondeployed era veterans. Multivariate logistic-regression analyses yielded ORs of less than 1 for ill-defined conditions for all 3 years. The authors noted that in an attempt to reduce the potential bias due to attrition, only members of the study population who remained on active duty for at least half the study period were included in the multivariate models.

A second hospitalization study expanding on Gray et al. (1996) study compared the postwar records of Gulf War-deployed veterans (n = 552,111) and nondeployed veterans (n = 1,479,751) from DoD's hospital-discharge data from August 1991 to April 1996 to search for admissions for unexplained illnesses in military hospitals (Knoke and Gray 1998). The study defined unexplained illnesses as diagnoses in 77 *ICD-9* diagnostic categories that comprised ill-defined conditions. The study examined only first hospitalizations to avoid overcounting medical conditions that required repeated hospitalizations of the subset of patients who had at least one unexplained illness coded on a discharge summary. Up to eight discharge diagnoses were examined per hospitalization. The authors found that deployed active-duty military members were less likely to have been hospitalized for unexplained illnesses than nondeployed (RR 0.93, 95% CI 0.91-0.96) (Knoke and Gray 1998). That finding included adjustment for a variety of covariates and removed the effect of participation in the CCEP after June 1994. Participants in the CCEP were more likely to have been hospitalized only for evaluation. This study has the advantage of a large sample that allowed detection of even minimal effects. Its major limitations are its inclusion of only active-duty personnel and its inability to detect illnesses that did not warrant hospitalization.

Although the previous studies demonstrated no increase in unexplained illness among active-duty Gulf War veterans, Gray et al. (2000) sought to expand their investigation of Gulf War veterans to include reserve and separated military personnel who may not have been treated in a DoD facility. They investigated hospitalization data from DoD, VA, and nonfederal hospitals in California for 1991-1994. Hospitalization rates could not be directly compared among the three sources, because of the unreliability of state-of-residence data in DoD and VA datasets. Therefore, PMRs of hospital-discharge diagnoses (14 diagnostic categories from *ICD-9*) were compared for deployed vs nondeployed veterans. For VA hospitals, but not for DoD or California hospitals, the PMR for the *ICD* code of symptoms, signs, and ill-defined diseases was increased for deployed vs nondeployed veterans (PMR 1.24, 95% CI 1.16-1.33).

A previous IOM report (IOM 2006) has carefully described and evaluated studies of unexplained illness and increased symptom self-reporting. Cluster or factor analysis has been used by several researchers (for example, Fukuda et al. 1998) to determine whether the many symptoms reported constituted a new syndrome or a variant of an existing syndrome. However, the 2006 IOM report concluded that outcomes based primarily on symptoms or self-reports constituted "no unique syndrome, unique illness, or unique symptom complex in deployed Gulf War veterans. Veterans of the Gulf War report higher rates of nearly all symptoms or sets of symptoms than their nondeployed counterparts; 29% of veterans meet a case definition of 'multisymptom illness,' as compared with 16% of nondeployed veterans" (IOM 2006).

Posttraumatic Stress Disorder and Unexplained Illness

Two studies of PTSD and unexplained illness were identified. In a nested case-control study drawn from a large, population-based study of Iowa veterans of the Gulf War, Barrett et al. (2002a) investigated the relationship between PTSD and perceived physical health. Of the 53 veterans who screened positive for PTSD (37 deployed and 16 nondeployed), over 50% had symptoms that corresponded with ill-defined conditions according to the *ICD-9* compared with less than 10% of the 3629 veterans without PTSD. The study was conducted by telephone interview 5 years after the Gulf War. The prevalence of PTSD among the Gulf War-deployed veterans was 3.4% and 1.4% for those who had participated in combat and for those who did not, respectively. The study is limited by the inclusion of both deployed and nondeployed veterans in the PTSD-positive group and the lack of specific data on the prevalence of various health outcomes.

A study of posttraumatic stress symptomatology (PTSS) and unexplained illness was conducted by Ford et al. (2001). They sought to determine whether there was an association between war-zone trauma or PTSS and illnesses reported by Gulf War veterans. Participants were randomly selected from a DoD database of 8603 eligible Gulf War veterans from Oregon or Washington who were deployed from August 1, 1990, through July 31, 1991. Of those deemed eligible and who completed questionnaires, 237 cases and 113 controls were identified by medical examination. A 4-hour test battery of 19 tests was administered to assess psychologic status and neurobehavioral function. Findings indicate that 13 of the 14 psychologic variables were significantly associated with case (vs control) status in unadjusted univariate logistic regression analyses. Case subjects reported significantly higher levels of somatic distress; health problems, fatigue, pain, and deterioration in physical health; global and specific psychiatric distress; negative effects of recent life events; and war-zone trauma exposure than controls. The study is limited by its retrospective analysis of war trauma and its lack of representativeness of the entire Gulf War veteran population.

Chronic Pain

Chronic pain, defined as "an unpleasant sensory and emotional experience, associated with actual or potential tissue damage or described in terms of such damage" that persists for 6 months or longer (Otis et al. 2003), is one of the most frequently reported symptoms in veteran populations. Such unexplained pain does not help the body to prevent injury. It can persist for weeks to years as pain signals continue to stimulate the nervous system. Common chronic pain complaints include headache, low-back pain, joint pain, neurogenic pain (pain resulting from damage to the peripheral nerves or to the central nervous system), and psychogenic pain (pain not due to disease, injury, or any visible sign of damage inside or outside the nervous system). Chronic pain is different from CWP (discussed earlier in the chapter with fibromyalgia) because it does not meet the ACR criteria necessary for a diagnosis of CWP. It has been estimated that 50 million Americans have serious chronic pain annually (American Pain Foundation 2007).

Studies of various types of unspecified and unexplained pain in deployed and nondeployed veteran groups invariably find that deployed veterans report significantly more pain symptoms—including joint pain, backache, chronic back pain, muscular pain, neck ache, neuralgia, and headache—than nondeployed troops (Gray et al. 1999; Kang et al. 2000b; Kelsall et al. 2006; Kuzma and Black 2006; Proctor et al. 1998, 2001; Simmons et al. 2004; Unwin et al. 1999). In a study of 970 OEF and OIF veterans seeking treatment at a VA medical center, 38% reported some level of pain; of those, 59% had pain that was clinically significant and likely to interfere with functional activities (Gironda et al. 2006). In over half the patients with chronic pain, the pain could not be attributed to any type of injury.

Thomas et al. (2006) conducted a meta-analysis of 20 studies that compared self-reports of pain in Gulf War-deployed veterans with era veterans. They found that deployment was most strongly associated with abdominal pain (six studies, OR 3.23, 95% CI 2.31-4.51), but deployment was also associated with reports of other pain, including muscle pain (eight studies, OR 3.06, 95% CI 2.18-4.30), joint pain (12 studies, OR 2.81, 95% CI 2.31-3.42), chest pain (seven studies, OR 2.52, 95% CI 2.23-2.85), and back pain (six studies, OR 1.58, 95% CI 1.23-

2.04). The authors commented on the potential effects of the survey procedures, response bias, symptom measurement, and confounding in each study. They noted that although the methodologic quality of the 20 studies varied considerably, all but one of the studies found more self-reports of pain in Gulf War-deployed than in nondeployed veterans.

The *DSM-IV* also has a category of somatoform disorders that includes pain disorder that has been studied in some veterans. Toomey et al. (2007) found that Gulf War veterans had substantially more pain disorders, as diagnosed with the CIDI using the *DSM-IV* criteria, than did nondeployed veterans (OR 91.66, 95% CI 10.52-798.21). Ikin et al. (2004) interviewed a random sample of Australian Gulf War veterans after the war to determine the prevalence of various psychiatric disorders using the CIDI. They found that deployed veterans (n = 1381) were no more likely than nondeployed veterans (n = 1377) to have any somatic disorder (OR 2.6, 95% CI 1.0-6.3) but not pain disorder (OR 1.4, 95% CI 0.2-16.4). ORs were adjusted for service type, rank, and age; for any somatic disorder, the OR was also adjusted for education and marital status.

Combat exposure has been linked to somatoform pain disorder (O'Toole et al. 1996a). The ORs for a current (1-month) diagnosis of somatoform pain disorder in Australian Vietnam veterans, based on the DIS, compared with each quartile increase in combat exposure (based on a 21-item combat index) were 1.00, 1.76, 3.07, and 5.08 ($p < 0.0005$); ORs for lifetime somatoform pain disorder and increasing combat exposure were 1.00, 1.05, 1.88, and 2.47 ($p < 0.001$).

Posttraumatic Stress Disorder and Chronic Pain

Although chronic pain is common in deployed veterans, veterans with PTSD are at particular risk. Chronic pain is one of the most commonly reported physical complaints of people (veterans and nonveterans) who have PTSD (McFarlane et al. 1994). And PTSD is common in people who have chronic pain as the result of an accident or trauma (Otis et al. 2003). Several studies that have examined the relationship between PTSD and chronic pain in veterans are discussed below.

Asmundson et al. (2004) reported on a sample of 221 female veterans who used a VA Health Center clinic in 1998-1999 for general health purposes. The women were identified as having PTSD on the basis of responses to a mailed questionnaire that included the PTSD Checklist-Civilian Version, the SF-36, and two additional questions about pain in the preceding 6 months. Female veterans with PTSD reported significantly greater pain—including bodily pain, pain interference, severe headache or migraine, and back pain—than did those without PTSD.

Beckham et al. (1997) investigated patterns of chronic pain in Vietnam veterans with PTSD. Of 129 combat veterans with PTSD, 80% reported chronic pain as determined by the Pain Disability Index, the McGill Pain Questionnaire, the Visual Analog Scale, and a pain drawing; PTSD was diagnosed with the CAPS. Combat veterans with PTSD and chronic pain reported significantly higher somatization, as measured by the hypochondriasis and hysteria subscales of the Minnesota Multiphasic Personality Inventory-2, than did combat veterans with PTSD but without chronic pain. In the sample of 103 veterans with PTSD and chronic pain, Minnesota Multiphasic Personality Inventory-2 hypochondriasis scores and PTSD symptoms from the re-experiencing symptom cluster were significantly related to pain disability, overall pain index, and current pain level.

Benedikt and Kolb (1986) examined case histories of 225 veterans who were referred to a VA pain clinic for the treatment of chronic pain between 1978 and 1984. Of the 225 patients, 22 later received a diagnosis of PTSD (two were World War II veterans, and 20 were Vietnam veterans); this suggests a high prevalence of PTSD (10%) in patients who have chronic pain.

Hoge et al. (2007) found that soldiers who screened positive for PTSD (n = 468) a year after their return from combat duty in Iraq reported more pain symptoms than those negative for PTSD (n = 2347). Half the soldiers with PTSD indicated that they were "bothered a lot" by pain in their arms, legs, or joints (OR 2.89, 95% CI 2.35-3.57); 40% were bothered by back pain (OR 3.36, 95% CI 2.72-4.16); and almost 32% had headaches (OR 4.25, 95% CI 3.32-5.42), compared with 26%, 22%, and 10%, respectively, of soldiers without PTSD. Several other studies report that Gulf War veterans with PTSD had more pain symptoms than did veterans without PTSD (Engel et al. 2000; Spiro et al. 2006).

It has been reported that one-fifth of U.S. Army soldiers returning from OIF have a diagnosis of migraines and that this group has nearly twice as high a risk of depression, PTSD, and other psychiatric disorders as returning soldiers who do not have migraines. When assessed within 90 days of their return from a 1-year tour of duty, 19% of the 2200 veterans had migraines, 32% had depression, 22% had PTSD, and 13% had anxiety. Of those with migraines, 50% were also depressed, 39% also had PTSD, and 22% also had anxiety disorders compared with 27%, 18%, and 10% of those who did not have migraines (Erickson and Diamond 2007).

Those studies suggest that PTSD and chronic pain are frequently comorbid and that each disorder has the potential to exacerbate the symptoms of the other (Otis et al. 2003).

Summary and Conclusions

Male and female veterans who have been deployed to a war zone, regardless of the war in which they served, report more symptoms and poorer health than do their nondeployed counterparts. Symptoms range from severe, such as chest pain and numbing in the extremities, to minor, such as loss of appetite. Combat exposure was associated with increased number and severity of symptoms.

The committee identified eight studies that assessed the prevalence of unexplained illness in Gulf War veterans compared with nondeployed veterans and found mixed results. Some researchers have attempted to cluster the symptoms into new diseases but in general the symptoms are too broad and nonspecific to suggest the presence of a new illness specific to the Gulf War (see IOM 2006). Fukuda et al. (1998) developed the case definition for chronic multisymptom illness based on an Air Force unit deployed to the Gulf War. A later study by Blanchard et al. (2006) found that deployed veterans reported higher rates of nearly all symptoms or sets of symptoms than their nondeployed counterparts 10 years after the war. Four other studies also found higher rates of unexplained illness in deployed Gulf War veterans than in nondeployed Gulf War veterans, but the use of self-reported symptoms introduced the possibility of reporting bias, and the low participation rates in some of the studies introduced the possibility of selection bias.

The three hospitalization studies did not find a consistent association between deployment and a diagnosis of unexplained illness. Although the Knoke and Gray (1998) and Gray et al. (1996) hospitalization studies did not demonstrate an increase in unexplained illness in active-duty Gulf War veterans, the Gray et al. (2000) study reviewed the hospital discharge diagnoses of Gulf War veterans and found an increase in hospitalization for unexplained illness in only one of the three hospital systems examined. The committee notes that symptoms of unexplained illness may not be severe enough to require hospitalization in many cases.

Chronic pain of unexplained origin is one symptom reported more frequently by deployed than nondeployed Gulf War veterans. A meta-analysis of 20 studies of Gulf War veterans found that deployment was most commonly associated with abdominal pain, but back, joint, and muscle pains were also frequently reported. One study of pain in Australian Vietnam veterans found that somatoform pain disorder, a psychiatric diagnosis, was associated with combat exposure.

PTSD is also associated with increased reporting of symptoms, medical conditions, and poor health in veterans, both male and female. Self-reports of more health problems in veterans with PTSD than in those without PTSD have also been confirmed by physical examination. Although combat exposure is associated with increased symptom reporting, PTSD appears to be an even stronger predictor of reports of poor health.

PTSD is widely associated with self-reports of pain in both civilian and veteran populations. Veterans of World War II, the Vietnam War, the Gulf War, and OIF and OEF who have PTSD all report more chronic pain than veterans without PTSD. The chronic pain is not specific; back pain, headaches (including migraines), and joint pain are all reported frequently by both male and female veterans.

The studies cited above have important limitations. Researchers used different terminology for symptoms, and definitions or descriptions of what was meant by the symptom, such as backache or cough, are lacking. Some asked veterans to indicate how much a symptom bothered them over a specific period; others simply asked for an indication of whether the veterans had ever had the symptom after the war. The onset and duration of the symptom were not always assessed or reported. For the studies of PTSD, the veterans were often not diagnosed but only screened for the disorder. And none of the studies indicated whether the veterans had had any of the symptoms before the war in which they were deployed. All those factors make it difficult to compare symptoms among studies.

The committee concludes that there is limited but suggestive evidence of an association between deployment to a war zone and increased symptom reporting, unexplained illness, and chronic pain.

TABLE 6-14 Symptom Reporting

Reference	Study Design	Population	Outcomes	Results	Adjustments	Comments
General symptoms and signs						
CDC 1988b VES	Retrospective cohort, prevalence, population-based, telephone interview followed by screening medical examination	2490 Vietnam-theater veterans, 1972 Vietnam-era veterans randomly selected from 7924 theater veterans and 7364 era veterans who had entered Army in 1965-1971	Perceived health status; somatic symptom; neurologic examination	Health status poor or fair OR 1.9, 95% CI excludes 1.0, $p < 0.05$; somatic symptoms OR 1.7, 95% CI excludes 1.0, $p < 0.05$; peripheral neuropathy symptoms OR 1.5, 95% CI 1.0-2.2	Age at enlistment, race, year of enlistment, enlistment status (volunteer vs draftee), score on general technical test, primary military occupational specialty	Low participation rate in control group, CI not given
Ishoy et al. 1999	Cross-sectional	686 Danish peacekeepers deployed to gulf in 1990-1997 vs 231 age- and sex-matched armed forces nondeployed controls	Health examination by physician, including lung function and self-report questionnaire	Prevalence: repeated headaches 19.2% vs 6.5%; balance disturbances or dizziness 13.65% vs 3.9%; concentration or memory difficulties 31.2% vs 8.2%; abnormal fatigue 26.4% vs 10.8%; sleep problems 19.8% vs 6.9%; feeling nervous, irritable, or agitated 21.0% vs 9.1%		Participation rate 83.6% deployed, 57.8% nondeployed
Unexplained illness						
Blanchard et al. 2006	Cross-sectional	1035 GW-deployed veterans, 1116 nondeployed veterans	CMI determined by medical examination in 1999-2001	CMI (all cases) OR 2.16, 95% CI 1.61-2.90; mild to moderate cases OR 1.92, 95% CI 1.41-2.63; severe cases OR 4.65, 95% CI 2.27-9.52	Age, sex, race, education, duty type, service branch, rank, income, combat exposure score, Khamisiyah exposure, psychiatric conditions and other conditions diagnosed before GW	

TABLE 6-14 Symptom Reporting

Reference	Study Design	Population	Outcomes	Results	Adjustments	Comments
Gray et al. 1996	Retrospective cohort, hospitalization	547,076 active-duty GW veterans, 618,335 non-GW veterans	Hospital-discharge diagnoses for ill-defined conditions for 1991-1993	All results for each year NS	Prewar hospitalization, sex, age, race, service branch, marital status, rank, length of service, salary, occupation	ORs statistically significantly below 1, but no values given; no separation of specific illnesses
Knoke and Gray 1998	Cross-sectional, military hospitalization	552,111 GW-deployed active-duty veterans, 1,479,751 nondeployed active-duty veterans followed from 1991 to March 1996	10 most common unexplained illnesses	Hospitalizations for all unexplained illnesses RR 1.06, 95% CI 1.03-1.09; when adjusted for CCEP participation RR 0.93, 95% CI 0.91-0.96	Race, rank, salary, branch of service, health-care worker status, prewar hospitalization, sex	Did not separate analyses for specific illnesses; adjusted for participation in CCEP after June 1994
Gray et al. 2000	Retrospective cohort, hospitalization	652,979 GW veterans, 652,922 randomly selected non-GW-deployed veterans	Hospital-discharge diagnoses for endocrine, nutritional, metabolic disease in three hospital systems: DoD, VA, COSHPD	DoD PMR 0.97, 95% CI 0.94-1.00 VA PMR 1.24, 95% CI 1.16-1.33 CA PMR 1.04, 95% CI 0.87-1.20	Age, sex, race	Able to assess only illnesses that resulted in hospitalization; possible undetected confounders

NOTE: CCEP = Comprehensive Clinical Evaluation Program, CI = confidence interval, CMI = chronic multisymptom illness, COSHPD = California Office of Statewide Health Planning and Development, DoD = Department of Defense, GW = Gulf War, NS = not significant, OR = odds ratio, PMR = proportional morbidity ratio, RR = relative risk, VA = Department of Veterans Affairs, VES = Vietnam Experience Study.

REFERENCES

Adams DP, Barton C, Mitchell GL, Moore AL, Einagel V. 1998. Hearts and minds: Suicide among United States combat troops in Vietnam, 1957-1973. *Social Science and Medicine* 47(11):1687-1694.

American Lung Association. 2007. *American Lung Association Site*. [Online]. Available: http://www.lungusa.org [accessed July 29, 2007].

American Pain Foundation. 2007. *American Pain Foundation: A United Voice of Hope and Power Over Pain*. [Online]. Available: http://www.painfoundation.org/ [accessed August 1, 2007].

Amital D, Fostick L, Polliack ML, Segev S, Zohar J, Rubinow A, Amital H. 2006. Posttraumatic stress disorder, tenderness, and fibromyalgia syndrome: Are they different entities? *Journal of Psychosomatic Research* 61(5):663-669.

Anderson R, Minino A, Hoyert D, Rosenberg H. 2001. Comparability of cause of death between ICD-9 and ICD-10: Preliminary estimates. *National Vital Statistics Reports* 49(2):1-32.

Ang DC, Peloso PM, Woolson RF, Kroenke K, Doebbeling BN. 2006. Predictors of incident chronic widespread pain among veterans following the first Gulf War. *The Clinical Journal of Pain* 22(6):554-563.

Araneta MR, Destiche DA, Schlangen KM, Merz RD, Forrester MB, Gray GC. 2000. Birth defects prevalence among infants of Persian Gulf War veterans born in Hawaii, 1989-1993. *Teratology* 62(4):195-204.

Araneta MR, Schlangen KM, Edmonds LD, Destiche DA, Merz RD, Hobbs CA, Flood TJ, Harris JA, Krishnamurti D, Gray GC. 2003. Prevalence of birth defects among infants of Gulf War veterans in Arkansas, Arizona, California, Georgia, Hawaii, and Iowa, 1989-1993. *Birth Defects Research* 67(4):246-260.

Archibald HC, Tuddenham RD. 1965. Persistent stress reaction after combat: A 20-year follow-up. *Archives of General Psychiatry* 12:475-481.

Asmundson GJ, Stein MB, McCreary DR. 2002. Posttraumatic stress disorder symptoms influence health status of deployed peacekeepers and nondeployed military personnel. *Journal of Nervous and Mental Disease* 190(12):807-815.

Asmundson GJ, Wright KD, Stein MB. 2004. Pain and PTSD symptoms in female veterans. *European Journal of Pain* 8(4):345-350.

Axelrod BN, Milner IB. 1997. Neuropsychological findings in a sample of Operation Desert Storm veterans. *Journal of Neuropsychiatry and Clinical Neurosciences* 9(1):23-28.

Baker DG, Mendenhall CL, Simbartl LA, Magan LK, Steinberg JL. 1997. Relationship between posttraumatic stress disorder and self-reported physical symptoms in Persian Gulf War veterans. *Archives of Internal Medicine* 157(18):2076-2078.

Barrett DH, Green ML, Morris R, Giles WH, Croft JB. 1996. Cognitive functioning and posttraumatic stress disorder. *American Journal of Psychiatry* 153(11):1492-1494.

Barrett DH, Doebbeling CC, Schwartz DA, Voelker MD, Falter KH, Woolson RF, Doebbeling BN. 2002a. Posttraumatic stress disorder and self-reported physical health status among U.S. military personnel serving during the Gulf War period: A population-based study. *Psychosomatics* 43(3):195-205.

Barrett DH, Gray GC, Doebbeling BN, Clauw DJ, Reeves WC. 2002b. Prevalence of symptoms and symptom-based conditions among Gulf War veterans: Current status of research findings. *Epidemiologic Reviews* 24(2):218-227.

Beckham JC, Crawford AL, Feldman ME, Kirby AC, Hertzberg MA, Davidson JR, Moore SD. 1997. Chronic posttraumatic stress disorder and chronic pain in Vietnam combat veterans. *Journal of Psychosomatic Research* 43(4):379-389.

Beckham JC, Moore SD, Feldman ME, Hertzberg MA, Kirby AC, Fairbank JA. 1998. Health status, somatization, and severity of posttraumatic stress disorder in Vietnam combat veterans with posttraumatic stress disorder. *American Journal of Psychiatry* 155(11):1565-1569.

Beckham JC, Feldman ME, Barefoot JC, Fairbank JA, Helms MJ, Haney TL, Hertzberg MA, Moore SD, Davidson JR. 2000. Ambulatory cardiovascular activity in Vietnam combat veterans with and without posttraumatic stress disorder. *Journal of Consulting and Clinical Psychology* 68(2):269-276.

Beckham JC, Vrana SR, Barefoot JC, Feldman ME, Fairbank J, Moore SD. 2002. Magnitude and duration of cardiovascular responses to anger in Vietnam veterans with and without posttraumatic stress disorder. *Journal of Consulting and Clinical Psychology* 70(1):228-234.

Beckham JC, Taft CT, Vrana SR, Feldman ME, Barefoot JC, Moore SD, Mozley SL, Butterfield MI, Calhoun PS. 2003. Ambulatory monitoring and physical health report in Vietnam veterans with and without chronic posttraumatic stress disorder. *Journal of Traumatic Stress* 16(4):329-335.

Beckham JC, Gehrman PR, McClernon FJ, Collie CF, Feldman ME. 2004. Cigarette smoking, ambulatory cardiovascular monitoring, and mood in Vietnam veterans with and without chronic posttraumatic stress disorder. *Addictive Behaviors* 29(8):1579-1593.

Beebe GW. 1975. Follow-up studies of World War II and Korean War prisoners. II. Morbidity, disability, and maladjustments. *American Journal of Epidemiology* 101(5):400-422.

Benedikt RA, Kolb LC. 1986. Preliminary findings on chronic pain and posttraumatic stress disorder. *American Journal of Psychiatry* 143(7):908-910.

Black DW, Carney CP, Forman-Hoffman VL, Letuchy E, Peloso P, Woolson RF, Doebbeling BN. 2004a. Depression in veterans of the first Gulf War and comparable military controls. *Annals of Clinical Psychiatry* 16(2):53-61.

Black DW, Carney CP, Peloso PM, Woolson RF, Schwartz DA, Voelker MD, Barrett DH, Doebbeling BN. 2004b. Gulf War veterans with anxiety: Prevalence, comorbidity, and risk factors. *Epidemiology* 15(2):135-142.

Blanchard EB, Kolb LC, Prins A, Gates S, McCoy GC. 1991. Changes in plasma norepinephrine to combat-related stimuli among Vietnam veterans with posttraumatic stress disorder. *The Journal of Nervous and Mental Disease* 179(6):371-373.

Blanchard MS, Eisen SA, Alpern R, Karlinsky J, Toomey R, Reda DJ, Murphy FM, Jackson LW, Kang HK. 2006. Chronic multisymptom illness complex in Gulf War I veterans 10 years later. *American Journal of Epidemiology* 163(1):66-75.

Boehmer TK, Flanders WD, McGeehin MA, Boyle C, Barrett DH. 2004. Postservice mortality in Vietnam veterans: 30-year follow-up. *Archives of Internal Medicine* 164(17):1908-1916.

Boscarino JA. 1995. Post-traumatic stress and associated disorders among Vietnam veterans: The significance of combat exposure and social support. *Journal of Traumatic Stress* 8(2):317-336.

Boscarino JA. 1997. Diseases among men 20 years after exposure to severe stress: Implications for clinical research and medical care. *Psychosomatic Medicine* 59(6):605-614.

Boscarino JA. 2004. Posttraumatic stress disorder and physical illness: Results from clinical and epidemiologic studies. *Annals of the New York Academy of Sciences* 1032:141-153.

Boscarino JA. 2005. Posttraumatic stress disorder and mortality among U.S. Army veterans 30 years after military service. *Annals of Epidemiology* 16(4):248-256.

Boscarino JA, Chang J. 1999. Electrocardiogram abnormalities among men with stress-related psychiatric disorders: Implications for coronary heart disease and clinical research. *Annals of Behavioral Medicine* 21(3):227-234.

Buckley TC, Kaloupek DG. 2001. A meta-analytic examination of basal cardiovascular activity in posttraumatic stress disorder. *Psychosomatic Medicine* 63(4):585-594.

Bullman TA, Kang HK. 1996. The risk of suicide among wounded Vietnam veterans. *American Journal of Public Health* 86(5):662-667.

Buske-Kirschbaum A, Geiben A, Hollig H, Morschhauser E, Hellhammer D. 2002. Altered responsiveness of the hypothalamus-pituitary-adrenal axis and the sympathetic adrenomedullary system to stress in patients with atopic dermatitis. *Journal of Clinical Endocrinology and Metabolism* 87(9):4245-4251.

Buske-Kirschbaum A, Kern S, Ebrecht M, Hellhammer DH. 2007. Altered distribution of leukocyte subsets and cytokine production in response to acute psychosocial stress in patients with psoriasis vulgaris. *Brain, Behavior, and Immunity* 21(1):92-99.

Buskila D. 2000. Fibromyalgia, chronic fatigue syndrome, and myofascial pain syndrome. *Current Opinion in Rheumatology* 12(2):113-123.

Caldwell BA, Redeker N. 2005. Sleep and trauma: An overview. *Issues in Mental Health Nursing* 26(7):721-738.

CDC (Centers for Disease Control and Prevention). 1987. Postservice mortality among Vietnam veterans. The Centers for Disease Control Vietnam Experience Study. *Journal of the American Medical Association* 257(6):790-795.

CDC. 1988a. Health status of Vietnam veterans. I. Psychosocial characteristics. The Centers for Disease Control Vietnam Experience Study. *Journal of the American Medical Association* 259(18):2701-2707.

CDC. 1988b. Health status of Vietnam veterans. II. Physical health. The Centers for Disease Control Vietnam Experience Study. *Journal of the American Medical Association* 259(18):2708-2714.

CDC. 1988c. Health status of Vietnam veterans. III. Reproductive outcomes and child health. The Centers for Disease Control Vietnam Experience Study. *Journal of the American Medical Association* 259(18):2715-2719.

CDC. 2007a. Chronic Fatigue Syndrome: The Revised Case Definition (abridged version). [Online]. Available at: http://www.cdc.gov/cfs/cfsdefinitionHCP.htm. [accessed August 31, 2007].

CDC. 2007b. Suicide Facts at a Glance. [Online]. Summer 2007. Available at: www.cdc.gov/injury [accessed August 31, 2007].

Chang L. 2006. Neuroendocrine and neuroimmune markers in IBS: Pathophysiological role or epiphenomenon? *Gastroenterology* 130(2):596-600.

Cherry N, Creed F, Silman A, Dunn G, Baxter D, Smedley J, Taylor S, Macfarlane GJ. 2001a. Health and exposures of United Kingdom Gulf war veterans. Part I: The pattern and extent of ill health. *Occupational and Environmental Medicine* 58(5):291-298.

Cherry N, Creed F, Silman A, Dunn G, Baxter D, Smedley J, Taylor S, Macfarlane GJ. 2001b. Health and exposures of United Kingdom Gulf War veterans. Part II: The relation of health to exposure. *Occupational and Environmental Medicine* 58(5):299-306.

Cosgrove DJ, Gordon Z, Bernie JE, Hami S, Montoya D, Stein MB, Monga M. 2002. Sexual dysfunction in combat veterans with post-traumatic stress disorder. *Urology* 60(5):881-884.

Cowan DN, DeFraites RF, Gray GC, Goldenbaum MB, Wishik SM. 1997. The risk of birth defects among children of Persian Gulf War veterans. *New England Journal of Medicine* 336(23):1650-1656.

Creed F, Levy R, Bradley L, Fransisconi C, Drossman D, Naliboff B. 2006. Psychosocial aspects of functional gastrointestinal disorders. In: Drossman D, Corazziari E, Delvaux M, Spiller R, Talley N, Thompson W, editors. *Rome III: The Functional Gastrointestinal Disorders*. 3rd Ed. McLean, VA: Degnon Associates, Inc.

Crowell TA, Kieffer KM, Siders CA, Vanderploeg RD. 2002. Neuropsychological findings in combat-related posttraumatic stress disorder. *The Clinical Neuropsychologist* 16(3):310-321.

Dagan Y, Lavie P, Bleich A. 1991. Elevated awakening thresholds in sleep stage 3-4 in war-related post-traumatic stress disorder. *Biological Psychiatry* 30(6):618-622.

Dalager NA, Kang HK, Thomas TL. 1995. Cancer mortality patterns among women who served in the military: The Vietnam experience. *Journal of Occupational and Environmental Medicine* 37(3):298-305.

David AS, Farrin L, Hull L, Unwin C, Wessely S, Wykes T. 2002. Cognitive functioning and disturbances of mood in UK veterans of the Persian Gulf War: A comparative study. *Psychological Medicine* 32(8):1357-1370.

David D, Woodward C, Esquenazi J, Mellman TA. 2004. Comparison of comorbid physical illnesses among veterans with PTSD and veterans with alcohol dependence. *Psychiatric Services* 55(1):82-85.

DeStefano F, Annest JL, Kresnow MJ, Schrader SM, Katz DF. 1989. Semen characteristics of Vietnam veterans. *Reproductive Toxicology* 3(3):165-173.

Dlugosz LJ, Hocter WJ, Kaiser KS, Knoke JD, Heller JM, Hamid NA, Reed RJ, Kendler KS, Gray GC. 1999. Risk factors for mental disorder hospitalization after the Persian Gulf War: U.S. Armed Forces, June 1, 1991-September 30, 1993. *Journal of Clinical Epidemiology* 52(12):1267-1278.

Dobie DJ, Kivlahan DR, Maynard C, Bush KR, Davis TM, Bradley KA. 2004. Posttraumatic stress disorder in female veterans: Association with self-reported health problems and functional impairment. *Archives of Internal Medicine* 164(4):394-400.

Dohrenwend B, Turner J, Turse N, Adams B, Koenen K, Marshal R. 2006. The pychological risks of Vietnam for U.S. veterans: A revisit with new data and methods. *Science* 313(5789):979-982.

Dow BM, Kelsoe JR Jr, Gillin JC. 1996. Sleep and dreams in Vietnam PTSD and depression. *Biological Psychiatry* 39(1):42-50.

Doyle P, Maconochie N, Davies G, Maconochie I, Pelerin M, Prior S, Lewis S. 2004. Miscarriage, stillbirth and congenital malformation in the offspring of UK veterans of the first Gulf war. *International Journal of Epidemiology* 33(1):74-86.

Drossman D. 2002. A biopsychosocial understanding of gastrointestinal illness and disease. In: Feldman M, Friedman LS, Sleisenger MH, editors. *Sleisenger and Fordtrans's Gastrointestinal and Liver Diseases*. 7th Ed. Philadelphia, PA: W.B. Saunders. Pp. 2372-2385.

Drossman D. 2006a. The functional gastrointestinal disorders and the Rome III process. In: Drossman D, Corazziari E, Delvaux M, Spiller R, Talley N, Thompson W, editors. *Rome III: The Functional Gastrointestinal Disorders*. 3rd Ed. McLean, VA: Degnon Associates, Inc.

Drossman D, Chang L. 2003. Psychosocial factors in the care of patients with GI disorders. In: Yamada T, editor. *Textbook of Gastroenterology*. Philadelphia, PA: Lippincott-Raven. Pp. 636-654.

Drossman D, Ringel Y. 2004. Psychosocial factors in ulcerative colitis and Crohn's disease. In: Sartor B, Sandborn W, editors. *Kirsner's Inflammatory Bowel Disease*. 6th ed. London, UK: W.B. Saunders. Pp. 340-356.

Drossman DA. 1998. Presidential address: Gastrointestinal illness and the biopsychosocial model. *Psychosomatic Medicine* 60(3):258-267.

Drossman DA. 1999. Mind over matter in the postinfective irritable bowel. *Gut* 44(3):306-307.

Drossman DA. 2006b. The functional gastrointestinal disorders and the Rome III process. *Gastroenterology* 130(5):1377-1390.

Drossman DA, Talley NJ, Leserman J, Olden KW, Barreiro MA. 1995. Sexual and physical abuse and gastrointestinal illness. Review and recommendations. *Annals of Internal Medicine* 123(10):782-794.

Drossman DA, Li Z, Leserman J, Tommey TC, Hu YJB. 1996. Health status by gastrointestinal diagnosis and abuse history. *Gastroenterology* 110(4):999-1007.

Drossman DA, Camilleri M, Mayer EA, Whitehead WE. 2002. AGA technical review on irritable bowel syndrome. *Gastroenterology* 123(6):2108-2131.

Dumitrascu DL, Baban A. 1991. Irritable bowel syndrome complaints following the uprising of December 1989 in Romania. *Medicine and War* 7(2):100-104.

Dunlop SP, Jenkins D, Neal KR, Spiller RC. 2003. Relative importance of enterochromaffin cell hyperplasia, anxiety, and depression in postinfectious IBS. *Gastroenterology* 125(6):1651-1659.

Dunphy RC, Bridgewater L, Price DD, Robinson ME, Zeilman CJ, 3rd, Verne GN. 2003. Visceral and cutaneous hypersensitivity in Persian Gulf war veterans with chronic gastrointestinal symptoms. *Pain* 102(1-2):79-85.

Eaton WW, Armenian H, Gallo J, Pratt L, Ford DE. 1996. Depression and risk for onset of type II diabetes. A prospective population-based study. *Diabetes Care* 19(10):1097-1102.

Eisen SA, Goldberg J, True WR, Henderson WG. 1991. A co-twin control study of the effects of the Vietnam War on the self-reported physical health of veterans. *American Journal of Epidemiology* 134(1):49-58.

Eisen SA, Griffith KH, Xian H, Scherrer JF, Fischer ID, Chantarujikapong S, Hunter J, True WR, Lyons MJ, Tsuang MT. 2004. Lifetime and 12-month prevalence of psychiatric disorders in 8,169 male Vietnam War era veterans. *Military Medicine* 169(11):896-902.

Eisen SA, Kang HK, Murphy FM, Blanchard MS, Reda DJ, Henderson WG, Toomey R, Jackson LW, Alpern R, Parks BJ, Klimas N, Hall C, Pak HS, Hunter J, Karlinsky J, Battistone MJ, Lyons MJ. 2005. Gulf War veterans' health: Medical evaluation of a U.S. cohort. *Annals of Internal Medicine* 142(11):881-890.

Engdahl BE, Eberly RE, Hurwitz TD, Mahowald MW, Blake J. 2000. Sleep in a community sample of elderly war veterans with and without posttraumatic stress disorder. *Biological Psychiatry* 47(6):520-525.

Engel CC Jr, Liu X, McCarthy BD, Miller RF, Ursano R. 2000. Relationship of physical symptoms to posttraumatic stress disorder among veterans seeking care for gulf war-related health concerns. *Psychosomatic Medicine* 62(6):739-745.

Erickson DJ, Wolfe J, King DW, King LA, Sharkansky EJ. 2001. Posttraumatic stress disorder and depression symptomatology in a sample of Gulf War veterans: A prospective analysis. *Journal of Consulting and Clinical Psychology* 69(1):41-49.

Erickson JC, Diamond S. 2007. *Presentation, Annual Meeting, American Academy of Neurology*. Boston, MA.

Escobar JI, Canino G, Rubio-Stipec M, Bravo M. 1992. Somatic symptoms after a natural disaster: A prospective study. *American Journal of Psychiatry* 149(7):965-967.

Falger PR, Op den Velde W, Hovens JE, Schouten EG, De Groen JH, Van Duijn H. 1992. Current posttraumatic stress disorder and cardiovascular disease risk factors in Dutch Resistance veterans from World War II. *Psychotherapy and Psychosomatics* 57(4):164-171.

Fiedler N, Ozakinci G, Hallman W, Wartenberg D, Brewer NT, Barrett DH, Kipen HM. 2006. Military deployment to the Gulf War as a risk factor for psychiatric illness among U.S. troops. *British Journal of Psychiatry* 188:453-459.

Fontana A, Rosenheck R. 1995a. Attempted suicide among Vietnam veterans: A model of etiology in a community sample. *American Journal of Psychiatry* 152(1):102-109.

Fontana A, Rosenheck R. 1995b. An etiological model of attempted suicide among Vietnam theater veterans: Prospective generalization to a treatment-seeking sample. *Journal of Nervous and Mental Disease* 183(6):377-383.

Ford JD, Campbell KA, Storzbach D, Binder LM, Anger WK, Rohlman DS. 2001. Posttraumatic stress symptomatology is associated with unexplained illness attributed to Persian Gulf War military service. *Psychosomatic Medicine* 63(5):842-849.

Forman-Hoffman VL, Carney CP, Sampson TR, Peloso PM, Woolson RF, Black DW, Doebbeling BN. 2005. Mental health comorbidity patterns and impact on quality of life among veterans serving during the first Gulf War. *Quality of Life Research: An International Journal of Quality of Life Aspects of Treatment, Care and Rehabilitation* 14(10):2303-2314.

Forman-Hoffman VL, Peloso PM, Black, DW, Woolson RF, Letuchy EM, Doebbeling BN. 2007. Chronic widespread pain in veterans of the first Gulf War: Impact of deployment status and associated health effects. [Online]. *Journal of Pain*. Available at: http://www.ampainsoc.org/pub/journal.

Freeman T, Roca V, Guggenhehn F, Kimbrell T, Griffin WST. 2005. Neuropsychiatric associations of apolipoprotein E alleles in subjects with combat-related posttraumatic stress disorder. *Journal of Neuropsychiatry and Clinical Neurosciences* 17(4):541-543.

Friedman M, Charney D, Deutch A. 1995. *Neurobiological and Clinical Consequences of Stress: from Normal Adaptation to Post-Traumatic Stress Disorder*. Philadelphia, PA: Lippincott-Raven Publishers.

Fu Q, Heath AC, Bucholz KK, Nelson EC, Glowinski AL, Goldberg J, Lyons MJ, Tsuang MT, Jacob T, True MR, Eisen SA. 2002. A twin study of genetic and environmental influences on suicidality in men. *Psychological Medicine* 32(1):11-24.

Fukuda K, Straus SE, Hickie I, Sharpe MC, Dobbins JG, Komaroff A. 1994. The chronic fatigue syndrome: A comprehensive approach to its definition and study. International Chronic Fatigue Syndrome Study Group. *Annals of Internal Medicine* 121(12):953-959.

Fukuda K, Nisenbaum R, Stewart G, Thompson WW, Robin L, Washko RM, Noah DL, Barrett DH , Randall B, Herwaldt BL, Mawle AC, Reeves WC. 1998. Chronic multisymptom illness affecting Air Force veterans of the Gulf War. *Journal of the American Medical Association* 280(11):981-988.

Fukudo S, Nomura T, Hongo M. 1998. Impact of corticotropin-releasing hormone on gastrointestinal motility and adrenocorticotropic hormone in normal controls and patients with irritable bowel syndrome. *Gut* 42(6):845-849.

Gander ML, von Kanel R. 2006. Myocardial infarction and post-traumatic stress disorder: Frequency, outcome, and atherosclerotic mechanisms. *European Journal of Cardiovascular Prevention and Rehabilitation* 13(2):165-172.

Gifford RK, Ursano RJ, Stuart JA, Engel CC. 2006. Stress and stressors of the early phases of the Persian Gulf War. *Philosophical Transactions of the Royal Society of London—Series B: Biological Sciences* 361(1468):585-591.

Gilbertson MW, Gurvits TV, Lasko NB, Orr SP, Pitman RK. 2001. Multivariate assessment of explicit memory function in combat veterans with posttraumatic stress disorder. *Journal of Traumatic Stress* 14(2):413-432.

Gironda RJ, Clark ME, Massengale JP, Walker RL. 2006. Pain among veterans of Operations Enduring Freedom and Iraqi Freedom. *Pain Medicine* 7(4):339-343.

Goldberg J, Eisen SA, True WR, Henderson WG. 1990. A twin study of the effects of the Vietnam conflict on alcohol drinking patterns. *American Journal of Public Health* 80(5):570-574.

Goss Gilroy Inc. 1998. *Health Study of Canadian Forces Personnel Involved in the 1991 Conflict in the Persian Gulf*. Ottawa, Canada: Goss Gilroy Inc. Department of National Defence.

Gray GC, Coate BD, Anderson CM, Kang HK, Berg SW, Wignall FS, Knoke JD, Barrett-Connor E. 1996. The postwar hospitalization experience of U.S. veterans of the Persian Gulf War. *New England Journal of Medicine* 335(20):1505-1513.

Gray GC, Kaiser KS, Hawksworth AW, Hall FW, Barrett-Connor E. 1999. Increased postwar symptoms and psychological morbidity among U.S. Navy Gulf War veterans. *American Journal of Tropical Medicine and Hygiene* 60(5):758-766.

Gray GC, Smith TC, Kang HK, Knoke JD. 2000. Are Gulf War veterans suffering war-related illnesses? Federal and civilian hospitalizations examined, June 1991 to December 1994. *American Journal of Epidemiology* 151(1):63-71.

Gray GC, Reed RJ, Kaiser KS, Smith TC, Gastanaga VM. 2002. Self-reported symptoms and medical conditions among 11,868 Gulf War-era veterans: The Seabee Health Study. *American Journal of Epidemiology* 155(11):1033-1044.

Grieger TA, Cozza SJ, Ursano RJ, Hoge C, Martinez PE, Engel CC, Wain HJ. 2006. Posttraumatic stress disorder and depression in battle-injured soldiers. *American Journal of Psychiatry* 163(10):1777-1783.

Grinker RR, Spiegel JP. 1945. *Men Under Stress.* Philadelphia, PA: Blakiston.

Haley RW, Vongpatanasin W, Wolfe GI, Bryan WW, Armitage R, Hoffmann RF, Petty F, Callahan TS, Charuvastra E, Shell WE, Marshall WW, Victor RG. 2004. Blunted circadian variation in autonomic regulation of sinus node function in veterans with Gulf War syndrome. *American Journal of Medicine* 117(7):469-478.

Harvey AG, Jones C, Schmidt DA. 2003. Sleep and posttraumatic stress disorder: A review. *Clinical Psychology Review* 23(3):377-407.

Helzer JE. 1984. The impact of combat on later alcohol use by Vietnam veterans. *Journal of Psychoactive Drugs* 16(2):183-191.

Higgins EM, Ismail K, Kant K, Harman K, Mellerio J, Du Vivier AWP, Wessely S. 2002. Skin disease in Gulf war veterans. *QJM: Monthly Journal of the Association of Physicians* 95(10):671-676.

Hoge CW, Castro CA, Messer SC, McGurk D, Cotting DI, Koffman RL. 2004. Combat duty in Iraq and Afghanistan, mental health problems, and barriers to care. *New England Journal of Medicine* 351(1):13-22.

Hoge CW, Auchterlonie JL, Milliken CS. 2006. Mental health problems, use of mental health services, and attrition from military service after returning from deployment to Iraq or Afghanistan. *Journal of the American Medical Association* 295(9):1023-1032.

Hoge CW, Terhakopian A, Castro CA, Messer SC, Engel CC. 2007. Association of posttraumatic stress disorder with somatic symptoms, health care visits, and absenteeism among Iraq War veterans. *American Journal of Psychiatry* 164(1):150-153.

Hollowell JG, Staehling NW, Flanders WD, Hannon WH, Gunter EW, Spencer CA, Braverman LE. 2002. Serum TSH, T4, and thyroid antibodies in the United States population (1988 to 1994): National Health and Nutrition Examination Survey (NHANES III). *Journal of Clinical Endocrinology and Metabolism* 87:489-499.

Hotopf M, David AS, Hull L, Ismail K, Palmer I, Unwin C, Wessely S. 2003a. The health effects of peace-keeping in the UK Armed Forces: Bosnia 1992-1996. Predictors of psychological symptoms. *Psychological Medicine* 33(1):155-162.

Hotopf M, David AS, Hull L, Nikalaou V, Unwin C, Wessely S. 2003b. Gulf war illness: Better, worse, or just the same? A cohort study. *British Medical Journal* 327(7428):1370-1372.

Hotopf M, Hull L, Fear NT, Browne T, Horn O, Iversen A, Jones M, Murphy D, Bland D, Earnshaw M , Greenberg N, Hughes JH, Tate AR, Dandeker C, Rona R, Wessely S. 2006. The health of UK military personnel who deployed to the 2003 Iraq war: A cohort study. *Lancet* 367(9524):1731-1741.

Hoyert D, Arias E, Smith B, Murphy S, Kochanek K. 2001. Deaths: Final data for 1999. *National Vital Statistics Reports* 49(8):1-116.

Hughes JW, Feldman ME, Beckham JC. 2006. Posttraumatic stress disorder is associated with attenuated baroreceptor sensitivity among female, but not male, smokers. *Biological Psychology* 71(3):296-302.

Hyams KC, Wignall FS, Roswell R. 1996. War syndromes and their evaluation: From the U.S. Civil War to the Persian Gulf War. *Annals of Internal Medicine* 125(5):398-405.

Ikin JF, Sim MR, Creamer MC, Forbes AB, McKenzie DP, Kelsall HL, Glass DC, McFarlane AC, Abramson MJ, Ittak P, Dwyer T, Blizzard L, Delaney KR, Horsley KW, Harrex WK, Schwarz H. 2004. War-related psychological stressors and risk of psychological disorders in Australian veterans of the 1991 Gulf War. *British Journal of Psychiatry* 185:116-126.

Inman DJ, Silver SM, Doghramji K. 1990. Sleep disturbance in post-traumatic stress disorder: A comparison with non-PTSD insomnia. *Journal of Traumatic Stress* 3(3): 429-437.

IOM (Institute of Medicine). 2006. *Gulf War and Health, Volume 4: Health Effects of Serving in the Gulf War*. Washington, DC: The National Academies Press.

IOM. 2007. *Gulf War and Health, Volume 5: Infectious Diseases*. Washington, DC: The National Academies Press.

Iowa Persian Gulf Study Group. 1997. Self-reported illness and health status among Gulf War veterans: A population-based study. *Journal of the American Medical Association* 277(3):238-245.

Irwin C, Falsetti SA, Lydiard RB, Ballenger JC, Brock CD, Brener W. 1996. Comorbidity of posttraumatic stress disorder and irritable bowel syndrome. *Journal of Clinical Psychiatry* 57(12):576-578.

Ishoy T, Suadicani P, Guldager B, Appleyard M, Hein HO, Gyntelberg F. 1999. State of health after deployment in the Persian Gulf. The Danish Gulf War Study. *Danish Medical Bulletin* 46(5):416-419.

Ishoy T, Suadicani P, Andersson AM, Guldager B, Appleyard M, Skakkebaek N, Gyntelberg F. 2001. Prevalence of male sexual problems in the Danish Gulf War Study. *Scandinavian Journal of Sexology* 4(1):43-55.

Jacobsen LK, Southwick SM, Kosten TR. 2001. Substance use disorders in patients with posttraumatic stress disorder: A review of the literature. *American Journal of Psychiatry* 158(8):1184-1190.

Janes GR, Goldberg J, Eisen SA, True WR. 1991. Reliability and validity of a combat exposure index for Vietnam era veterans. *Journal of Clinical Psychology* 47(1):80-86.

Johnson FY. 1989. Post-traumatic stress disorder. *Papua and New Guinea Medical Journal* 32(2):87-88.

Jones E, Hodgins-Vermaas R, McCartney H, Everitt B, Beech C, Poynter D, Palmer I, Hyams K, Wessely S. 2002. Post-combat syndromes from the Boer war to the Gulf war: A cluster analysis of their nature and attribution. *British Medical Journal* 324(7333):321-324.

Jones M, Rona RJ, Hooper R, Wesseley S. 2006. The burden of psychological symptoms in UK Armed Forces. *Occupational Medicine (Oxford)* 56(5):322-328.

Jordan BK, Schlenger WE, Hough R, Kulka RA, Weiss D, Fairbank JA, Marmar CR. 1991. Lifetime and current prevalence of specific psychiatric disorders among Vietnam veterans and controls. *Archives of General Psychiatry* 48(3):207-215.

Kagan BL, Leskin G, Haas B, Wilkins J, Foy D. 1999. Elevated lipid levels in Vietnam veterans with chronic posttraumatic stress disorder. *Biological Psychiatry* 45(3):374-377.

Kang HK, Bullman TA. 1996. Mortality among U.S. veterans of the Persian Gulf War. *New England Journal of Medicine* 335(20):1498-1504.

Kang HK, Bullman TA. 2001. Mortality among U.S. veterans of the Persian Gulf War: 7-year follow-up. *American Journal of Epidemiology* 154(5):399-405.

Kang HK, Mahan CM, Lee KY, Magee CA, Mather SH, Matanoski G. 2000a. Pregnancy outcomes among U.S. women Vietnam veterans. *American Journal of Industrial Medicine* 38(4):447-454.

Kang HK, Mahan CM, Lee KY, Magee CA, Murphy FM. 2000b. Illnesses among United States veterans of the Gulf War: A population-based survey of 30,000 veterans. *Journal of Occupational and Environmental Medicine* 42(5):491-501.

Kang HK, Mahan CM, Lee KY, Magee CA, Selvin S. 2000c. Prevalence of gynecologic cancers among female Vietnam veterans. *Journal of Occupational and Environmental Medicine* 42(11):1121-1127.

Kang HK, Natelson BH, Mahan CM, Lee KY, Murphy FM. 2003. Post-traumatic stress disorder and chronic fatigue syndrome-like illness among Gulf War veterans: A population-based survey of 30,000 veterans. *American Journal of Epidemiology* 157(2):141-148.

Kaplan MS, Huguet N, McFarland BH, Newsom JT. 2007. Suicide among male veterans: A prospective population-based study. *Journal of Epidemiology and Community Health* 61(7):619-624.

Kardiner A, Spiegel H. 1947. *War Stress and Neurotic Illness*. New York: Paul B. Hoeber.

Karlinsky JB, Blanchard M, Alpern R, Eisen SA, Kang H, Murphy FM, Reda DJ. 2004. Late prevalence of respiratory symptoms and pulmonary function abnormalities in Gulf War I Veterans. *Archives of Internal Medicine* 164(22):2488-2491.

Karlovic D, Martinac M, Buljan D, Zoricic Z. 2004. Relationship between serum lipid concentrations and posttraumatic stress disorder symptoms in soldiers with combat experiences. *Acta Medica Okayama* 58(1):23-27.

Kawakami A, Nagasaka S, Rokkaku K, Nakamura T, Kusaka I, Yajima Y, Ishikawa S, Saito T. 1999. Pseudohypoparathyroidism, obesity, and type 2 diabetes. A hypothesis. *Diabetes Care* 22(3):523.

Kellow JE, Azpiroz F, Delvaux M, Gebhart GF, Mertz HR, Quigley EM, Smout AJ. 2006a. Applied principles of neurogastroenterology: Physiology/motility sensation. *Gastroenterology* 130(5):1412-1420.

Kellow J, Azpiroz F, Delvaux M, Gebhart G, Mertz H, Quigley E. 2006b. Principles of applied neurogastroenterology: Physiology/motility-sensation. In: Drossman D, Corazziari E, Delvaux M, Spiller R, Talley N, Thompson W, editors. *Rome III: The Functional Gastrointestinal Disorders*. 3rd Ed. McLean, VA: Degnon Associates, Inc.

Kelsall H, Sim M, McKenzie D, Forbes A, Leder K, Glass D, Ikin J, McFarlane A. 2006. Medically evaluated psychological and physical health of Australian Gulf War veterans with chronic fatigue. *Journal of Psychosomatic Research* 60(6):575-584.

Kelsall HL, Sim MR, Forbes AB, Glass DC, McKenzie DP, Ikin JF, Abramson MJ, Blizzard L, Ittak P. 2004a. Symptoms and medical conditions in Australian veterans of the 1991 Gulf War: Relation to immunisations and other Gulf War exposures. *Occupational and Environmental Medicine* 61(12):1006-1013.

Kelsall HL, Sim MR, Forbes AB, McKenzie DP, Glass DC, Ikin JF, Ittak P, Abramson MJ. 2004b. Respiratory health status of Australian veterans of the 1991 Gulf War and the effects of exposure to oil fire smoke and dust storms. *Thorax* 59(10):897-903.

Kelsall HL, Sim MR, Ikin JF, Forbes AB, McKenzie DP, Glass DC, Ittak P. 2007. Reproductive health of male Australian veterans of the 1991 Gulf War. *BMC Public Health* 7(1):79.

Kessler RC, Sonnega A, Bromet E, Hughes M, Nelson CB. 1995. Posttraumatic stress disorder in the National Comorbidity Survey. *Archives of General Psychiatry* 52(12):1048-1060.

Kessler RC, Berglund P, Demler O, Jin R, Merikangas KR, Walters EE. 2005a. Lifetime prevalence and age-of-onset distributions of DSM-IV disorders in the National Comorbidity Survey Replication. *Archives of General Psychiatry* 62(6):593-602.

Kessler RC, Chiu WT, Demler O, Merikangas KR, Walters EE. 2005b. Prevalence, severity, and comorbidity of 12-month DSM-IV disorders in the National Comorbidity Survey Replication. *Archives of General Psychiatry* 62(6):617-627.

Knoke JD, Gray GC. 1998. Hospitalizations for unexplained illnesses among U.S. veterans of the Persian Gulf War. *Emerging Infectious Diseases* 4(2):211-219.

Knoke JD, Gray GC, Garland FC. 1998. Testicular cancer and Persian Gulf War service. *Epidemiology* 9(6):648-653.

Koenen KC, Lyons MJ, Goldberg J, Simpson J, Williams WM, Toomey R, Eisen SA, True W, Tsuang MT. 2003a. Co-twin control study of relationships among combat exposure, combat-related PTSD, and other mental disorders. *Journal of Traumatic Stress* 16(5):433-438.

Koenen KC, Lyons MJ, Goldberg J, Simpson J, Williams WM, Toomey R, Eisen SA, True WR, Cloitre M, Wolfe J, Tsuang MT. 2003b. A high risk twin study of combat-related PTSD comorbidity. *Twin Research* 6(3):218-226.

Koso M, Hansen S. 2006. Executive function and memory in posttraumatic stress disorder: A study of Bosnian war veterans. *European Psychiatry* 21(3):167-173.

Kramer TL, Lindy JD, Green BL, Grace MC, Leonard AC. 1994. The comorbidity of post-traumatic stress disorder and suicidality in Vietnam veterans. *Suicide and Life-Threatening Behavior* 24(1):58-67.

Kubzansky LD, Koenen KC, Spiro A, 3rd, Vokonas PS, Sparrow D. 2007. Prospective study of posttraumatic stress disorder symptoms and coronary heart disease in the Normative Aging Study. *Archives of General Psychiatry* 64(1):109-116.

Kulka RA, Schlenger WE, Fairbank JA, Hough RL, Jordan BK, Marmar CR, Weiss DS. 1990. *Trauma and the Vietnam War Generation: Report of Findings from the National Vietnam Veterans Readjustment Study*. New York: Brunner/Mazel Publishers.

Kuzma JM, Black DW. 2006. Chronic widespread pain and psychiatric disorders in veterans of the first Gulf War. *Current Pain and Headache Reports* 10(2):85-89.

Lambert MT, Fowler DR. 1997. Suicide risk factors among veterans: Risk management in the changing culture of the Department of Veterans Affairs. *Journal of Mental Health Administration* 24(3):350-358.

Lauterbach D, Vora R, Rakow M. 2005. The relationship between posttraumatic stress disorder and self-reported health problems. *Psychosomatic Medicine* 67(6):939-947.

Lavie P, Hefez A, Halperin G, Enoch D. 1979. Long-term effects of traumatic war-related events on sleep. *American Journal of Psychiatry* 136(2):175-178.

Lavie P, Katz N, Pillar G, Zinger, Y. 1998. Elevated awaking thresholds during sleep: Characteristics of chronic war-related posttraumatic stress disorder patients. *Biological Psychiatry* 44(10):1060-1065.

Lee KA, Vaillant GE, Torrey WC, Elder GH. 1995. A 50-year prospective study of the psychological sequelae of World War II combat. *American Journal of Psychiatry* 152(4):516-522.

Leung DY. 2000. Atopic dermatitis: New insights and opportunities for therapeutic intervention. *Journal of Allergy and Clinical Immunology* 105(5):860-876.

Leung DY, Soter NA. 2001. Cellular and immunologic mechanisms in atopic dermatitis. *Journal of the American Academy of Dermatology* 44(1 Suppl):S1-S12.

Levine PH, Young HA, Simmens SJ, Rentz D, Kofie VE, Mahan CM, Kang HK. 2005. Is testicular cancer related to Gulf War deployment? Evidence from a pilot population-based study of Gulf War era veterans and cancer registries. *Military Medicine* 170(2):149-153.

Levy RL, Whitehead WE, Von Korff MR, Feld AD. 2000. Intergenerational transmission of gastrointestinal illness behavior. *American Journal of Gastroenterology* 95(2):451-456.

Levy RL, Olden KW, Naliboff BD, Bradley LA, Francisconi C, Drossman DA, Creed F. 2006. Psychosocial aspects of the functional gastrointestinal disorders. *Gastroenterology* 130(5):1447-1458.

Lieberman HR, Bathalon GP, Falco CM, Kramer FM, Morgan CA, 3rd, Niro P. 2005a. Severe decrements in cognition function and mood induced by sleep loss, heat, dehydration, and undernutrition during simulated combat. *Biological Psychiatry* 57(4):422-429.

Lieberman HR, Bathalon GP, Falco CM, Morgan CA, 3rd, Niro PJ, Tharion WJ. 2005b. The fog of war: Decrements in cognitive performance and mood associated with combat-like stress. *Aviation Space and Environmental Medicine* 76(7 Suppl):C7-C14.

Lindauer RT, van Meijel EP, Jalink M, Olff M, Carlier IV, Gersons BP. 2006. Heart rate responsivity to script-driven imagery in posttraumatic stress disorder: Specificity of response and effects of psychotherapy. *Psychosomatic Medicine* 68(1):33-40.

Lindem K, White RF, Heeren T, Proctor SP, Krengel M, Vasterling J, Wolfe J, Sutker PB, Kirkley S, Keane TM. 2003. Neuropsychological performance in Gulf War era veterans: Motivational factors and effort. *Journal of Psychopathology and Behavioral Assessment* 25(2):129-138.

Longstreth GF, Thompson WG, Chey WD, Houghton LA, Mearin F, Spiller RC. 2006a. Functional bowel disorders. *Gastroenterology* 130(5):1480-1491.

Longstreth G, Thompson W, Chey W, Houghton L, Mearin F, Spiller R. 2006b. Functional bowel disorders. In: Drossman D, Corazziari E, Delvaux M, Spiller R, Talley N, Thompson W, editors. *Rome III: The Functional Gastrointestinal Disorders*. 3rd Ed. McLean, VA: Degnon Associates, Inc.

Macfarlane GJ, Thomas E, Cherry N. 2000. Mortality among UK Gulf War veterans. *Lancet* 356(9223):17-21.

Macfarlane GJ, Biggs AM, Maconochie N, Hotopf M, Doyle P, Lunt M. 2003. Incidence of cancer among UK Gulf war veterans: Cohort study. *British Medical Journal* 327(7428):1373.

Macfarlane GJ, Hotopf M, Maconochie N, Blatchley N, Richards A, Lunt M. 2005. Long-term mortality amongst Gulf War Veterans: Is there a relationship with experiences during deployment and subsequent morbidity? *International Journal of Epidemiology* 34(6):1403-1408.

Maconochie N, Doyle P, Davies G, Lewis S, Pelerin M, Prior S, Sampson P. 2003. The study of reproductive outcome and the health of offspring of UK veterans of the Gulf war: Methods and description of the study population. *BMC Public Health* 3(1):4.

Maconochie N, Doyle P, Carson C. 2004. Infertility among male UK veterans of the 1990-1 Gulf war: Reproductive cohort study. *British Medical Journal* 329(7459):196-201.

Mason J, Southwick S, Yehuda R, Wang S, Riney S, Bremner D, Johnson D, Lubin H, Blake D, Zhou G, Gusman F, Charney D. 1994. Elevation of serum free triiodothyronine, total triiodothyronine, thyroxine-binding globulin, and total thyroxine levels in combat-related posttraumatic stress disorder. *Archives of General Psychiatry* 51(8):629-641.

Mayer EA. 2006. Commentary on peripheral and central contributions to hyperalgesia in irritable bowel syndrome. *Journal of Pain* 7(8):539-543.

McCauley LA, Joos SK, Barkhuizen A, Shuell T, Tyree WA, Bourdette DN. 2002a. Chronic fatigue in a population-based study of Gulf War veterans. *Archives of Environmental Health* 57(4):340-348.

McCauley LA, Lasarev M, Sticker D, Rischitelli DG, Spencer PS. 2002b. Illness experience of Gulf War veterans possibly exposed to chemical warfare agents. *American Journal of Preventive Medicine* 23(3):200-206.

McEwen BS. 2002. Protective and damaging effects of stress mediators: The good and bad sides of the response to stress. *Metabolism* 51(6 Suppl 1):2-4.

McEwen BS. 2004. Protection and damage from acute and chronic stress: Allostasis and allostatic overload and relevance to the pathophysiology of psychiatric disorders. *Annals of the New York Academy of Sciences* 1032:1-7.

McFarlane AC. 1997. The prevalence and longitudinal course of PTSD. Implications for the neurobiological models of PTSD. *Annals of the New York Academy of Sciences* 821:10-23.

McFarlane AC, Atchison M, Rafalowicz E, Papay P. 1994. Physical symptoms in post-traumatic stress disorder. *Journal of Psychosomatic Research* 38(7):715-726.

McKeown ES, Parry SD, Stansfield R, Barton JR, Welfare MR. 2006. Postinfectious irritable bowel syndrome may occur after non-gastrointestinal and intestinal infection. *Neurogastroenterology and Motility* 18(9):839-843.

McLeod D, Koenen KC, Meyer JM, Lyons MJ, Eisen S, True W, Goldberg J. 2001. Genetic and environmental influences on the relationship among combat exposure, posttraumatic stress disorder symptoms, and alcohol use. *Journal of Traumatic Stress* 14(2):259-275.

Mellman TA, Randolph CA, Brawman-Mintzer O, Flores LP, Milanes FJ. 1992. Phenomenology and course of psychiatric disorders associated with combat-related posttraumatic stress disorder. *American Journal of Psychiatry* 149(11):1568-1574.

Mellman TA, Kulick-Bell R, Ashlock LE, Nolan B. 1995a. Sleep events among veterans with combat-related posttraumatic stress disorder. *American Journal of Psychiatry* 152(1):110-115.

Mellman TA, Kumar A, Kulick-Bell R, Kumar M, Nolan B. 1995b. Nocturnal/daytime urine noradrenergic measures and sleep in combat-related PTSD. *Biological Psychiatry* 38(3):174-179.

Mellman TA, Nolan B, Hebding J, Kulick-Bell R, Dominguez R. 1997. A polysomnographic comparison of veterans with combat-related PTSD, depressed men, and non-ill controls. *Sleep* 20(1):46-51.

MHAT (Mental Health Advisory Team). 2006a. *Mental Health Advisory Team (MHAT) III Operation Iraqi Freedom 04-06: Final Report.* [Washington, DC]: Office of the Surgeon Multinational Force-Iraq and Office of the Surgeon General United States Army Medical Command. 29 May 2006. [Online]. Available: http://www.armymedicine.army.mil/news/mhat/mhat_iii/mhat-iii.cfm.

MHAT. 2006b. *Mental Health Advisory Team (MHAT) IV Operation Iraqi Freedom 05-07: Final Report.* [Washington, DC]: Office of the Surgeon Multinational Force-Iraq and Office of the Surgeon General United States Army Medical Command. 17 November 2006. [Online]. Available: http://www.armymedicine.army.mil/news/mhat/mhat_iv/MHAT_IV_Report_17NOV06.pdf.

Mizokami T, Wu Li A, El-Kaissi S, Wall JR. 2004. Stress and thyroid autoimmunity. *Thyroid* 14(12):1047-1055.

Mooy JM, de Vries H, Grootenhuis PA, Bouter LM, Heine RJ. 2000. Major stressful life events in relation to prevalence of undetected type 2 diabetes: The Hoorn Study. *Diabetes Care* 23(2):197-201.

Morgan CA, 3rd, Wang S, Mason J, Southwick SM, Fox P, Hazlett G, Charney DS, Greenfield G. 2000. Hormone profiles in humans experiencing military survival training. *Biological Psychiatry* 47(10):891-901.

Muraoka MY, Carlson JG, Chemtob CM. 1998. Twenty-four-hour ambulatory blood pressure and heart rate monitoring in combat-related posttraumatic stress disorder. *Journal of Traumatic Stress* 11(3):473-484.

Murburg MM, McFall ME, Lewis N, Veith RC. 1995. Plasma norepinephrine kinetics in patients with posttraumatic stress disorder. *Biological Psychiatry* 38(12):819-825.

Murphy FM, Kang H, Dalager NA, Lee KY, Allen RE, Mather SH, Kizer KW. 1999. The health status of Gulf War veterans: Lessons learned from the Department of Veterans Affairs Health Registry. *Military Medicine* 164(5):327-331.

Murray CD, Flynn J, Ratcliffe L, Jacyna MR, Kamm MA, Emmanuel AV. 2004. Effect of acute physical and psychological stress on gut autonomic innervation in irritable bowel syndrome. *Gastroenterology* 127(6):1695-1703.

National Heart Lung and Blood Institute. 2007. *Sleep Disorders Information.* [Online]. Available: http://www.nhlbi.nih.gov/health/prof/sleep/ [accessed July 26, 2007].

Neylan TC, Marmar CR, Metzler TJ, Weiss DS, Zatzick DF, Delucchi KL, Wu RM, Schoenfeld FB. 1998. Sleep disturbances in the Vietnam generation: Findings from a nationally representative sample of male Vietnam veterans. *American Journal of Psychiatry* 155(7):929-933.

Nisenbaum R, Barrett DH, Reyes M, Reeves WC. 2000. Deployment stressors and a chronic multisymptom illness among Gulf War veterans. *Journal of Nervous and Mental Disease* 188(5):259-266.

Office of the Surgeon Multinational Force-Iraq, Office of the Surgeon General United States Army Medical Command. 2006. *Mental Health Advisory Team (MHAT) IV Operation Iraqi Freedom 05-07. Final Report.*

Orr SP, Meyerhoff JL, Edwards JV, Pitman RK. 1998. Heart rate and blood pressure resting levels and responses to generic stressors in Vietnam veterans with posttraumatic stress disorder. *Journal of Traumatic Stress* 11(1):155-164.

Orr SP, Metzger LJ, Lasko NB, Macklin ML, Hu FB, Shalev AY, Pitman RK. 2003. Physiologic responses to sudden, loud tones in monozygotic twins discordant for combat exposure: Association with posttraumatic stress disorder. *Archives of General Psychiatry* 60(3):283-288.

Otis JD, Keane TM, Kerns RD. 2003. An examination of the relationship between chronic pain and post-traumatic stress disorder. *Journal of Rehabilitation Research and Development* 40(5):397-405.

O'Toole BI, Marshall RP, Grayson DA, Schureck RJ, Dobson M, French M, Pulvertaft B, Meldrum L, Bolton J, Vennard J. 1996a. The Australian Vietnam Veterans Health Study: III. Psychological health of Australian Vietnam veterans and its relationship to combat. *International Journal of Epidemiology* 25(2):331-340.

O'Toole BI, Marshall RP, Grayson DA, Schureck RJ, Dobson M, French M, Pulvertaft B, Meldrum L, Bolton J, Vennard J. 1996b. The Australian Vietnam Veterans Health Study: II. Self-reported health of veterans compared with the Australian population. *International Journal of Epidemiology* 25(2):319-330.

O'Toole BI, Marshall RP, Schureck RJ, Dobson M. 1998. Posttraumatic stress disorder and comorbidity in Australian Vietnam veterans: Risk factors, chronicity and combat. *Australian and New Zealand Journal of Psychiatry* 32(1):32-42.

Ouimette PC, Wolfe J, Chrestman KR. 1996. Characteristics of posttraumatic stress disorder-alcohol abuse comorbidity in women. *Journal of Substance Abuse* 8(3):335-346.

Ozakinci G, Hallman WK, Kipen HM. 2006. Persistence of symptoms in veterans of the First Gulf War: 5-year follow-up. *Environmental Health Perspectives* 114(10):1553-1557.

Palatini P, Julius S. 1997. Heart rate and the cardiovascular risk. *Journal of Hypertension* 15(1):3-17.

Pallmeyer TP, Blanchard EB, Kolb LC. 1986. The psychophysiology of combat-induced post-traumatic stress disorder in Vietnam veterans. *Behaviour Research and Therapy* 24(6):645-652.

Papageorgiou AC, Silman, AJ, Macfarlane GJ. 2002. Chronic widespread pain in the population: A seven year follow up study. *Annals of the Rheumatic Diseases* 61:1071-1074.

Pierce PF. 1997. Physical and emotional health of Gulf War veteran women. *Aviation Space and Environmental Medicine* 68(4):317-321.

Pizarro J, Silver RC, Prause J. 2006. Physical and mental health costs of traumatic war experiences among Civil War veterans. *Archives of General Psychiatry* 63(2):193-200.

Price RK, Risk NK, Haden AH, Lewis CE, Spitznagel EL. 2004. Post-traumatic stress disorder, drug dependence, and suicidality among male Vietnam veterans with a history of heavy drug use. *Drug and Alcohol Dependence* 76(Suppl):S31-S43.

Prigerson HG, Maciejewski PK, Rosenheck RA. 2002. Population attributable fractions of psychiatric disorders and behavioral outcomes associated with combat exposure among U.S. men. *American Journal of Public Health* 92(1):59-63.

Proctor SP, Heeren T, White RF, Wolfe J, Borgos MS, Davis JD, Pepper L, Clapp R, Sutker PB, Vasterling JJ, Ozonoff D. 1998. Health status of Persian Gulf War veterans: Self-reported symptoms, environmental exposures and the effect of stress. *International Journal of Epidemiology* 27(6):1000-1010.

Proctor SP, White RF, Heeren T, Debes F, Gloerfelt-Tarp B, Appleyard M, Ishoy T, Guldager B, Suadicani P, Gyntelberg F, Ozonoff DM. 2003. Neuropsychological functioning in Danish Gulf War veterans. *Journal of Psychopathology and Behavioral Assessment* 25(2):85-93.

Proctor SP, Harley R, Wolfe J, Heeren T, White RF. 2001. Health-related quality of life in Persian Gulf War veterans. *Military Medicine* 166(6):510-519.

Putnam SD, Sanders JW, Frenck RW, Monteville M, Riddle MS, Rockabrand DM, Sharp TW, Frankart C, Tribble DR. 2006. Self-reported description of diarrhea among military populations in operations Iraqi Freedom and Enduring Freedom. *Journal of Travel Medicine* 13(2):92-99.

Reid S, Hotopf M, Hull L, Ismail K, Unwin C, Wessely S. 2001. Multiple chemical sensitivity and chronic fatigue syndrome in British Gulf War veterans. *American Journal of Epidemiology* 153(6):604-609.

Reifman A, Windle M. 1996. Vietnam combat exposure and recent drug use: A national study. *Journal of Traumatic Stress* 9(3):557-568.

Ries L, Eisner M, Kosary C, Hankey B, Miller B, Clegg L, Mariotto A, Feuer E, Edwards B. 2005. *SEER Cancer Statistics Review, 1975-2002*. [Online]. Available: http://caonline.amcancersoc.org/cgi/reprint/56/1/9.pdfseer.cancer.gov/csr/1975_2002/ [accessed June 2006].

Ro BI, Dawson TL. 2005. The role of sebaceous gland activity and scalp microfloral metabolism in the etiology of seborrheic dermatitis and dandruff. *Journal of Investigative Dermatology Symposium Proceedings* 10(3):194-197.

Robins LN, Davis DH, Nurco DN. 1974. How permanent was Vietnam drug addiction? *American Journal of Public Health* 64(Suppl 12):38-43.

Ryan MA, Ness RB, Wells TS, O'Donnell FL. 2004. Birth defects among infants of Gulf War veterans, 1989-1993. *Birth Defects Research* 70(1):47.

Schnurr PP, Jankowski MK. 1999. Physical health and post-traumatic stress disorder: Review and synthesis. *Seminars in Clinical Neuropsychiatry* 4(4):295-304.

Schnurr PP, Spiro A. 1999. Combat exposure, posttraumatic stress disorder symptoms, and health behaviors as predictors of self-reported physical health in older veterans. *Journal of Nervous and Mental Disease* 187(6):353-359.

Schnurr PP, Spiro A, 3rd, Paris AH. 2000. Physician-diagnosed medical disorders in relation to PTSD symptoms in older male military veterans. *Health Psychology* 19(1):91-97.

Selected Cancers Cooperative Study Group. 1990a. The association of selected cancers with service in the U.S. military in Vietnam. I. Non-Hodgkin's lymphoma. *Archives of Internal Medicine* 150(12):2473-2483.

Selected Cancers Cooperative Study Group. 1990b. The association of selected cancers with service in the U.S. military in Vietnam. II. Soft-tissue and other sarcomas. *Archives of Internal Medicine* 150(12):2485-2492.

Selected Cancers Cooperative Study Group. 1990c. The association of selected cancers with service in the U.S. military in Vietnam. III. Hodgkin's disease, nasal cancer, nasopharyngeal cancer, and primary liver cancer. *Archives of Internal Medicine* 150(12):2495-2505.

Shalev AY, Sahar T, Freedman S, Peri T, Glick N, Brandes D, Orr SP, Pitman RK. 1998. A prospective study of heart rate response following trauma and the subsequent development of posttraumatic stress disorder. *Archives of General Psychiatry* 55(6):553-539.

Sharafkhaneh A, Giray N, Richardson P, Young T, Hirshkowitz M. 2005. Association of psychiatric disorders and sleep apnea in a large cohort. *Sleep* 28(11):1405-1411.

Shipherd JC, Stafford J, Tanner LR. 2005. Predicting alcohol and drug abuse in Persian Gulf War veterans: What role do PTSD symptoms play? *Addictive Behaviors* 30(3):595-599.

Simmons R, Maconochie N, Doyle P. 2004. Self-reported ill health in male UK Gulf War veterans: A retrospective cohort study. *BMC Public Health* 4(1):27.

Sloan P, Arsenault L, Hilsenroth MJ. 2005. Impact of Event Scale prediction of DSM-IV PTSD and physical symptoms in Gulf War veterans. *Stress, Trauma and Crisis: An International Journal* 8(4):215-228.

Smith TC, Gray GC, Knoke JD. 2000. Is systemic lupus erythematosus, amyotrophic lateral sclerosis, or fibromyalgia associated with Persian Gulf War service? An examination of Department of Defense hospitalization data. *American Journal of Epidemiology* 151(11):1053-1059.

Snow BR, Stellman JM, Stellman SD, Sommer JF Jr. 1988. Post-traumatic stress disorder among American Legionnaires in relation to combat experience in Vietnam: Associated and contributing factors. *Environmental Research* 47(2):175-192.

Solter V, Thaller V, Karlovic D, Crnkovic D. 2002. Elevated serum lipids in veterans with combat-related chronic posttraumatic stress disorder. *Croatian Medical Journal* 43(6):685-689.

Sostek MB, Jackson S, Linevsky JK, Schimmel EM, Fincke BG. 1996. High prevalence of chronic gastrointestinal symptoms in a National Guard Unit of Persian Gulf veterans. *American Journal of Gastroenterology* 91(12):2494-2497.

Spiller R, Campbell E. 2006. Post-infectious irritable bowel syndrome. *Current Opinions in Gastroenterology* 22(1):13-17.

Spiro A, 3rd, Hankin CS, Mansell D, Kazis LE. 2006. Posttraumatic stress disorder and health status: The veterans health study. *Journal of Ambulatory Care Management* 29(1):71-86.

Steele L. 2000. Prevalence and patterns of Gulf War illness in Kansas veterans: Association of symptoms with characteristics of person, place, and time of military service. *American Journal of Epidemiology* 152(10):992-1002.

Stermer E, Bar H, Levy N. 1991. Chronic functional gastrointestinal symptoms in Holocaust survivors. *American Journal of Gastroenterology* 86(4):417-422.

Stimpson NJ, Unwin C, Hull L, David T, Wessely S, Lewis G. 2006. Prevalence of reported pain, widespread pain, and pain symmetry in veterans of the Persian Gulf War (1990-1991): The use of pain manikins in Persian Gulf War health research. *Military Medicine* 171(12):1181-1186.

Straus SE. 1991. History of chronic fatigue syndrome. *Reviews of Infectious Diseases* 13(Suppl 1):S2-S7.

Stretch RH, Bliese PD, Marlowe DH, Wright KM, Knudson KH, Hoover CH. 1995. Physical health symptomatology of Gulf War-era service personnel from the states of Pennsylvania and Hawaii. *Military Medicine* 160(3):131-136.

Sutker PB, Allain AN Jr, Winstead DK. 1993a. Psychopathology and psychiatric diagnoses of World War II Pacific theater prisoner of war survivors and combat veterans. *American Journal of Psychiatry* 150(2):240-245.

Sutker PB, Uddo M, Brailey K, Allain AN. 1993b. War-zone trauma and stress-related symptoms in Operation Desert Shield/Storm (ODS) returnees. *Journal of Social Issues* 49(4):33-50.

Taft CT, Stern AS, King LA, King DW. 1999. Modeling physical health and functional health status: The role of combat exposure, posttraumatic stress disorder, and personal resource attributes. *Journal of Traumatic Stress* 12(1):3-23.

Thomas HV, Stimpson NJ, Weightman A, Dunstan F, Lewis G. 2006. Pain in veterans of the Gulf War of 1991: A systematic review. *BMC Musculoskeletal Disorders* 7:74.

Thomas TL, Kang HK, Dalager NA. 1991. Mortality among women Vietnam veterans, 1973-1987. *American Journal of Epidemiology* 134(9):973-980.

Thompson R, Kane VR, Sayers SL, Brown GK, Coyne JC, Katz IR. 2002. An assessment of suicide in an urban VA Medical Center. *Psychiatry* 65(4):327-337.

Toomey R, Kang HK, Karlinsky J, Baker DG, Vasterling JJ, Alpern R, Reda DJ, Henderson WG, Murphy FM, Eisen SA. 2007. Mental health of U.S. Gulf War veterans 10 years after the war. *British Journal of Psychiatry* 190:385-393.

Uddo M, Vasterling JJ, Brailey K, Sutker PB. 1993. Memory and attention in combat-related post-traumatic stress disorder (PTSD). *Journal of Psychopathology and Behavioral Assessment* 15(1):43-52.

Unwin C, Blatchley N, Coker W, Ferry S, Hotopf M, Hull L, Ismail K, Palmer I, David A, Wessely S. 1999. Health of UK servicemen who served in Persian Gulf War. *Lancet* 353(9148):169-178.

Vasterling JJ, Rogers C, Kaplan E. 2000. Qualitative block design analysis in posttraumatic stress disorder. *Assessment* 7(3):217-226.

Vasterling JJ, Duke LM, Brailey K, Constans JI, Allain AN Jr, Sutker PB. 2002. Attention, learning, and memory performances and intellectual resources in Vietnam veterans: PTSD and no disorder comparisons. *Neuropsychology* 16(1):5-14.

Vasterling JJ, Brailey K, Constans JI, Sutker PB. 1998. Attention and memory dysfunction in posttraumatic stress disorder. *Neuropsychology* 12(1):125-133.

Vasterling JJ, Proctor SP, Amoroso P, Kane R, Gackstetter G, Ryan MA, Friedman MJ. 2006. The Neurocognition Deployment Health Study: A prospective cohort study of Army Soldiers. *Military Medicine* 171(3):253-260.

Vasterling JJ, Brailey K, Tomlin H, Rice J, Sutker PB. 2003. Olfactory functioning in Gulf War-era veterans: Relationships to war-zone duty, self-reported hazards exposures, and psychological distress. *Journal of the International Neuropsychological Society* 9(3):407-418.

Vieweg WV, Julius DA, Benesek J, Satterwhite L, Fernandez A, Feuer SJ, Pandurangi AK. 2006. Posttraumatic stress disorder and body mass index in military veterans. Preliminary findings. *Progress in Neuro-Psychopharmacology and Biological Psychiatry* 30(6):1150-1154.

Villa VM, Harada ND, Washington D, Damron-Rodriquez J. 2002. Health and functioning among four war ears of U.S. veterans: Examining the impact of war cohort membership, socioeconomic status, mental health, and disease prevalence. *Military Medicine* 167(9):783-789.

Wang S, Mason J. 1999. Elevations of serum T3 levels and their association with symptoms in World War II veterans with combat-related posttraumatic stress disorder: Replication of findings in Vietnam combat veterans. *Psychosomatic Medicine* 61(2):131-138.

Wang S, Mason J, Southwick S, Johnson D, Lubin H, Charney D. 1995. Relationships between thyroid hormones and symptoms in combat-related posttraumatic stress disorder. *Psychosomatic Medicine* 57(4):398-402.

Watanabe KK, Kang HK. 1995. Military service in Vietnam and the risk of death from trauma and selected cancers. *Annals of Epidemiology* 5(5):407-412.

Weiss DS, Marmar CR, Schlenger WE, Fairbank JA, Jordan BK, Hough RL, Kulka RA. 1992. The prevalence of lifetime and partial post-traumatic stress disorder in Vietnam theater veterans. *Journal of Traumatic Stress* 5(2):365-376.

Wells TS, Wang LZ, Spooner CN, Smith TC, Hiliopoulos KM, Kamens DR, Gray GC, Sato PA. 2006. Self-reported reproductive outcomes among male and female 1991 Gulf War era U.S. military veterans. *Maternal and Child Health Journal* 10(6):501-510.

Werler MM, Sheehan JE, Mitchell AA. 2005. Gulf War veterans and hemifacial microsomia. *Birth Defects Research* 73(1):50-52.

Wessely S. 2005. Risk, psychiatry and the military. *British Journal of Psychiatry* 186:459-466.

White RF, Proctor SP, Heeren T, Wolfe J, Krengel M, Vasterling J, Lindem K, Heaton KJ, Sutker P, Ozonoff DM. 2001. Neuropsychological function in Gulf War veterans: Relationships to self-reported toxicant exposures. *American Journal of Industrial Medicine* 40(1):42-54.

Whitehead WE, Palsson O, Jones KR. 2002. Systematic review of the comorbidity of irritable bowel syndrome with other disorders: What are the causes and implications? *Gastroenterology* 122(4):1140-1156.

Wills TA, Yaeger AM, Sandy JM. 2003. Buffering effect of religiosity for adolescent substance use. *Psychology of Addictive Behaviors* 17(1):24-31.

Wolfe F. 1989. Fibromyalgia: The clinical syndrome. *Rheumatic Diseases Clinics of North America* 15(1):1-18.

Wolfe F, Smythe HA, Yunus MB, Bennett RM, Bombardier C, Goldenberg DL, Tugwell P, Campbell SM, Abeles M, Clark P, Fam AG, Farber SJ, Fiechtner JJ, Franklin MC, Gatter RA, Hamaty D, Lesserd J, Lichtbroun AS, Masi AT, McCain GA, Reynolds WJ, Romano TJ, Russel IJ, Sheon RP. 1990. The American College of Rheumatology 1990 Criteria for the Classification of Fibromyalgia. Report of the Multicenter Criteria Committee. *Arthritis and Rheumatism* 33(2):160-172.

Wolfe J, Schnurr PP, Brown PJ, Furey J. 1994. Posttraumatic stress disorder and war-zone exposure as correlates of perceived health in female Vietnam War veterans. *Journal of Consulting and Clinical Psychology* 62(6):1235-1240.

Wolfe J, Proctor SP, Davis JD, Borgos MS, Friedman MJ. 1998. Health symptoms reported by Persian Gulf War veterans two years after return. *American Journal of Industrial Medicine* 33(2):104-113.

Wolfe J, Proctor SP, Erickson DJ, Heeren T, Friedman MJ, Huang MT, Sutker PB, Vasterling JJ, White RF. 1999. Relationship of psychiatric status to Gulf War veterans' health problems. *Psychosomatic Medicine* 61(4):532-540.

Wolfe J, Proctor SP, Erickson DJ, Hu H. 2002. Risk factors for multisymptom illness in U.S. Army veterans of the Gulf War. *Journal of Occupational and Environmental Medicine* 44(3):271-281.

Woodward SH, Murburg MM, Bliwise DL. 2000. PTSD-related hyperarousal assessed during sleep. *Physiology and Behavior* 70(1-2):197-203.

Writer JV, DeFraites RF, Brundage JF. 1996. Comparative mortality among U.S. military personnel in the Persian Gulf region and worldwide during Operations Desert Shield and Desert Storm. *Journal of the American Medical Association* 275(2):118-121.

Yarvis JS, Bordnick PS, Spivey CA, Pedlar D. 2005. Subthreshold PTSD: A comparison of alcohol, depression, and health problems in Canadian peacekeepers with different levels of traumatic stress. *Stress, Trauma and Crisis: An International Journal* 8(2-3):195-213.

Yehuda R, Southwick SM, Giller EL, Ma X, Mason JW. 1992. Urinary catecholamine excretion and severity of PTSD symptoms in Vietnam combat veterans. *Journal of Nervous and Mental Disease* 180(5):321-325.

Yehuda R, Keefe RS, Harvey PD, Levengood RA, Gerber DK, Geni J, Siever LJ. 1995. Learning and memory in combat veterans with posttraumatic stress disorder. *American Journal of Psychiatry* 152(1):137-139.

Yehuda R, Siever LJ, Teicher MH, Levengood RA, Gerber DK, Schmeidler J, Yang RK. 1998. Plasma norepinephrine and 3-methoxy-4-hydroxyphenylglycol concentrations and severity of depression in combat posttraumatic stress disorder and major depressive disorder. *Biological Psychiatry* 44(1):56-63.

Zalewski C, Thompson W, Gottesman I. 1994. Comparison of neuropsychological test performance in PTSD, generalized anxiety disorder, and control Vietnam veterans. *Assessment* 1(2):133-142.

Zatzick DF, Marmar CR, Weiss DS, Browner WS, Metzler TJ, Golding JM, Stewart A, Schlenger WE, Wells KB. 1997a. Posttraumatic stress disorder and functioning and quality of life outcomes in a nationally representative sample of male Vietnam veterans. *American Journal of Psychiatry* 154(12):1690-1695.

Zatzick DF, Weiss DS, Marmar CR, Metzler TJ, Wells K, Golding JM, Stewart A, Schlenger WE, Browner WS. 1997b. Post-traumatic stress disorder and functioning and quality of life outcomes in female Vietnam veterans. *Military Medicine* 162(10):661-665.

Zhang Q, Zhou XD, Denny T, Ottenweller JE, Lange G, LaManca JJ, Lavietes MH, Pollet C, Gause WC, Natelson BH. 1999. Changes in immune parameters seen in Gulf War veterans but not in civilians with chronic fatigue syndrome. *Clinical and Diagnostic Laboratory Immunology* 6(1):6-13.

7

PSYCHOSOCIAL EFFECTS

Evidence from World War II, the Vietnam War, the 1991 Gulf War, and now Operation Enduring Freedom (OEF) in Afghanistan and Operation Iraqi Freedom (OIF) in Iraq suggests that many military personnel deployed to war zones suffer not only long-term health effects (see Chapter 6) but also adverse psychosocial effects. According to the Oxford English Dictionary, one definition of psychosocial refers to the interrelationship of behavior and social factors (http://dictionary.oed.com). Veterans on return from deployment, especially those suffering from posttraumatic stress disorder (PTSD), anxiety, and depression, might find reintegration into family, social, and occupational settings difficult.

Given the complexity of the psychosocial factors in the lives of veterans and their families, the committee addresses the following issues in this chapter: connections between deployment to a war zone and marital and family conflict, including intimate partner violence and adverse effects on children; employment; incarceration; and homelessness. As in Chapter 6, the committee describes the epidemiologic literature that compares deployed veterans from the Gulf War and other wars with their nondeployed counterparts.

MARITAL AND FAMILY CONFLICT

Marital and family conflict includes divorce, separation, infidelity, and abuse. Abuse is considered in the section on interpersonal violence. In this section, the committee evaluates the evidence on marital and family conflict and deployment. The potential influence of deployment on rates of divorce is also discussed.

Gimbel and Booth (1994), in a historical overview of how the experiences encountered by soldiers in combat adversely affect marital relations, noted that typically each war in the last century was followed by an increase in the divorce rate. The most recent report issued by the Department of Defense (DoD) Mental Health Advisory Team of the Office of the Surgeon Multinational Force-Iraq and the Office of the Surgeon General U.S. Army Medical Command (MHAT 2006) noted that marital satisfaction, in general, was high among soldiers and Marines deployed to Iraq although there had been a downward trend during 2006. The number of deployed soldiers experiencing severe stress or emotional, alcohol, or family concerns increased from 7% in 2003 to 13% in 2006. During this time, the proportion of soldiers reporting a good marriage dropped from 81% to 71%, the proportion planning a divorce or separation rose from 11% to 20%, problems with infidelity rose from 4% to 15%, and marital problems more than doubled, from 12% to 27%.

The committee identified four primary papers and several secondary papers that assessed marital conflict and deployment. The committee also considered additional papers on the effects of parental deployment on children. Several of the studies considered the effects of deployment on marital stability of veterans with and without PTSD, and these are included in the discussions of both primary and secondary studies. The primary studies for marital conflict are summarized in Table 7-1.

Primary Studies

Gimbel and Booth (1994) assessed the degree of marital adversity, combat exposure, and premilitary factors in a sample of 2101 Vietnam veterans who had participated in the Vietnam Experience Study (VES) conducted by the Centers for Disease Control and Prevention. The VES was conducted in two stages: first, a random sample of 17,867 Vietnam-era veterans was interviewed by telephone, of these veterans, 7748 were randomly selected for in-person testing and medical examinations. Of those selected, 4462 participated in the examinations which were conducted in 1985-1965. The 2101 veterans were selected from the ever-married examination participants who had served in the Vietnam theater; all the men were of enlisted rank and had only served one tour of duty in Vietnam. Combat exposure was found to be moderately related (standardized regression coefficient 0.109, $p \leq 0.01$) with marital adversity (divorce, separation, abuse, or infidelity). Premilitary characteristics, such as early emotional problems and problems in school, when factored into the model, reduced the impact of combat by about one-third (standardized regression coefficient 0.073, $p \leq 0.01$). The impact of combat on marital adversity was also mediated by two postmilitary factors: posttraumatic stress symptoms and antisocial behavior. When both those postmilitary factors were in the model, the impact of combat itself became insignificant and did not have a direct relationship with marital quality and stability. Furthermore, it appeared that the influence of postmilitary stress symptoms was mediated by antisocial behavior, as was the effect of combat stress. Thus, the authors concluded that combat exposure creates stress that leads to postcombat antisocial behavior and ultimately to adversity in marriage. Although the low participation rate (60%) in the VES and the retrospective nature of the early-life experience data represent limitations in this cross-sectional study, the representativeness of the sample and thoroughness of the data analysis lend credence to the conclusions.

The National Survey of the Vietnam Generation (NSVG) and the Spouse/Partner Interview (also called the Family Interview) components of the National Vietnam Veterans Readjustment Study (NVVRS) have been used by several researchers assessing impact of serving in Vietnam on the veterans' marital and family status and intimate partner violence. In the NVVRS, male Vietnam-theater veterans with PTSD were compared with theater veterans without PTSD. In the NSVG, 1200 Vietnam-theater veterans were randomly selected from all military personnel who had served in the Vietnam theater between August 1964 and May 1975; 432 female Vietnam-theater veterans, and 412 male and 304 female era veterans were also included in the study. Most male veterans were middle-aged and married at the time of the interview; over 50% had some college education. About 17% of veterans were of black or Hispanic backgrounds. PTSD symptom level at the time of the interview was assessed with the Mississippi Scale for Combat-Related PTSD; a study cutoff score of 94 was used as a threshold for an assessment of current PTSD. A diagnosis of PTSD was confirmed in a subset of the veterans using the Structured Clinical Interview for *DSM-III* (SCID). Psychiatric comorbidity was diagnosed with the Diagnostic Interview Schedule (DIS). The veterans participated in face-to-face interviews and medical examinations in 1986-1988. The response rate for the NSVG was 83% for Vietnam-theater veterans. Of the 1200 theater veterans who were interviewed, 862 were selected for followup on the basis of PTSD classification. The followup group also contained an oversampling of veterans without PTSD who indicated they had had high combat exposure or high levels of nonspecific psychological distress. Of these veterans, 585 were living with a female spouse or partner at the time of the survey and 376 of these women were selected to participate in the 1-hour Spouse/Partner Interview; the response rate was 80%. PTSD in the veterans was determined based on the DIS and the Mississippi Scale for Combat-Related PTSD; the clinical examination portion of the NVVRS also included the SCID and the Minnesota Multiphasic Personality Inventory (MMPI) PTSD Scale. The PTSD cases for the following studies were identified based on the Mississippi Scale and adjusted for the bias relative to the clinical interview assessments.

Based on responses to the NSVG, Jordan et al. (1992) selected all households of theater veterans who appeared to have PTSD, and the households of a subset of veterans who did not appear to have PTSD, to determine the effects of PTSD on family adjustment and marital conflict. The 1200 Vietnam veterans and 376 of their spouses or partners completed the Marital Problems Index (MPI), the Parental Problems Index (PPI), the Family Adjustment Index, the Level of Functioning Index, the Social Isolation Index, the Child Behavior Checklist, and the Index of Subjective Well-Being. Of the veterans who were married or cohabitating at the time of the survey, the 231 veterans with PTSD, compared with the 736 veterans without PTSD, reported significantly ($p < 0.001$) more marital and relationship problems (mean MPI score 2.54 vs 1.74), more parenting problems (mean PPI score 2.61 vs 1.93), and poorer family adjustment (54.8% vs 19.3% reporting extreme problems). Veterans with PTSD were six times as likely to have the most martial and relationship problems (that is to score in the high range on the MPI) (48.9% vs 8.7%), three times as likely to fall in the highest category on the PPI (54.7% vs 17.3%), and two times as likely to report extreme family adjustment issues (49.2% vs 21.9%) as veterans without PTSD. The 122 partners and spouses of veterans with PTSD were significantly more likely to report lower levels of happiness and life satisfaction (11.2% vs 1.9%), and higher demoralization scores (42.7% vs 15.4%) than the 252 spouses or partners of veterans without PTSD. Along similar lines, children of veterans with PTSD were substantially more likely to have a behavior problem than those of veterans without PTSD (20.5% vs 12.0%). The authors suggest that a veteran's PTSD is a major source of family dysfunction.

Two studies (Call and Teachman 1991, 1996) used data from the Career Development Study (CDS). In the CDS, a stratified sample of 6729 young men and women in public high schools in the state of Washington who completed a questionnaire in 1965-1966 (time 1) were contacted again in 1979-1980 (time 2) by telephone to gather information on life experiences since high school. The response rate at the followup was 90.6%.

Call and Teachman (1991) classified the CDS cohort of 2901 men responding at time 2 into 627 Vietnam-combat veterans, 586 Vietnam-era veterans, and 1688 nonveterans. The men were about 30-31 years old at time 2. As of 1980, 87.2%, 82.1%, and 79.9%, of the men, respectively, had been married. The authors used multivariate analysis to determine the probability of divorce and the influence of combat service on marital stability. The authors found that being in combat in Vietnam vs serving in the military but not in Vietnam, had no impact on the probability of being divorced. They also found that combat service had a positive impact on marriage duration.

Using a subsample of 2369 men from the CDS who had married by the age of 30 years, Call and Teachman (1996) embarked on a study of 610 Vietnam-combat veterans, 581 Vietnam-era veterans, and 1666 nonveterans. The study assessed the rates and timing of marriage and the association between deployment and marital stability. A multivariate analysis was used to account for variation in the duration of martial disruption, specifically divorce. By 1980, the prevalence of divorce was 28% in nonveterans, 34% in veterans (both theater and era) who married before military service (less then 10% of the sample), 28% in veterans who married during service, and 21% in veterans who married after service. Combat exposure had no significant effect on the likelihood of being divorced. Marrying for the first time after military service increased marital stability.

Although both those CDS studies provided complex multivariate analyses with comparisons between deployed and nondeployed veterans, they had some methodologic limitations. The sample consisted only of white men whose families had slightly higher socioeconomic status and higher educational achievement than other such studies and there were no minorities in the sample, so the studies lacked representativeness.

Secondary Studies

Several secondary studies have reported an association between deployment and marital conflict and dissatisfaction. Several studies that assessed the relationship between PTSD and marital conflict in veteran populations are also briefly discussed. Finally, the committee reviewed four additional secondary studies that reported positive findings that specifically address the role of deployment-related marital and family conflict in psychosocial effects on children.

Two studies that yielded negative findings regarding the association between deployment and marital functioning were published in 1996. The survey by Schumm et al. (1996b) of 806 married active-duty soldiers inquired about marital satisfaction at the time of the survey in 1991-1992, and in 1990 before the invasion of Kuwait. Soldiers who had deployed in the Gulf War showed no significant overall changes with respect to marital satisfaction; this suggested that the effect of deployment was neutral for couples who remained married for 18 months after the conflict, regardless of their predeployment marital satisfaction. Limitations of the study included lack of presentation of results, the absence of a comparison nondeployed group, and the retrospective nature of the predeployment marriage assessment.

The second study was conducted by Schumm et al. (1996a) in August 1993. They examined the perceived effects of stressors on marital satisfaction in civilian wives of enlisted soldiers deployed to Somalia for 6 months from December 1992 to July 1993. Marital stability was a strong predictor of marital satisfaction. The results suggest that being stressed during a husband's deployment by being pregnant, experiencing loneliness or missing the spouse, having problems in communication with the spouse, or having a close friend or family member die did not result in more marital dissatisfaction a month after the return of the spouse. However, those results must be interpreted with caution because the survey was conducted during the "honeymoon" period (that is, the first 3 months after return), the deployments were relatively short and uneventful, and many of the soldiers and spouses were familiar with the deployment experience.

Prigerson et al. (2001) conducted a cross-sectional survey of a subsample of the 1990-1992 National Comorbidity Study to explore the risk factors for veterans with PTSD symptoms. Of the sample of 1703 men who indicated that they had experienced a trauma, 96 reported combat as their most traumatic experience, and 42% of the 96 met the criteria for PTSD at some time in their lives. PTSD was diagnosed with the DIS or Composite International Diagnostic Interview (CIDI). Following combat, the trauma next-most likely to result in PTSD was ever having been raped or sexually molested. Men with combat trauma were the most likely to be divorced (39%) or to be physically abusive to their spouses (15%).

The association between PTSD and parenting satisfaction was explored by Samper et al. (2004), who assessed a sample of 250 male Vietnam veterans, part of the NVVRS cohort, for depression, intimate partner violence, PTSD, and parenting satisfaction. Results indicated that the PTSD severity and symptoms of numbness and avoidance were significantly negatively associated with parenting satisfaction.

Reports on a clinical sample of 270 Australian Vietnam veterans suffering with chronic PTSD showed the influences of PTSD-related symptoms on family functioning (Evans et al. 2003). In particular, PTSD symptoms of avoidance, affect dysregulation, and heightened anger led to more dissension in families of veterans with PTSD. Veterans reported that their avoidance behavior contributed to poor family functioning, and the arousal symptoms of PTSD were associated with angry reactions that also adversely affected family functioning.

The perceptions of 951 U.S. Army male and female peacekeepers deployed to Bosnia were queried by Newby et al. (2005). Although most of the soldiers (77%) reported favorable consequences of their deployment, married soldiers were more than twice as likely as single soldiers to report adverse consequences, primarily being away from family and missing important events.

Intimate Partner Violence

To define intimate partner violence, the committee considered the definition developed by the DoD Task Force on Domestic Violence (DoD 2004):

- A pattern of behavior resulting in emotional or psychologic abuse, economic control, and/or interference with personal liberty and that is directed toward a current or former spouse, a person with whom the abuser shares a child in common; or a current or former intimate partner.
- The use, attempted use, or threatened use of physical force, violence, a deadly weapon, sexual assault, or the intentional destruction of property.
- Behavior that has the intent or impact of placing a victim in fear of physical injury.

Most intimate partner violence involves perpetration of violence by men against women. Findings of past-year prevalence in the general U.S. population vary from 0.5% in the 2001 National Crime Victimization Survey to 11.6% in the 1985 National Family Violence Re-Survey; the prevalence of severe violence was estimated to be 3.4% in the latter survey. Surveys that are based on crime statistics and criminal-offense records tend to yield a lower prevalence of intimate partner violence because the report of offenses is voluntary, whereas national surveys of randomly selected couples are generally more accurate and yield a higher prevalence if such instruments as the Conflict Tactics Scale (CTS) are used (Clark et al. 2006). The CTS is an 18-item self-report inventory that assesses conflict tactics as functional (for example, calmly discussing a problem), verbally abusive, or physically abusive.

Heyman and Neidig (1999) addressed the prevalence of intimate partner violence in the U.S. Army (n = 33,762) and the general population (n = 3044) and found a higher prevalence of severe husband-against-wife violence in the military population than in the general population whether reported by men (2.5% vs 0.7%, respectively) or by women (4.4 % vs 2.0%, respectively). Rates of moderate violence committed by military men and women were higher (10.8% and 13.1%, respectively) than by civilian men and women (9.9% and 10.0%, respectively).

The committee reviewed ten papers related to the associations between deployment and intimate partner violence. Two studies (Jordan et al. 1992; McCarroll et al. 2000) met the criteria for a primary study as described in Chapter 2. The Jordan et al. (1992) study focused on the effects of PTSD on intimate partner violence using data from the NVVRS. Studies by Orcutt et al. (2003) and by Taft et al. (2005) provided additional analyses of the Jordan data. The primary studies for intimate partner violence are summarized in Table 7-1.

Primary Studies

McCarroll et al. (2000) conducted a cross-sectional survey in 1990-1994 of a randomly chosen sample of about 15% of the married, active-duty Army men and women at each of 47 Army installations; civilian spouses were not included in the survey. A modified version of the CTS, a widely used self-report instrument, was used to assess aggression in the past year by the military spouse toward the nonmilitary spouse. Responses were categorized as no, moderate, or severe physical aggression. Of the 37,514 surveys received, 26,835 were deemed eligible: 25,520 from men and 1315 from women. Dual military couples were excluded from the survey, and an analysis of responders and nonresponders found no pattern of bias. During the year prior to the survey, 11,540 soldiers had been deployed: 6195 of them for less than 3 months, 3944 for between 3 and 6 months, and 1402 for between 6 and 12 months; 15,294 soldiers had not been deployed. The nature and location of the deployments was not provided. Using multinomial logistic modeling, the researchers found that the predicted probability of moderate and severe aggression increased with increasing length of deployment. For moderate aggression the probability was 0.1762 for nondeployed, 0.1776 for less than 3 month deployments, 0.1793 for 3-6 month deployments, and 0.1850 for 6-12 month deployments; the probabilities for severe aggression were 0.0367, 0.0425, 0.0464, and 0.0495, respectively. The model was controlled for deployment, age, race, sex, rank, and children living with the respondent. A comparison of the predicted probabilities for moderate and severe aggression with no aggression found that the ratios increased with deployment length, although only the difference in ratios for severe aggression were significant ($p < 0.05$). For severe aggression, ratios of no deployment vs deployment were: 1.1580 (deployed less than 3 months, 95% CI 1.1370-1.1791), 1.2643 (deployed 3-6 months, 95% CI 1.2415-1.2872); and 1.3488 (deployed 6-12 months, 95% CI 1.3245-1.3731). For moderate aggression the ratios were: 1.0079 (95% CI 0.8431-1.1728), 1.0176 (5% CI 0.8518-1.1834), and 1.0499 (95% CI 0.8808-1.2190), respectively. The researchers note that although the increases were significant for severe aggression the changes represented small absolute values of probability. Although there are limitations inherent in a cross-sectional design, this study demonstrates a clear association between deployment and increased spousal aggression.

Intimate partner violence was studied by three research groups using information from the NVVRS discussed above. Based on responses to the NSVG, Jordan et al. (1992) selected all households of theater veterans who appeared to have PTSD and the households of a subset of veterans who did not appear to have PTSD to determine the effects of PTSD on family adjustment and marital conflict, including intimate partner violence. Of those without PTSD, the researchers oversampled for veterans who indicated they had had high combat exposure or high levels of nonspecific psychological distress. Family violence in the past year was assessed with the Standard Family Violence Measure, an eight-item subscale of the CTS, and an Alternate Family Violence Measure, which is the total number of violent acts committed or threatened in the past year; scores were categorized as low, medium-low, medium-high, or high violence. Both measures were completed by the veteran as a self-report and by the spouse/partner of the veteran. Family violence, perpetrated by the veteran or by the spouse or partner, was significantly more prevalent in families of veterans with PTSD, with about a third of the veterans with PTSD having engaged in some level of family violence in the past year compared with 15% of those without PTSD. The mean score on the Standard Family Violence Index for the 736 veterans with PTSD was 2.08 vs 0.54 for the 231 veterans without PTSD ($p = 0.002$), scores for the spouses or partners were 1.57 and 0.51, respectively ($p = 0.001$). In all, 372 spouses or partners were interviewed. The 122 spouses or partners of veterans with PTSD reported up to four times as much medium-high to very-high family violence perpetrated by the veteran as did the 252 spouses or partners of veterans without PTSD (7-12% vs 3%, standard error 1.4-3.9, $p < 0.01$) on both the Standard Family Violence Index and the Alternate Family Violence Index. The mean number of violent acts committed or threatened by veterans in the past year was 4.86 for those with PTSD vs 1.32 for those without PTSD; for spouses or partners of the veterans the mean number of violent acts was 3.03 and 0.96, respectively. Over 9% of the veterans with PTSD had committed 13 or more acts of violence in the past year. The analyses were weighted to compensate for differences in selection probabilities so that the data provide unbiased national estimates for all male theater veterans with a spouse or partner. Age, sex, race or ethnicity, and nonresponse were used to stratify the weights. Strengths of this study are the reporting of family violence perpetrated by both the veteran and the spouse or partner and the use of a nationally representative sample of veterans.

In a further analysis of the same 376 Vietnam veteran couples who had participated in NSVG, Orcutt et al. (2003) used structural-equation modeling to assess the influence of early-life stressors, war-zone stressors, and PTSD symptom severity on intimate partner severity. The modeling showed that there were four direct influences on intimate partner violence in male Vietnam veterans: a poor relationship with mother, combat exposure, perceived threat in the war zone, and PTSD symptom severity. All the influences resulted in more intimate partner violence except for combat exposure. Increasing combat exposure was related to less violence against a spouse or partner. The model also suggests that retrospective reports of a stressful early family-life and antisocial behavior during childhood acted indirectly on intimate partner violence via war-zone stressors and PTSD symptom severity.

Taft et al. (2005) also assessed the NSVG subsample of the 376 veterans and spouses or partners who had participated in the family interview. Veterans with a lifetime history of physical violence toward their spouse or partner but with none reported for the past year were excluded. In all, 40 male veterans were classified as both PTSD-positive and partner violent (one or more episodes of partner violence in the past year), 41 were PTSD-negative but partner violent, and 28 were PTSD-positive but nonviolent. Data analysis showed that PTSD severity did not differ significantly between the two PTSD groups, nor did violence severity between the two partner-violent groups. The PTSD-positive and partner-violent group scored higher for all the following factors than did the PTSD-positive/nonviolent or PTSD-negative/partner-violent groups: psychiatric disorders (antisocial personality disorder, major depressive disorder, and alcohol and drug-use/dependence), violence between the veteran's parents, relationship variables (marital adjustment, family adaptability, family cohesion), and war-zone variables (combat exposure, perceived threat, atrocities exposure). However, the PTSD-positive/nonviolent group had the most childhood abuse (49%), over twice that of the other groups (21-23%). Both PTSD-positive groups both had more combat exposure than the PTSD-negative group; the PTSD-positive/partner-violent group had more exposure to combat and particularly to atrocities than the PTSD-positive/nonviolent group.

Secondary Studies

In addition to the primary studies that support the association between deployment and intimate partner violence after deployment, there are numerous supportive secondary studies. Studies that assess deployed vs nondeployed veterans are discussed first, followed by studies of intimate partner violence in veterans with and without PTSD.

McCarroll et al. (2003) surveyed a group of 313 male U.S. Army soldiers assigned to peacekeeping functions in Bosnia for 6 months from September 1998 to April 1999 and compared them with 712 male soldiers who had not deployed. The research team used the CTS to explore the incidence of intimate partner violence at two times: prior to September 1998, and April-June 1999. There were no significant demographic differences between the two groups; all participants were married, and deployed soldiers had been home from deployment for 90-113 days at the time of the survey. The rates of predeployment intimate partner violence did not differ between deployed and nondeployed soldiers (11.5% vs 10.3%) and deployment was not a significant predictor of later moderate or severe domestic violence (6.7% deployed vs 7.4% nondeployed). The strongest predictor of postdeployment domestic violence was a previous history of domestic violence (OR 4.56, 95% CI 2.60-8.00); the next-strongest was living off post (OR 2.71, 95% CI 1.39-5.32), which was followed by being nonwhite (OR 1.69, 95% CI 1.03-2.76). Although this study had a reasonably representative sample and deployment to a single area, behavior was assessed for the "honeymoon period," which typically is not accompanied by heightened intimate partner violence, so the study may underestimate the degree of intimate partner violence that may later develop.

Several other secondary studies highlight the association between PTSD and intimate partner violence after deployment. Several of the studies of veterans with PTSD and intimate partner violence involved treatment populations; all were of Vietnam veterans, and, like the studies discussed above, many used data from the NVVRS.

Prigerson et al. (2002) used data from the 1990-1992 National Comorbidity Survey that sought to determine the prevalence of psychiatric disorders in a nationally representative sample of 2578 men 18-54 years old, of whom 1337 were currently married or cohabitating. Participants were asked about possible combat exposure and the CIDI was used to diagnose psychiatric disorders, except for PTSD, which was assessed for the previous 12 months with the DIS. The married or cohabiting men were asked about abuse of spouses or partners, and those who responded with "never" or "rarely" were counted as nonabusive. Combat exposure was associated with current spouse or partner abuse (relative risk [RR] 4.40, 95% CI 1.68-10.49, $p = 0.004$; adjusted for age, race, urbanicity, and low socioeconomic status in family of origin). Path analysis suggested that the effect of combat exposure on current spouse or partner abuse was indirect and mediated through PTSD.

Savarese et al. (2001) also analyzed the NSVG data on the 376 male Vietnam veterans and their female partners discussed above (Jordan et al. 1992) to examine the joint effects of drinking frequency, drinking quantity, and the severity of the hyperarousal symptoms of PTSD on marital abuse and violence. Of the 376 men, 315 (84%) indicated that they had engaged in at least one or more act of psychologic violence toward their partners in the preceding year, and 21% had engaged in physical violence; men who engaged in psychologic abuse are more likely also to engage in physical abuse. Both physical and psychologic abuse were associated with hyperarousal symptoms and this association was exacerbated when excessive alcohol was consumed on an occasion. However, frequent consumption of small quantities of alcohol, even during high hyperarousal conditions, does not increase, and may even mitigate, husband-to-wife violence.

Beckham et al. (1997) conducted two studies to explore PTSD, intimate partner violence, and their correlates in Vietnam-combat veterans. The first study assessed 37 male outpatients at a VA medical center: 17 help-seeking combat veterans with PTSD and 20 combat veterans without PTSD recruited from all veterans who had attended the VA center within the past year. The second study involved 118 male Vietnam veterans who were also outpatients at the PTSD clinic. The SCID or Clinician-Administered PTSD Scale (CAPS) was used to diagnose PTSD. In the first study all veterans and a family member or friend completed the Standard Family Violence Index of the CTS; in the second study only the veterans completed the Standard Family Violence Index and they also completed the CAGE screening questionnaire for alcohol use. In the first study, veterans with PTSD reported significantly greater occurrences of violent behavior during the preceding year than veterans without PTSD (22 acts vs 0.2 acts of violence). Both PTSD and combat exposure had a significant main effect on interpersonal violence ($\chi2 = 9.4$, $p = 0.002$, and $\chi2 = 4.2$, $p = 0.04$, respectively). In the second study, risk factors for increased intimate partner violence, in order of importance, were lower socioeconomic status ($\chi2 = 6.0$, $p = 0.01$), increased aggressiveness ($\chi2 = 5.7$, $p = 0.02$), and greater PTSD severity ($\chi2 = 4.4$, $p = 0.04$). Current problems with alcohol abuse were not associated with intimate partner violence.

An association between PTSD in veterans and heightened violence was demonstrated in a study by McFall et al. (1999). They compared 228 Vietnam-combat veterans seeking inpatient treatment for PTSD at a VA medical center with 64 psychiatric inpatients without PTSD who had served during the Vietnam War but not served in a war zone. An additional comparison was with 273 community-dwelling Vietnam veterans with PTSD (assessed with the Mississippi Scale for Combat-Related PTSD), who had never been hospitalized for the disorder. PTSD was diagnosed with a standard clinical interview by a psychiatrist. The sample of community-dwelling PTSD veterans was derived from the NVVRS data set; veterans were selected to have a level of combat exposure comparable with that of the inpatient PTSD veterans. Data from the NVVRS, CTS, and clinician interviews were used to assess the level of violence engaged in by the veterans. PTSD inpatients were significantly more likely to report having engaged in one or more acts of violence in the preceding month than the psychiatric inpatients (OR 7.40, $p < 0.001$), particularly having destroyed property, threatened others with or without a weapon, or been involved in a physical fight. Comparison with the community sample of veterans who had PTSD yielded similar findings except that the community veterans were more likely than the PTSD inpatients to have destroyed property. Symptom severity and, to a lesser degree, substance abuse were correlated with violence among the PTSD inpatients. It should be noted that this study did not include intimate partner violence as a violence endpoint.

Deployment Impacts on Families and Children

Young families are at greatest risk for coping with children who are distressed by deployment of one of their parents. The distress may be related to anxieties or worries about separation from a parent or may be caused by the parent's PTSD symptoms of avoidance or hyperarousal. In general, boys and younger children appear to be more vulnerable to symptoms of depression related to the parent's deployment. Results of several studies support an association between deployment and adverse psychosocial effects on children.

Jensen et al. (1996) conducted a study of 480 families with children 4-17 years old, randomly selected from a sample of families living on a military base near Washington, DC; 383 families completed all or part of the survey. Although the study emphasized the children's reactions to their parents' deployment for Operation Desert Storm, it also considered the effect of deployment on the caretaker parents and the marriages. Almost all the parents were married (94.4%), and the racial distribution of the families was 52.5% non-Hispanic white, 30.9% black, and 9.0% Hispanic. Both of the parents and the children completed a wide array of surveys and questionnaires that assessed behavior, depression, anxiety, and social assets. Families were divided into those with a soldier-parent who was deployed to the Gulf War and those with a soldier-parent who was not deployed and remained on the military base. The researchers also compared the results of the assessments with an assessment of some of the same families a year earlier, before deployment. Prior to deployment of any parents, there were no meaningful differences in terms of the children's or parent's self-reported behaviors and parent or family functioning between families where a parent would deploy and those where no parent deployed. Children whose parents had deployed scored moderately higher on the Children's Depression Inventory than those with nondeployed parents (8.06 vs 5.33), but there were no other significant differences in reports of the children's anxiety level or behavior. Boys had more dysfunction than girls, regardless of the girl's parent's deployment status and boys with a deployed parent were more likely to have increased dysfunction than boys with a nondeployed parent. Deployment itself rarely provoked pathologic symptoms in otherwise healthy children. Parents with deployed spouses reported more depression and higher levels of life stressors than those parents whose spouses had not deployed. The same differences seen between caretaking parents' reports of depression for those with and without a deployed spouse were again found after control for level of depression before deployment ($p \leq 0.001$). Likewise, there continued to be significant predeployment and postdeployment differences in reported stress levels of the caretaking parent. There were no predeployment and postdeployment differences in marital adjustment, social supports, or coping. The data indicate that it is deployment itself, rather than pre-existing differences in the parents' levels of depression or stress, that is related to the caregiving parents' increase in stress and depression during their spouses' deployment. The authors suggest that many young families have particular difficulty with even temporary-duty separations, perhaps because they also have less experience with a military lifestyle. The authors note that the findings do not suggest that the caretaking parents cause their children's symptoms of depression; instead, the interrelationships between caretaking parent, child, and absent deployed parent contribute to a complex outcome.

Rosen et al. (1993) explored caretaker parents' reactions to the responses of 1601 children to questions about their other parents' Gulf War deployment. Results were similar to those of Jensen et al. (1996). Although the children expressed sadness and had eating and sleeping problems, among other symptoms of distress, the most important predictor of a child's symptoms was the expression of symptoms of distress by other members of the household. This study lacked direct input from the children themselves, but the findings support an association between deployment and adverse psychologic effects on children, which association seems to be mediated by its effect on the parent.

Family dysfunction was also found by Rosenheck and Fontana (1998), who explored the transgenerational effects of abusive violence on the children of Vietnam combat veterans in the NVVRS. Children of veterans who had participated in abusive violence or had high war-zone stress during the war, scored significantly higher (worse) on the Child Behavior Checklist than did children of other Vietnam veterans ($p < 0.01$). That study showed that children of veterans who exhibited abusive violence had more behavior problems themselves even 15-20 years after their fathers' deployment.

Rentz et al. (2007) examined the rate of child maltreatment in military families. The design involved a time-series analysis of Texas child-maltreatment data from the 2000-2003 National Child Abuse and Neglect Data System to examine changes in the occurrence of child maltreatment over time and the effect of recent increases in deployment. Substantiated child maltreatment in military families was twice as frequent between October 2002 (the 1-year anniversary of the September 11, 2001, attacks) and June 2003, than in the period between October 2002 and October 2001 (rate ratio 2.15, 95% CI 1.85-2.50). Between January 2000 and September 2002, the rate of child maltreatment in military families was 37% lower than in nonmilitary families (rate ratio 0.67, 95% CI 0.62-0.72) but after October 2002, the rate was 22% higher (rate ratio 1.22, 95% CI 1.10-1.36). After December 2002, child maltreatment was found to increase by about 30% for every 1% increase in the number of active-duty personnel who departed for or returned from operational deployments. The results suggest that both departures for, and returns from, deployment impose stress on military families and increase rates of child maltreatment. Maltreated children in military families were more likely to be non-Hispanic whites less than 4 years old. The study's cross-sectional design has limitations, but its strengths include comparisons of deployed and nondeployed soldier-parents.

One study focused on veteran populations who sought treatment for PTSD. For example, Glenn et al. (2002) assessed the degree of violence and hostility in 31 Vietnam veterans who had a diagnosis of PTSD (using the CAPS) and their spouses or partners and 29 of their older adolescent or adult children. The veterans, their spouses or partners, and their children reported a moderate to moderate-high level of violent behavior based on responses to the Childhood Physical Punishment Scale, Cook-Medley Hostility Scale, and the Violent Behavior Index. Veterans' reports of PTSD symptoms were associated with reports of hostility and violence towards their children. Veterans' violent behavior was also correlated with their children's violent behavior. Although this study suffers from the absence of a representative sample, the findings highlight the disruptive effects of PTSD on all members of a family.

Summary and Conclusions

The collective findings of the primary and secondary studies of marital and family conflict, including intimate partner violence, indicate that many veterans and their families will experience significant stress after the return of the veterans from deployment. The impact of deployment on marital and family conflict is mixed. Two primary studies indicated that exposure to combat alone did not result in increased marital conflict, particularly divorce, for Vietnam theater veterans. The two secondary studies considered by the committee also found that exposure to combat alone did not increase postdeployment marital conflict for Gulf War veterans. However, the two primary and three secondary studies of Vietnam veterans with combat-related PTSD all found that marital conflict and family adjustment problems were significantly increased in these veterans and that the problems persisted for years after the war.

Six studies explored the associations between deployment and adverse psychosocial outcomes in children of veterans. The one primary study, by Jensen et al. (1996), found that children who had a parent who had been deployed to the Gulf War had more behavioral dysfunction and that boys were at greater risk for depression associated with their parents' deployment than were girls; a secondary study found similar results. Three secondary studies also support an association between deployment to war zone and veterans' violent behavior toward their children, particularly if the veterans have PTSD. One secondary study found that children of veterans who had PTSD and were physically abusive also exhibited violent behavior even 15-20 years after their fathers had returned from the Vietnam War.

There is an extensive literature on the effect of deployment on the perpetration of intimate partner violence by veterans against spouses and partners. One large primary study conducted in the early 1990s found an association between deployment and heightened intimate partner violence perpetrated by active-duty soldiers and found that the aggression increased with the length of deployment. Three other studies, all of which used data from a survey of spouses and partners of Vietnam veterans who participated in the NVVRS, found an association between combat-related PTSD and increased intimate partner violence. Four secondary studies lend additional support to the findings of primary studies. Virtually all the studies of veterans and intimate partner violence have been conducted in Vietnam veterans. In particular, veterans with PTSD score higher on various indexes of anger and, given the link between anger and aggression, are therefore more likely to engage in intimate partner violence. Although most of the studies have focused on intimate partner violence, other studies have shown that deployed veterans have more interpersonal violence outside intimate partner violence than nondeployed veterans. The committee therefore based it conclusions on the association between deployment and heightened marital and family conflict, including increased intimate partner violence.

There also appears to be more depression in children of deployed veterans and more aggression against children perpetrated by veterans. Of the 7 primary studies, 5 showed a positive association and 2 no association; of the 18 secondary studies, 15 showed a positive association and 3 no association. The association was particularly strong for veterans with PTSD, almost all of whom were Vietnam-combat veterans.

The committee concludes that there is sufficient evidence of an association between deployment to a war zone and later marital and family conflict, including intimate partner violence. The association is especially strong when a veteran has a diagnosis of PTSD.

TABLE 7-1 Marital and Family Conflict

Reference	Study Design	Population	Outcomes	Results	Adjustments	Comments
Jordan et al. 1992 (Derived from NVVRS)	Cross-sectional survey, NSVG	871 male Vietnam theater veterans without PTSD vs 319 with PTSD from the NSVG 252 spouses or partners of veterans without PTSD vs 122 spouses of veterans with PTSD	Marital and family-adjustment patterns associated with PTSD prevalence Measures included -Mississippi Scale for Combat-Related PTSD, DIS-PTSD module, and detailed assessment of exposure to traumatic events -Parental Problems Index -Level of Functioning Index -Family-Violence subscale of CTS -Index of Subjective Well-Being -PERI Demoralization Scale -Social Isolation Index -alcohol problems -nervous breakdown -Child Behavior Checklist	Men with PTSD are more likely to report: marital or relationship problems; higher levels of parenting problems; higher levels of family violence Partners and spouses of theater veterans with PTSD were significantly more likely to report lower levels of happiness and life satisfaction and to have higher demoralization scores than spouses or partners of theater veterans without PTSD Children of veterans with PTSD were substantially more likely to have a problem score in the clinical range than children of veterans without PTSD	None	Strengths: -nationally representative population -deployed vs nondeployed status -plethora of measures and interview -long-term effects Limitations: -study was conducted 15 years after Vietnam War ended -no adjustments
McCarroll et al. 2000	Cross-sectional survey in 1990-1994	Randomized sample of 11,541 GW-deployed vs 15,294 nondeployed married active-duty Army men and women (95% men, 5% women)	Probability of spousal aggression in association with deployment CTS to measure self-reports of behaviors exhibited in marital conflict	Probability of severe aggression in preceding year significantly greater in deployed (4.25%-4.95%) vs nondeployed soldiers (3.67%) Probability of severe aggression increased with length of deployment from 15.8% (< 3 months) to 34.9% (6-12 months)	Age, race, sex, rank, and number of children living with respondent	Causal relationship between deployment and spousal aggression cannot be determined

TABLE 7-1 Marital and Family Conflict

Reference	Study Design	Population	Outcomes	Results	Adjustments	Comments
Orcutt et al. 2003 (Derived from NVVRS)	Cross-sectional survey	376 Vietnam veterans and their spouses or partners based on NSVG	Association of trauma exposure in war zone and spousal violence Measures included -four measures of family dysfunction -DIS -Mississippi Scale for Combat-Related PTSD -CTS	PTSD symptom severity highly associated with increased IPV Combat exposure associated with decreased IPV	Family dysfunction, relationship with mother and father, childhood antisocial behavior, perceived threat	Possible recall and response bias Inability to determine causality Other possible risk factors not controlled for
Taft et al. 2005 (Derived from NVVRS)	Cross-sectional survey	109 male Vietnam veterans and their spouses or partners from NSVG	Association between PTSD and various war-zone exposures (combat exposure, atrocity exposure) and IPV	Men with PTSD and history of IPV report more atrocity exposure than men without PTSD but with history of IPV and more than men with PTSD but without history of IPV ($p < 0.05$)	Childhood abuse, interparental violence, antisocial personality disorder, major depressive episode, alcohol dependence, drug dependence	Relatively small sample Possible recall bias Inability to determine causality
Call and Teachman 1991	Cohort; Career Development Study	2,901 white men who graduated from Washington state high schools in 1966 and 1967, 627 Vietnam combat veterans, 586 noncombat Vietnam veterans, 1688 civilians	Association between combat service and marital status Original data collected by questionnaire in 1965-1966 in high schools; in 1979-1980, telephone interview yielded event history data on 88.8 % of original 1966 panel members	Young men in military service during Vietnam War were most likely to marry No long-term evidence of destructive effect of combat service on life-course sequencing or veterans' first marriages	Education, birth, military life-history data	Limited generalizability

TABLE 7-1 Marital and Family Conflict

Reference	Study Design	Population	Outcomes	Results	Adjustments	Comments
Call and Teachman 1996	Cohort	Part 1: 2857 white males who graduated from Washington state high schools in 1966 and 1967 Part 2: subsample of 2369 men who married by age of 30 years	Association between military service and marital status Part I questionnaire and Part II telephone interview about school, family military and work experiences in Pacific Northwest	Marriages initiated during military service in Vietnam did not have a significant adverse effect on long-term marital stability Marrying for first time after military service increased marital stability	Age at first marriage, marital conception of first child, education level	Limited generalizability
Gimbel and Booth 1994	Cross-sectional survey	2101 Vietnam veterans who served in Army in 1965-1971	Military service in Vietnam and marital difficulties Measures include scales to assess marital adversity, combat, premilitary problems	Combat exposure has statistically significant relationship with marital adversity (including divorce, separation, abuse, and infidelity) Combat itself does not have direct relationship with marital quality and stability; instead, combat creates stress and antisocial behavior, but only antisocial behavior has direct effect on marital adversity Combat directly increases violent and unlawful (antisocial) behavior and stress, which then affect marital stability and quality	Age, intelligence, race, early emotional problems	Limited generalizability Possible recall bias Inability to determine causality

TABLE 7-1 Marital and Family Conflict

Reference	Study Design	Population	Outcomes	Results	Adjustments	Comments
Jensen et al. 1996	Cross-sectional survey	383 children and remaining caretaking parent, drawn from random sample of 480 families living on military post near Washington, DC, with at least one child 4-17 years old; almost all parents were married (94.4%)	Association of children's mental health status and parental deployment Parents: Child Behavior Checklist, CES Depression Scale, Dyadic Adjustment Scale, Live Events Record, Social Assets Scale Children: Children's Inventory, Revised Children's Manifest Anxiety Scale	Children of deployed personnel experienced increased self-reported symptoms of depression, as did their parents Families of deployed personnel reported significantly more intervening stressors than children and families of nondeployed personnel Deployment itself rarely provoked pathologic symptoms in otherwise healthy children	Sex, age	No control for other factors, including halo effects, pre-existing parental characteristics predisposing them toward deployment Limited generalizability Inability to determine causality

NOTE: CES = Combat Exposure Scale, CTS = Conflict Tactics Scale, DIS = Diagnostic Interview Schedule, GW = Gulf War, IPV = intimate partner violence, NSVG = National Survey of the Vietnam Generation, NVVRS = National Vietnam Veterans Readjustment Study, PTSD = posttraumatic stress disorder.

HOMELESSNESS

For some, homelessness is a temporary condition; but for others, homelessness is a more permanent situation. The National Law Center on Homelessness and Poverty estimates that about 1% of the U.S. population experiences homelessness in any year. Homeless people may be living on the streets, in shelters, or with relatives or friends. Most homeless people live in urban areas. VA reports that about one-third of the adult homeless population in the United States served in the armed forces at some point. That means that on any given day, 200,000 men (and women) veterans are in need of shelter, food, medical care, and other essentials. Many homeless veterans are Vietnam-era veterans, although veterans of other periods are also homeless or at risk of being homeless. It is estimated that almost half the homeless veterans have some form of mental disorder, almost 70% have a substance-use disorder, and over half are black or Hispanic (VHA 2006).

The committee reviewed 10 studies regarding deployment and homelessness. Three were designated as primary and seven secondary. The primary studies are summarized in Table 7-2.

Primary Studies

The three studies that were designated as primary used data from the NVVRS (Rosenheck and Fontana 1994) or from community surveys (Gamache et al. 2001; Rosenheck et al. 1994). Subjects were viewed as more representative of U.S. veterans than subjects in the secondary studies. The secondary studies—Gamache et al. (2000, 2003), Mares and Rosenheck (2004), Rosenheck et al. (1991, 1992), Tessler et al. (2002), and Wenzel et al. (1993)—relied primarily on homeless subjects who were mentally ill.

Rosenheck and Fontana (1994) reanalyzed data from the NVVRS on 1460 male Vietnam veterans to model the risk of homelessness on the basis of premilitary personal experiences, exposure to war-zone stress, current PTSD, other psychiatric disorders, and substance abuse. Veterans surveyed in the NVVRS who had never been homeless served as a control group for comparison with the 8.4% of the sample who did report homelessness since the war. Structural-equation modeling was used to determine the influence of 18 hypothesized risk factors. Risk ratios ranged from a low of 1.0 (95% CI 0.7-1.4) for being a member of a minority racial or ethnic group to the three highest risk ratios: 5.0 (95% CI 3.5-7.2) for PTSD, 5.3 (95% CI 2.0-14.2) for being in foster care when young, and 6.5 (95% CI 1.9-22.5) for having psychiatric treatment before age 18. The modeling showed that four postmilitary factors—psychiatric disorder other than PTSD, not being married, substance abuse, and low levels of support—were directly related to homelessness, but PTSD was not; its effect was mediated through other psychiatric disorders. Combat exposure and participation in atrocities were associated with increased risk of homelessness—risk ratios were 2.1 (95% CI 1.5-3.0) and 2.7 (95% CI 1.9-3.8), respectively—but their effects on homelessness were also mediated through psychiatric disorders. Social support during the year after discharge was the most important variable in risk of homelessness in the model.

Rosenheck et al. (1994) used data from four community surveys to determine whether male veterans, in general, were disproportionately represented among homeless people or whether vulnerability to homelessness was peculiar to one age or race cohort of veterans. Secondary analyses were performed on data from the Urban Institute's 1987 national survey of homeless-service users (n = 1140) and from single-city surveys conducted in Los Angeles (n =

270), Baltimore (n = 295), and Chicago (n = 486) in 1985-1987. It assessed whether veterans were more likely to be homeless than men who were not veterans. Among homeless men, 41% reported military service, compared with 34% of men in the general U.S. population. Comparing veterans with nonveterans showed that those 35-44 years old (those who were most likely to have served in Vietnam) had an odds ratio (OR) for homelessness of 1.01 (95% CI 0.85-1.21). Among both white and black veterans, the cohorts 20-34 and 45-54 years old had a greater likelihood of homelessness (OR 3.95, 95% CI 3.39-4.58; and OR 1.75, 95% CI 1.45-2.15, respectively). The youngest veterans in the 1987 Third Survey of Veterans, a nationally representative sample of 9442 noninstitutionalized veterans, had served after Vietnam in the all-volunteer Army, and only 7% had seen combat. Most of the veterans 45-54 years old had served between the Korean War and the Vietnam War, and 17% of them had seen combat; among veterans who served during the Vietnam War era, 40% reported combat exposure. The much higher prevalence of psychiatric illness, substance abuse, and antisocial personality disorder among white veterans 20-34 years old seemed to be a more likely contributor to the greater vulnerability of this group than combat exposure. Homeless veterans in the most vulnerable groups were the least likely to have served during wartime or combat, and this reduces the role that could be attributed to combat stress in the genesis of homelessness among veterans.

Gamache et al. (2001) conducted a followup of the study by Rosenheck et al. (1994) to determine whether the exceptionally high risk of homelessness among post-Vietnam-era, largely noncombat veterans first observed in 1987 was still evident one decade later. Data on 1841 current male clients of homeless assistance programs throughout the U.S. gathered by the 1996 National Survey of Homeless Assistance Providers were compared with information on the general population from the 1996 Current Population Survey. The homeless clients, who were interviewed face-to-face, came from the 28 largest metropolitan statistical areas (MSAs), 24 randomly chosen small and medium-sized MSAs, and 24 randomly chosen rural counties. The relative probability of homelessness for veteran vs nonveteran was determined for defined age and race groups. As of 1996, the proportion of veterans in the adult male homeless population had declined from 41% to 33%, although this proportion was still greater than the 28% in the general population. The especially high risk of homelessness among veterans of the immediate post-Vietnam era who had been aged 20-34 in 1987 was sustained 10 years later (OR 3.17, 95% CI 2.69-3.73), although the youngest cohort of veterans also showed a significant risk of homelessness (OR 2.04, 95% CI 1.59-2.64).

Secondary Studies

The secondary studies that were reviewed provided mixed findings as to whether deployment to a war zone increased the risk of homelessness.

Winkleby and Fleshin (1993) compared three groups of homeless men residing in three California shelters: 173 combat-exposed veterans, 250 veterans without combat exposure, and 585 nonveterans. The prevalence of psychiatric hospitalizations and physical injuries before homelessness was approximately 1.5-2 times as high in combat veterans as in nonveterans or veterans who had not experienced combat. The time between military discharge and first being homeless was more than a decade for 76% of the homeless combat veterans.

Rosenheck et al. (1991) compared data on 10,524 veterans participating in the VA Homeless Chronically Mentally Ill Veterans Program with veterans in the general population. Of the participating veterans, 50% had served in the military during the Vietnam War era, 45% had served in the Vietnam theater, and 41% had been exposed to combat. Only 29% of the total U.S.

veteran population served during the Vietnam War era. However, because the proportion of homeless veterans who served in combat and served in the Vietnam theater was about the same for the veterans who were not homeless, the authors interpreted that finding to suggest that the risk of homelessness could be attributed more to age—that is, being 30-44 years old (an age of specific vulnerability of men to homelessness)—than to combat exposure.

Rosenheck et al. (1992), in a study of the relationship between combat stress and homelessness, compared data on 627 Vietnam veterans who were evaluated in a VA clinical program for homeless mentally-ill veterans with data on Vietnam veterans assessed in a national epidemiologic study. Some 43% of the 627 veterans in the VA program showed evidence of combat stress that was associated with more severe psychiatric and substance-abuse problems.

Wenzel et al. (1993) assessed 343 homeless male veterans receiving treatment for physical, mental, or substance-abuse disorders and compared the long-term homeless (more than 12 months) with the short-term homeless (12 months or less). The long-term homeless were more likely to be white, to have symptoms of mental and substance-abuse disorders, and to have weaker social support.

A 2001-2003 survey of 631 homeless veterans enrolled in a VA clinical demonstration project designed to evaluate a vocational rehabilitation model, found that 31% of the veterans thought that military service had increased their risk of being homeless (Mares and Rosenheck 2004). Among all the homeless veterans, 19% had received hostile or friendly fire in a combat zone. Only 15% of those who did not think that being in the military had increased their risk of homelessness had received such fire, compared with 25% of those who perceived being in the military as a risk factor. Logistic regression showed that each additional childhood problem reported before military life also almost doubled the likelihood of perceiving that military service increased the risk of homelessness.

Gamache et al. (2000), in the only study of homeless women, estimated the proportions of veterans and nonveterans. Subjects were drawn primarily from a program for homeless persons with mental illness, but the results showed that the risk of homelessness overall was 2-4 times greater for veterans than for nonveterans. Although Vietnam-era women were at greatest risk for homelessness in this sample, the study did not distinguish between Vietnam-theater veterans and Vietnam-era veterans.

Tessler et al. (2002) compared homeless veterans with homeless nonveterans; all were enrolled in an outreach program for persons suffering from serious mental illness. The introduction of an all-volunteer military force did not appear to have changed the composition of the adult male homeless population. Similar results had been obtained by Gamache et al. (2001).

Summary and Conclusions

The primary and secondary studies reviewed by the committee yielded mixed results with respect to the effect of deployment, particularly combat, on the risk of homelessness in veterans. Of the three primary studies, only one (Rosenheck and Fontana 1994) showed an association between combat exposure and homelessness in Vietnam veterans. The other two studies were equivocal. The secondary studies were also mixed and in general showed that homelessness was related more to the presence of psychiatric disorders than to combat exposure itself. Nevertheless, as the committee concluded in Chapter 6, deployment to a war zone does increase the risk of psychiatric disorders among veterans, so there may be an indirect effect on homelessness.

The committee concludes that there is inadequate/insufficient evidence to determine whether an association exists between deployment to a war zone and homelessness.

TABLE 7-2 Homelessness

Reference	Study Design	Population	Outcomes	Results	Adjustments	Comments
Rosenheck and Fontana 1994 (Derived from NVVRS)	Retrospective cohort; NSVG	1460 male Vietnam theater and era veterans discharged from military before 1979	DIS, Mississippi Scale for Combat-Related PTSD (collected in NVVRS), Combat Exposure Scale, association of multiple risk factors and vulnerability to homelessness	High combat exposure: OR 2.1, 95% CI 1.5-3.0 Participation in atrocities: OR 2.7, 95% CI 1.9-3.8	Race, age, rank, year of birth, childhood poverty, parental mental illness, childhood abuse, other childhood trauma, adult nonmilitary trauma, social support, marital status, substance abuse, psychiatric disorders	Limited recall bias, low generalizability
Rosenheck et al. 1994	Cross-sectional (four surveys administered in 1985-1987)	Homeless men from Urban Institute survey (n = 1140), Baltimore (n = 295), Chicago (n = 486), Los Angeles (n = 270) vs general population (from 1987 CPS)	Prevalence of homelessness in male veteran vs general population	All ages: OR 1.38, 95% CI 1.05-1.85 Age 20-34: OR 3.95, 95% CI 3.39-4.58 Age 35-44: OR 1.01, 95% CI 0.85-1.21 Age 45-54: OR 1.75, 95% CI 1.45-2.15	Includes whites, blacks, others	
Gamache et al. 2001 (Followup of Rosenheck et al. 1994)	Cross-sectional, study	1841 homeless males vs general population (data from 1996 CPS)	Prevalence of homeless veterans in each population	All ages: OR 1.25, 95% CI 1.13-1.38 Age 20-34: OR 2.04, 95% CI 1.59-2.64 Age 35-44: OR 3.17, 95% CI 2.69-3.73 Age 45-54: OR 1.39, 95% CI 1.14-1.71	Includes both white, blacks, and others	

NOTE: CI = confidence interval, CPS = Current Population Survey, DIS = Diagnostic Interview Schedule, NSVG = National Survey of the Vietnam Generation, NVVRS = National Vietnam Veterans Readjustment Study, OR = odds ratio, PTSD = posttraumatic stress disorder.

INCARCERATION

As of 1998, over 225,000 veterans were in prison or jail in the United States, more than half for violent offenses. Of the incarcerated veterans, about 20% had served in combat duty in the Vietnam War or the Gulf War (Mumola 2000). The committee reviewed six studies regarding the relationship between deployment to a war zone and incarceration. Two (Black et al. 2005; Yager et al. 1984) met the criteria for primary studies, and the other four (Boivin 1987; Hiley-Young et al. 1995; Kulka et al. 1990; Shaw et al. 1987) were designated as secondary studies. The primary studies involved a population-based survey of military personnel who had listed Iowa as their place of residence at enlistment for the Gulf War (Black et al. 2005) and a national sample of men who were of military age during the Vietnam War (Yager et al. 1984). Three of the secondary studies did not have representative samples: Hiley-Young et al. (1995) studied only PTSD inpatients, Shaw et al. (1987) studied Vietnam veterans who had been incarcerated in the state prisons of Iowa, and Boivin (1987) studied a group of incarcerated Vietnam veterans in the maximum-security section of a state prison. Kulka et al. (1990) did not use a validated instrument to determine Vietnam veterans' involvement with the criminal justice system. Because of the small number of studies considered for this psychosocial effect, primary and secondary studies are treated together here; the two primary studies are summarized in Table 7-3.

Black et al. (2005) investigated the prevalence of incarceration and its association with deployment among veterans who had been on active duty during the Gulf War. The study covered military personnel residing in Iowa in 1995-1996 who had deployed to the gulf and a comparison sample of nondeployed military personnel. A total of 4886 subjects were randomly drawn from four study domains: Gulf War regular military (n = 985), Gulf War National Guard and reserve (n = 911), non-Gulf War regular military (n = 968), and non-Gulf War National Guard and reserve (n = 831). A structured telephone interview consisting of validated questions, validated instruments, and investigator-derived questions regarding relevant medical and psychiatric conditions was used. Instruments included the PRIME-MD, the PTSD Checklist, and the Marlowe-Crowne Social Desirability Scale. The sample included 3695 participants (76% of eligible subjects), and a valid telephone number was identified for 91% of them. Of the 3695, 22.9% (845) reported that they had been incarcerated at some point in their lives, 14.5% had been incarcerated at least once before their deployment, and 8.3% had been incarcerated only during or after their deployment. The prevalence of incarceration only after August 1990 for Gulf War veterans vs nondeployed veterans was 8.1% (SE 0.7) and 8.4% (0.8), respectively (OR 0.71, 95% CI 0.5-1.0). In a multivariate model adjusted for age, gender, race, branch of service, and military status, the association between combat experience and being incarcerated only after the Gulf War was significant (OR 1.6, 95% CI 1.0-2.5), suggesting that combat was modestly associated with subsequent incarceration.

Yager et al. (1984) studied a sample of 1342 American men who were of draft-eligible age during the Vietnam War. Respondents were chosen on a stratified-probability basis at 10 sites, including big cities, small cities, and rural areas in various regions of the United States. The combined dataset included 629 nonveterans and 713 veterans, 350 of whom served in Vietnam. Subjects were interviewed 6-15 years after the veterans left the service (1977-1979). Respondents were asked whether they had ever been arrested, when it had occurred, what the charge had been, and whether they had been convicted. Vietnam-theater veterans who did not experience combat or participate in abusive violence had lower conviction rates than era controls. However, if the veteran experienced combat or abusive violence, the results showed impressive effects of heavy combat exposure on arrests and convictions. The arrest rate increased by an average of 2.32 percentage points and the conviction rate by 1.23 percentage points for every point increase on the Combat Exposure Scale. When preservice background factors were statistically controlled for, combat exposure continued to show an association with arrests and convictions (generally for nonviolent offenses). The authors concluded that arrests in the years after service, including arrests that led to conviction, increased sharply with exposure to combat. Of the Vietnam veterans with heavy combat exposure who were arrested after discharge, 19.6% had been arrested for nonviolent offenses and 4.9% for violent offenses, compared with 17.7% and 2.1%, respectively, of veterans with moderate combat exposure and 5.7% and 0.6% of those with light combat exposure.

In the 1986-1987 NVVRS, Kulka et al. (1990) found that the 406 Vietnam theater veterans with high levels of war-zone stress were more likely to have been arrested or jailed than the 783 theater veterans with moderate-low war-zone stress (39.1% vs 27.7%) and were almost 3 times as likely (8.8% vs 2.8%) to have been convicted of a felony. Involvement with the criminal-justice system was based on self-reports of number of times arrested since the age of 18 years, nights spent in jail or prison (since the age of 18 years), and number of lifetime convictions for a felony offense and on whether the veteran was in jail or prison at the time of the interview. Of the 319 Vietnam theater veterans with current PTSD, 45.7% had been arrested or jailed more than once in their lives compared with 11.6% of the 871 theater veterans without PTSD; 11.5% of the veterans with PTSD had been convicted of a felony. PTSD symptom level at the time of the interview was assessed with the Mississippi Scale for Combat-Related PTSD; a study cutoff score of 94 was used as a threshold for an assessment of current PTSD. A diagnosis of PTSD was validated in a subsample of the veterans with the SCID. Black theater veterans were more likely to be involved in the criminal-justice system than whites or Hispanics, but black and Hispanic theater veterans with low war-zone stress were less likely to be involved in the criminal-justice system than black or Hispanic era veterans.

In contrast, the other three secondary studies were less likely to attribute incarceration to deployment. In a small study of 61 Vietnam veterans (31 incarcerated and 30 not) in Iowa state prisons, Shaw et al. (1987) concluded that previous personal characteristics, such as a history of antisocial behavior, and not wartime experiences best explained incarceration. Combat stress was similar in both groups although high stress was associated with the development of PTSD. Incarcerated veterans were found to have a higher prevalence of antisocial personality disorder than the community sample (36% vs 7%) and a higher prevalence of alcohol and drug abuse. In the study by Hiley-Young et al. (1995) of 177 Vietnam combat veterans who were receiving treatment for PTSD as inpatients at a VA hospital, high levels of combat exposure were not found to predict criminal activities. A strength of this study is that the authors verified combat status with military records.

Boivin (1987), studying incarcerated male Vietnam veterans in a maximum-security section of a Michigan state prison, found that incarcerated veterans (n = 46) were more likely to be black, to have come from a less supportive family background, to have been assigned to an Army infantry combat unit, and to have been injured in combat than incarcerated nonveterans at the same prison (n = 19), nonincarcerated Vietnam veterans from a Vietnam Veterans of America chapter (n = 28), and nonincarcerated non-Vietnam veterans from a National Guard group at a local college (n = 28). The incarcerated veterans were also more likely to have been involved in killing enemy soldiers, prisoners, or civilians and to have flashbacks of those events. The author attributed their incarceration, however, to having been poor prospects with respect to their social, economic, and interpersonal well-being before being sent to Vietnam.

Summary and Conclusions

The two primary studies, one of Gulf War veterans and one of Vietnam veterans, found that exposure to heavy combat increased the likelihood of being incarcerated after release from military service. However, veterans who were deployed but did not experience heavy combat were less likely to be incarcerated than those exposed to heavy combat and were not any more likely to be incarcerated than nondeployed veterans. The secondary studies, conducted mainly with Vietnam veterans, were mixed and tended to show that having a psychiatric disorder increased the risk of a veteran being incarcerated.

The committee concludes that there is limited but suggestive evidence of an association between deployment to a war zone and later incarceration.

TABLE 7-3 Incarceration

Reference	Study Design	Population	Outcomes	Results	Adjustments	Comments
Black et al. 2005	Cross-sectional survey conducted in 1995-1996	985 Gulf War regular military, 911 Gulf War National Guard or reserve, 968 nondeployed regular military, 831 nondeployed National Guard or reserve veterans drawn as a random sample from 4886 Iowa-based veterans	Structured telephone interview to assess prevalence of incarceration in Gulf War vs non-Gulf War veterans	Deployed vs nondeployed veterans incarcerated after August 1990: OR 0.71, 95% CI 0.5-1.0; ever incarcerated: OR 1.04, 95% CI 0.9-1.3	Age, sex, race, rank, branch of service, military status	Recall bias, limited generalizability, lack of specificity of details of incarceration
Yager et al. 1984	Cross-sectional survey conducted 6-15 years after leaving service (1977-1979)	350 Vietnam-theater veterans, 363 era veterans, 629 nonveterans	Interview about war experience variable Combat Exposure Scale Incarceration prevalence between Vietnam theater and era veterans	Arrest rate increased by average of 2.32 percentage points and conviction rate by average of 1.23 percentage points for every point increase on Combat Exposure Scale ($p < 0.01$) Prevalence of being arrested after discharge: -heavy combat exposed, 19.6% nonviolent offenses, 4.9% violent offenses -moderate combat exposure, 17.7% and 2.1%, respectively -light combat exposure, 5.7% and 0.6%, respectively	Age, race, drug use, alcohol use	Recall bias, limited generalizability

NOTE: CI = confidence interval, OR = odds ratio.

EMPLOYMENT

Closely related to the disabling effects of PTSD on a person's ability to function is its effect on the ability to find and maintain employment. The committee reviewed five studies regarding the effect of deployment to a war zone on employment and earnings. The two that were designated as primary studies used data from the NVVRS, a nationally representative sample of male Vietnam veterans. Of the three secondary studies, two were based on data from the National Comorbidity Survey (NCS) and these were considered secondary because the subjects were selected nonrandomly and because there was no control or comparison group. The third secondary study had a nonrepresentative sample consisting only of veterans in treatment for PTSD. Primary studies are summarized in Table 7-4.

Zatzick et al. (1997a,b) studied the relationship between PTSD and functioning and quality of life. One sample included male Vietnam veterans, and the other, female Vietnam veterans. The authors used archival data from the NVVRS NSVG, a study that was completed in 1988 and included a cohort of 1200 male and 432 female Vietnam-theater veterans, and 412 male and 304 female era veterans. Most male veterans were middle-aged and married at the time of the interview; over 50% had some college education. About 17% of veterans were of black or Hispanic backgrounds. PTSD symptom level at the time of the interview was assessed with the Mississippi Scale for Combat-Related PTSD; a study cutoff score of 94 and 89 was used to define current PTSD in the men and women, respectively. Psychiatric comorbidity was diagnosed with the DIS. A single question assessed the subjects' ability to function in a particular role on the job, at home, or at school. Male veterans who were gainfully employed (n = 1033), active with schoolwork (n = 2), or engaged in housework (n = 2) were categorized as working. Logistic models were used to determine the association between PTSD and outcome; adjustment was made for demographic characteristics and comorbid psychiatric and other medical conditions. The results showed that veterans with PTSD (n = 242) were more likely not to be working at the time of the survey than veterans without PTSD (n = 948), for an OR of 3.3 (95% CI 1.5-7.6) adjusted for age, ethnicity, marital status, educational attainment, region of country, and comorbidity; 10 veterans did not complete the scale and were not included in the analyses.

The study of 432 female Vietnam veterans also used archival data from the NVVRS (Zatzick et al. 1997b). Aside from the use of a cutoff of 89 for a PTSD diagnosis, the methods for this study were the same as for the study of male veterans. About 8.9% (37) women were estimated to have PTSD. Once again, logistic models were used to determine the association between PTSD and various outcomes, including employment. Adjusted for age, ethnicity, marital status, educational attainment, region of country, and comorbidity, PTSD was associated with approximately 10 times greater odds of not working (OR 10.4, 95% CI 1.8-61.9). This was the strongest association found between PTSD and the various outcomes, which also included subjective well-being and self-reported physical health status. A limitation of both Zatzick et al. studies is that they were cross-sectional, making it impossible to determine the extent to which PTSD may have caused this functional impairment.

Savoca and Rosenheck (2000) also used data from the NVVRS NSVG to explore the influence of psychiatric disorders on the civilian labor-market experiences of 1417 Vietnam-era veterans. The authors used the NSVG lifetime diagnoses of major depression, anxiety disorders, substance abuse or dependence, constructed with the DIS and combat-related PTSD based on the

Mississippi Scale for Combat-Related PTSD. The employment probability equation was estimated by using a probit: hourly earnings and hour-worked were estimated via ordinary least squares conditioned on being employed. The comparison group was white veterans without a history of psychiatric disorder, who had served in the military, but not in Southeast Asia, for less than one year and had low levels of war-related stress. The presence of any of four psychiatric diagnoses had a statistically significant negative effect on the probability of being employed: anxiety disorder, -0.415 ($p < 0.01$); substance abuse or dependence, -0.233 ($p < 0.01$); major depression, -0.390 ($p < 0.01$); and PTSD -0.498 ($p < 0.01$). However, none of the psychiatric disorders had an effect on the usual number of hours worked per week. Veterans with lifetime PTSD were 8.6% less likely to be working and, if working, earned 16% less per hour than veterans without PTSD. Veterans with major depression or substance use or dependence, but not anxiety disorders, also had lower hourly wages, although the lower wages are not significant for those with substance abuse or dependence. For men with depression, there was as 45% decrease in hourly wages ($p \leq 0.01$), whereas for men with anxiety disorders, there was a 31% increase ($p \leq 0.01$). In summary, combat-related PTSD significantly lowered the likelihood of working and the hourly wage. The authors noted that PTSD had a greater effect on reducing the likelihood of working and on the hourly wage than did deployment to Vietnam itself.

Similar results were seen by Jordan et al. (1992). Using data from the NVVRS, they found that Vietnam veterans with PTSD were five times more likely to be unemployed than veterans without PTSD (13.3% vs 2.5%).

The three secondary studies (Prigerson et al. 2001, 2002; Smith et al. 2005) reported similar results. Prigerson et al. (2001) used a subsample of 1703 men from the 1990-1992 NCS who reported experiencing a traumatic event to assess the impact of combat exposure on employment. They found that the 96 men who reported combat as their worst trauma had the highest rates of unemployment (20%) or having been fired in the last year (13%) compared with the highest rates for men who reported one of eight other traumas as their worst (13.4% and 9.7%, respectively). Using a different subsample of 2248 men from NCS, 179 of whom reported combat exposure data, Prigerson et al. (2002) estimated that 11.7% of 12-month job loss (relative risk 2.90, 95% CI 1.70-4.70, $p < 0.001$) and 8.9% of current unemployment (relative risk 2.37, 95% CI 1.55-3.44, $p < 0.001$) could be attributed to combat exposure.

Among 325 male Vietnam-era veterans being treated in 10 VA medical centers for severe or very severe PTSD symptoms, veterans with more severe PTSD symptoms (based on responses to the CAPS) were more likely to work part-time or not at all. A 10-point increase in CAPS score was associated with an almost 6% increase in the probability of not working, a 2% decrease in the likelihood of part-time work, and almost a 4% decrease in having full-time work (Smith et al. 2005).

Summary and Conclusions

Both primary studies considered by the committee indicated that veterans with PTSD are at greater risk for being unemployed and, if they are employed, are at risk for receiving lower wages than their counterparts without PTSD. However, the conclusions that can be drawn from the studies are limited in that they did not assess whether deployment itself had the same effect. Furthermore, all the primary studies were conducted in Vietnam veterans; none assessed the effect of Gulf War or other deployment on the later employment status of veterans. The secondary studies also indicated that veterans with combat exposure had poorer employment outcomes than those who experienced other or no traumas, particularly if they had PTSD.

The committee concludes that there is inadequate/insufficient evidence to determine whether an association exists between deployment to a war zone and adverse employment outcomes.

TABLE 7-4 Adverse Employment Outcomes

Reference	Study Design	Population	Outcomes	Results	Adjustments	Comments
Zatzick et al. 1997a (Derived from NVVRS)	Cross-sectional survey; archival analysis of data from NVVRS	1200 male Vietnam-theater veterans; 242 veterans with PTSD vs 948 without PTSD	Not working vs working associated with PTSD	OR 3.3, 95% CI 1.5-7.6	Demographic characteristics, other medical disorders	Unable to determine causality, employment status determined with single question, possible recall bias due to self-reports
Zatzick et al. 1997b (Derived from NVVRS)	Cross-sectional survey; archival analysis of data from NVVRS	432 female Vietnam theater veterans, mostly nurses; 37 with PTSD	Not working vs working associated with PTSD	OR 10.4, 95% CI 1.8-61.9	Demographic characteristics, other medical disorders	Unable to determine causality, employment status determined with single question, possible recall bias due to self-reports
Savoca and Rosenheck 2000 (Derived from NVVRS)	Cross-sectional survey	1417 Vietnam-era veterans Comparison group is white veterans with no history of psychiatric disorders and deployed elsewhere	Estimates of hourly wages and probability of employment	Theater veteran: 60% higher chance of employment ($p < 0.01$); 50% higher wages (NS) PTSD: 50% lower chance of employment; 16% lower wages	Demographic characteristics, length of service, other psychiatric disorders, difficulty of job	Unable to determine causality, comparison group is nonrepresentative

NOTE: CI = confidence interval, NS = nonsignificant, NVVRS = National Vietnam Veterans Readjustment Study, OR = odds ratio, PTSD = posttraumatic stress disorder.

REFERENCES

Beckham JC, Feldman ME, Kirby AC, Hertzberg MA, Moore SD. 1997. Interpersonal violence and its correlates in Vietnam veterans with chronic posttraumatic stress disorder. *Journal of Clinical Psychology* 53(8):859-869.

Black DW, Carney CP, Peloso PM, Woolson RF, Letuchy E, Doebbeling BN. 2005. Incarceration and veterans of the first Gulf War. *Military Medicine* 170(7):612-618.

Boivin MJ. 1987. Forgotten warriors: An evaluation of the emotional well-being of presently incarcerated Vietnam veterans. *Genetic, Social, and General Psychology Monographs* 113(1):109-125.

Call VR, Teachman JD. 1991. Military service and stability in the family life course. *Military Psychology* 3(4):233-250.

Call VR, Teachman JD. 1996. Life-course timing and sequencing of marriage and military service and their effects on marital stability. *Journal of Marriage and the Family* 58(1):219-226.

Clark JC, Messer SC, Castro CAE, Adler ABE, Britt TWE. 2006. Intimate partner violence in the U.S. military: Rates, risks, and responses. *Military Life: The Psychology of Serving in Peace and Combat* 3:193-219.

DoD (Department of Defense). 2004. *Task Force Report on Care for Victims of Sexual Assault.* Washington, DC.

Evans L, McHugh T, Hopwood M, Watt C. 2003. Chronic posttraumatic stress disorder and family functioning of Vietnam veterans and their partners. *Australian and New Zealand Journal of Psychiatry* 37(6):765-772.

Gamache G, Rosenheck R, Tessler R. 2000. Military discharge status of homeless veterans with mental illness. *Military Medicine* 165(11):803-808.

Gamache G, Rosenheck R, Tessler R. 2001. The proportion of veterans among homeless men: A decade later. *Social Psychiatry and Psychiatric Epidemiology* 36(10):481-485.

Gamache G, Rosenheck R, Tessler R. 2003. Overrepresentation of women veterans among homeless women. *American Journal of Public Health* 93(7):1132-1136.

Gimbel C, Booth A. 1994. Why does military combat experience adversely affect marital relations? *Journal of Marriage and the Family* 56(3):691-703.

Glenn DM, Beckham JC, Feldman ME, Kirby AC, Hertzberg MA, Moore SD. 2002. Violence and hostility among families of Vietnam veterans with combat-related posttraumatic stress disorder. *Violence and Victims* 17(4):473-489.

Heyman RE, Neidig PH. 1999. A comparison of spousal aggression prevalence rates in U.S. Army and civilian representative samples. *Journal of Consulting and Clinical Psychology* 67(2):239-242.

Hiley-Young B, Blake DD, Abueg FR, Rozynko V, Gusman FD. 1995. Warzone violence in Vietnam: An examination of premilitary, military, and postmilitary factors in PTSD in-patients. *Journal of Traumatic Stress* 8(1):125-141.

Jensen PS, Martin D, Watanabe H. 1996. Children's response to parental separation during operation desert storm. *Journal of the American Academy of Child and Adolescent Psychiatry* 35(4):433-441.

Jordan BK, Marmar CR, Fairbank JA, Schlenger WE, Kulka RA, Hough RL, Weiss DS. 1992. Problems in families of male Vietnam veterans with posttraumatic stress disorder. *Journal of Consulting and Clinical Psychology* 60(6):916-926.

Kulka RA, Schlenger WE, Fairbank JA, Hough RL, Jordan BK, Marmar CR, Weiss DS. 1990. *Trauma and the Vietnam War Generation: Report of Findings from the National Vietnam Veterans Readjustment Study*. New York: Brunner/Mazel Publishers.

Mares AS, Rosenheck RA. 2004. Perceived relationship between military service and homelessness among homeless veterans with mental illness. *Journal of Nervous and Mental Disease* 192(10):715-719.

McCarroll JE, Ursano RJ, Liu X, Thayer LE, Newby JH, Norwood AE, Fullerton CS. 2000. Deployment and the probability of spousal aggression by U.S. Army soldiers. *Military Medicine* 165(1):41-44.

McCarroll JE, Ursano RJ, Newby JH, Liu X, Fullerton CS, Norwood AE, Osuch EA. 2003. Domestic violence and deployment in U.S. Army soldiers. *Journal of Nervous and Mental Disease* 191(1):3-9.

McFall M, Fontana A, Raskind M, Rosenheck R. 1999. Analysis of violent behavior in Vietnam combat veteran psychiatric inpatients with posttraumatic stress disorder. *Journal of Traumatic Stress*. 12(3):501-517.

MHAT (Mental Health Advisory Team). 2006. *Mental Health Advisory Team (MHAT) IV Operation Iraqi Freedom 05-07: Final Report*. [Washington, DC]: Office of the Surgeon Multinational Force-Iraq and Office of the Surgeon General United States Army Medical Command. 17 November 2006. [Online]. Available: http://www.armymedicine.army.mil/news/mhat/mhat_iv/MHAT_IV_Report_17NOV06.pdf.

Mumola CJ. 2000. *Veterans in Prison or Jail*. [Online]. Available: http://www.ojp.usdoj.gov/bjs/pub/ascii/vpj.txt [accessed July 31, 2007].

Newby JH, McCarroll JE, Ursano RJ, Fan Z, Shigemura J, Tucker-Harris Y. 2005. Positive and negative consequences of a military deployment. *Military Medicine* 170(10):815-819.

Orcutt HK, King LA, King DW. 2003. Male-perpetrated violence among Vietnam veteran couples: Relationships with veteran's early life characteristics, trauma history, and PTSD symptomatology. *Journal of Traumatic Stress* 16(4):381-390.

Prigerson HG, Maciejewski PK, Rosenheck RA. 2001. Combat trauma: Trauma with highest risk of delayed onset and unresolved posttraumatic stress disorder symptoms, unemployment, and abuse among men. *Journal of Nervous and Mental Disease* 189(2):99-108.

Prigerson HG, Maciejewski PK, Rosenheck RA. 2002. Population attributable fractions of psychiatric disorders and behavioral outcomes associated with combat exposure among U.S. men. *American Journal of Public Health* 92(1):59-63.

Rentz ED, Marshall SW, Loomis D, Casteel C, Martin SL, Gibbs DA. 2007. Effect of deployment on the occurrence of child maltreatment in military and nonmilitary families. *American Journal of Epidemiology* 165(10):1199-1206.

Rosen LN, Teitelbaum JM, Westhuis DJ. 1993. Children's reactions to the Desert Storm deployment: Initial findings from a survey of Army families. *Military Medicine* 158(7):465-469.

Rosenheck R, Fontana A. 1994. A model of homelessness among male veterans of the Vietnam War generation. *American Journal of Psychiatry* 151(3):421-427.

Rosenheck R, Fontana A. 1998. Transgenerational effects of abusive violence on the children of Vietnam combat veterans. *Journal of Traumatic Stress* 11(4):731-742.

Rosenheck R, Gallup P, Leda CA. 1991. Vietnam era and Vietnam combat veterans among the homeless. *American Journal of Public Health* 81(5):643-646.

Rosenheck R, Leda C, Gallup P. 1992. Combat stress, psychosocial adjustment, and service use among homeless Vietnam veterans. *Hospital and Community Psychiatry* 43(2):145-149.

Rosenheck R, Frisman L, Chung AM. 1994. The proportion of veterans among homeless men. *American Journal of Public Health* 84(3):466-469.

Samper RE, Taft CT, King DW, King LA. 2004. Posttraumatic stress disorder symptoms and parenting satisfaction among a national sample of male Vietnam veterans. *Journal of Traumatic Stress* 17(4):311-315.

Savarese VW, Suvak MK, King LA, King DW. 2001. Relationships among alcohol use, hyperarousal, and marital abuse and violence in Vietnam veterans. *Journal of Traumatic Stress* 14(4):717-732.

Savoca E, Rosenheck R. 2000. The civilian labor market experiences of Vietnam-era veterans: The influence of psychiatric disorders. *Journal of Mental Health Policy and Economics* 3(4):199-207.

Schumm WR, Bell DB, Knott B, Rice RE. 1996a. The perceived effect of stressors on marital satisfaction among civilian wives of enlisted soldiers deployed to Somalia for Operation Restore Hope. *Military Medicine* 161(10):601-606.

Schumm WR, Hemesath K, Bell D, Palmer-Johnson C, Elig TW. 1996b. Did Desert Storm reduce marital satisfaction among Army enlisted personnel? *Psychological Reports* 78(3 Pt 2):1241-1242.

Shaw DM, Churchill CM, Noyes R Jr, Loeffelholz PL. 1987. Criminal behavior and post-traumatic stress disorder in Vietnam veterans. *Comprehensive Psychiatry* 28(5):403-411.

Smith MW, Schnurr PP, Rosenheck RA. 2005. Employment outcomes and PTSD symptom severity. *Mental Health Services Research* 7(2):89-101.

Taft CT, Pless AP, Stalans LJ, Koenen KC, King LA, King DW. 2005. Risk factors for partner violence among a national sample of combat veterans. *Journal of Consulting and Clinical Psychology* 73(1):151-159.

Tessler R, Rosenheck R, Gamache G. 2002. Comparison of homeless veterans with other homeless men in a large clinical outreach program. *Psychiatric Quarterly* 73(2):109-119.

VHA (Veterans Health Administration). 2006. *Overview of Homelessness*. [Online]. Available: http://www1.va.gov/homeless/page.cfm?pg=1 [accessed August 14, 2007].

Wenzel SL, Gelberg L, Bakhtiar L, Caskey N, Hardie E, Redford C, Sadler N. 1993. Indicators of chronic homelessness among veterans. *Hospital and Community Psychiatry* 44(12):1172-1176.

Winkleby MA, Fleshin D. 1993. Physical, addictive, and psychiatric disorders among homeless veterans and nonveterans. *Public Health Reports* 108(1):30-36.

Yager T, Laufer R, Gallops M. 1984. Some problems associated with war experience in men of the Vietnam generation. *Archives of General Psychiatry* 41(4):327-333.

Zatzick DF, Marmar CR, Weiss DS, Browner WS, Metzler TJ, Golding JM, Stewart A, Schlenger WE, Wells KB. 1997a. Posttraumatic stress disorder and functioning and quality of life outcomes in a nationally representative sample of male Vietnam veterans. *American Journal of Psychiatry* 154(12):1690-1695.

Zatzick DF, Weiss DS, Marmar CR, Metzler TJ, Wells K, Golding JM, Stewart A, Schlenger WE, Browner WS. 1997b. Post-traumatic stress disorder and functioning and quality of life outcomes in female Vietnam veterans. *Military Medicine* 162(10):661-665.

8

CONCLUSIONS AND RECOMMENDATIONS

The committee was established to review, evaluate, and summarize the peer-reviewed scientific and medical literature regarding the association between deployment-related stress and long-term health effects in Gulf War veterans. This chapter summarizes what the literature collectively tells us about physiologic, psychologic, and psychosocial effects seen in veterans as a result of deployment.

QUALITY OF THE STUDIES

The epidemiologic and other studies reviewed by the committee varied in quality. A major limitation in virtually all the studies reviewed by the committee, except some studies on posttraumatic stress disorder (PTSD), was the lack of an assessment of the perception of stress experienced by the military personnel during deployment to a war zone. The studies that assessed deployment stressors tended to use scales, such as the Combat Exposure Scale, that ascertain whether an exposure to a given stressor occurred (and possibly how frequently), but such assessment tools do not query veterans about their perception of the stressor, for example, whether they were very stressed, somewhat stressed, or not stressed at all. The committee is aware that using deployment as a surrogate for deployment-related stress is a less than perfect method for assessing the long-term health effects of deployment to a war zone, but no other acceptable approaches to the problem were evident. The exception is the use of deployment- or combat-related PTSD to indicate exposure to a war-zone trauma.

Few studies met the criteria established by the committee for a primary study. The requirement that the disease or other adverse effect in question be diagnosed through an appropriate examination or diagnostic instrument meant that many studies, although large and representative of the veteran population, were considered not to be primary studies because they relied on self-reports of symptoms or medical conditions. Other well-done studies involved small sample sizes or used nonstandardized measures. Prior life experiences known to be modifiers of health effects were infrequently assessed. Researchers that compared the accuracy of self-reports with objective measures, such as physical examinations or medical records, often found conflicting results; and the correlation between self-reports and objective measures or diagnoses was sufficiently poor that the committee decided that, although self-reports provided valuable information, a self-report alone was not sufficient to show an association between deployment and a specific health effect. Furthermore, some of the veterans studied were not representative of the entire veteran population being studied, for example, some were receiving medical treatment.

Many of the studies were cross-sectional and so could not fully assess symptom duration and chronicity, latency of onset, and prognosis; this is an important limitation because many of the long-term outcomes assessed in this report, such as coronary heart disease and cancer, have latent periods of decades. Some studies of veterans of World War II, the Korean War, and the Vietnam War were longitudinal and allowed an assessment of the health of veterans over time. Finally, many of the studies looked at a variety of exposures of deployed personnel, particularly those of the Gulf War, and this makes it difficult to distinguish specific effects from any one of the multitude of exposures. The committee did not consider the effect of many co-occurring exposures of Gulf War veterans, such as exposure to oil-well fires, pyridostigmine bromide, and vaccines and, for Vietnam veterans, Agent Orange. Therefore, because this report considered the agent of interest—deployment to a war zone—as the only exposure, it may have reached conclusions different from those of other *Gulf War and Health* reports, particularly *Volume 4: Health Effects of Serving in the Gulf War*, and *Veterans and Agent Orange* reports.

Several large-scale, nationally representative studies of veterans have been conducted, most notably the Vietnam Experience Study (CDC 1988), which compared Vietnam theater and Vietnam-era veterans for a multitude of health and psychosocial end points; the National Vietnam Veterans Readjustment Study, which made similar comparisons (Jordan et al. 1992; Kulka et al. 1990); the National Health Survey of Gulf War Era Veterans and Their Families (Eisen et al. 2005; Kang et al. 2000); the studies of Australian Gulf War veterans (Ikin et al. 2004; Kelsall et al. 2004) and Danish Gulf War peacekeepers (Ishoy et al. 1999); the hospitalization studies of Gulf War veterans (Gray et al. 1996, 2000); and the Department of Veterans Affairs (VA) Normative Aging Study, which has followed World War II and Korean War veterans since 1961. Those and other studies that evaluated specific health effects formed the backbone of the committee's assessment of the association between deployment-related stress and various health effects.

Many other studies also dealt with large populations of veterans, such as the study of Canadian Gulf War veterans by Goss Gilroy Inc. (1998) and several studies of UK Gulf War veterans, but, although helpful, they used self-reports of symptoms and medical conditions to reach their conclusions. The committee did not consider symptom reporting alone to be sufficient evidence of a health effect in veterans; it required objective measures of a medical condition or a physician's diagnosis or assessment.

OVERVIEW OF HEALTH EFFECTS

The experimental literature on stress in both animals and humans suggests that exposure to a stressor initiates a cascade of biologic mechanisms that result in short-term and long-term consequences. In most people, once the stressor is removed, the stress response ceases and the body returns to normal; we consider such a stress response "adaptive." In some people, however, the stress response does not turn off when the stressor is no longer present, and it becomes "maladaptive" because the body continues to produce stress hormones and other chemical mediators that eventually result in deterioration of normal physiologic processes. The prolonged or chronic stress response can affect virtually all organ systems. Most research has focused on effects in the brain, the cardiovascular system, the gastrointestinal tract, the endocrine system, and the immune system, and the literature on the effects of stress in the general population suggests that chronic stress results in adverse health effects. The epidemiologic literature reviewed by the committee, however, did not demonstrate the array of effects seen in the experimental literature.

The epidemiologic literature on deployed vs nondeployed veterans yielded sufficient evidence of an association between deployment to a war zone and psychiatric disorders, including posttraumatic stress disorder (PTSD), other anxiety disorders, and depression; alcohol abuse; accidental death and suicide in the first few years after return from deployment; and marital and family conflict, including interpersonal violence. For several health and psychosocial effects—such as unexplained illness, drug abuse, chronic fatigue syndrome, gastrointestinal symptoms consistent with functional gastrointestinal disorders, skin diseases, incarceration, and fibromyalgia and chronic widespread pain—there was limited and suggestive evidence of an association. For the majority of health effects, the epidemiologic data were insufficient or too inconsistent to determine whether an association existed. The committee also found that deployed veterans report more symptoms and medical conditions and poorer health than veterans who were not deployed, particularly those deployed veterans with PTSD. The prevalence and severity of PTSD was associated with increased exposure to combat.

The conclusions reached by the committee regarding various health and psychosocial effects are presented in Table 8-1.

TABLE 8-1 Summary of Findings Regarding the Association Between Deployment to a War Zone and Specific Health and Psychosocial Effects

Sufficient Evidence of a Causal Association

Evidence from available studies is sufficient to conclude that there is a causal relationship between deployment to a war zone and a specific health outcome in humans. The evidence is supported by experimental data and fulfills the guidelines for sufficient evidence of an association (below). The evidence must be biologically plausible and satisfy several of the guidelines used to assess causality, such as strength of association, dose-response relationship, consistency of association, and temporal relationship.

- No effects.

Sufficient Evidence of an Association

Evidence from available studies is sufficient to conclude that there is a positive association. That is, a consistent positive association has been observed between deployment to a war zone and a specific health outcome in human studies in which chance and bias, including confounding, could be ruled out with reasonable confidence. For example, several high-quality studies report consistent positive associations, and the studies are sufficiently free of bias and include adequate control for confounding.

- Psychiatric disorders, including PTSD, other anxiety disorders, and depressive disorders.
- Alcohol abuse.
- Accidental death in the early years after deployment.
- Suicide in the early years after deployment.
- Marital and family conflict.

TABLE 8-1 Continued

Limited but Suggestive Evidence of an Association

Evidence from available studies is suggestive of an association between deployment to a war zone and a specific health outcome, but the body of evidence is limited by the inability to rule out chance and bias, including confounding, with confidence. For example, at least one high-quality study reports a positive association that is sufficiently free of bias, including adequate control for confounding, and other corroborating studies provide support for the association (corroborating studies might not be sufficiently free of bias, including confounding). Alternatively, several studies of lower quality show consistent positive associations, and the results are probably not due to bias, including confounding.

- Drug abuse.
- Chronic fatigue syndrome.
- Gastrointestinal symptoms consistent with functional gastrointestinal disorders, such as irritable bowel syndrome or functional dyspepsia.
- Skin disorders.
- Fibromyalgia and chronic widespread pain.
- Increased symptom reporting, unexplained illness, and chronic pain.
- Incarceration.

Inadequate/Insufficient Evidence to Determine Whether an Association Exists

Evidence from available studies is of insufficient quantity, quality, or consistency to permit a conclusion regarding the existence of an association between deployment to a war zone and a specific health outcome in humans.

- Cancer.
- Diabetes mellitus.
- Thyroid disease.
- Neurocognitive and neurobehavioral effects.
- Sleep disorders or objective measures of sleep disturbance.
- Hypertension.
- Coronary heart disease.
- Chronic respiratory effects.
- Structural gastrointestinal diseases.
- Reproductive effects.
- Homelessness.
- Adverse employment outcomes.

Limited/Suggestive Evidence of No Association

Evidence from well-conducted studies is consistent in not showing a positive association between exposure to a specific agent and a specific health effect after exposure of any magnitude. A conclusion of no association is inevitably limited to the conditions, magnitudes of exposure, and length of observation in the available studies. The possibility of a very small increase in risk after exposure studied cannot be excluded.

- No effects.

RECOMMENDATIONS

The committee acknowledges that the VA and the Department of Defense (DoD) have expended enormous effort and resources in attempts to address the numerous health issues related to veterans. The information obtained from those efforts, however, has not been sufficient to determine conclusively the origins, extent, and long-term implications of health problems associated with veterans' participation in war. The difficulty in obtaining useful answers, as noted by numerous past Institute of Medicine committees and the present committee, is due largely to inadequacies in predeployment and postdeployment screening and medical examinations and to lack of recording of stressors to which deployed personnel are exposed.

The committee recommends that DoD conduct comprehensive, standardized predeployment and postdeployment evaluations of medical conditions, psychiatric symptoms and diagnoses, and psychosocial status and trauma history. Predeployment evaluation would serve two purposes. First, it would help to identify at-risk personnel who might benefit from targeted intervention programs during deployment—such as marital counseling, medication for psychiatric or other disorders, or psychologic counseling and therapy—which might eliminate or minimize future problems. Second, such evaluations would establish a baseline against which later health and psychosocial effects could be measured.

Postdeployment assessment would also serve two purposes. First, it would provide data that could be analyzed to determine the long-term consequences of deployment-related stress and its modifiers; the committee recommends that postdeployment assessments be made shortly after deployment and at regular intervals thereafter (such as every 5 years) to measure the health and psychosocial status of veterans as they age. Second, such assessments would allow VA and DoD to implement intervention programs to assist veterans in adjusting to postdeployment life. The initial assessment after deployment should also ask the veterans what situations, events, or conditions they found to be most stressful during deployment. Knowing which veterans experienced the most stress and recognizing the possible modifiers and consequences of that stress would enable VA and DoD to target prevention and intervention programs to those at greatest risk for adverse effects. The committee further recommends that any longitudinal assessments also be conducted in a representative group of nondeployed veterans to allow appropriate comparisons between deployed and nondeployed veterans regarding health and psychosocial effects.

REFERENCES

CDC (Centers for Disease Control and Prevention). 1988. Health status of Vietnam veterans. I. Psychosocial characteristics. The Centers for Disease Control Vietnam Experience Study. *Journal of the American Medical Association* 259(18):2701-2707.

Eisen SA, Kang HK, Murphy FM, Blanchard MS, Reda DJ, Henderson WG, Toomey R, Jackson LW, Alpern R, Parks BJ, Klimas N, Hall C, Pak HS, Hunter J, Karlinsky J, Battistone MJ, Lyons MJ. 2005. Gulf War veterans' health: Medical evaluation of a U.S. cohort. *Annals of Internal Medicine* 142(11):881-890.

Goss Gilroy Inc. 1998. *Health Study of Canadian Forces Personnel Involved in the 1991 Conflict in the Persian Gulf.* Ottawa, Canada: Goss Gilroy Inc. Department of National Defence.

Gray GC, Coate BD, Anderson CM, Kang HK, Berg SW, Wignall FS, Knoke JD, Barrett-Connor E. 1996. The postwar hospitalization experience of U.S. veterans of the Persian Gulf War. *New England Journal of Medicine* 335(20):1505-1513.

Gray GC, Smith TC, Kang HK, Knoke JD. 2000. Are Gulf War veterans suffering war-related illnesses? Federal and civilian hospitalizations examined, June 1991 to December 1994. *American Journal of Epidemiology* 151(1):63-71.

Ikin JF, Sim MR, Creamer MC, Forbes AB, McKenzie DP, Kelsall HL, Glass DC, McFarlane AC, Abramson MJ, Ittak P, Dwyer T, Blizzard L, Delaney KR, Horsley KW, Harrex WK, Schwarz H. 2004. War-related psychological stressors and risk of psychological disorders in Australian veterans of the 1991 Gulf War. *British Journal of Psychiatry* 185:116-126.

Ishoy T, Suadicani P, Guldager B, Appleyard M, Hein HO, Gyntelberg F. 1999. State of health after deployment in the Persian Gulf. The Danish Gulf War Study. *Danish Medical Bulletin* 46(5):416-419.

Jordan BK, Marmar CR, Fairbank JA, Schlenger WE, Kulka RA, Hough RL, Weiss DS. 1992. Problems in families of male Vietnam veterans with posttraumatic stress disorder. *Journal of Consulting and Clinical Psychology* 60(6):916-926.

Kang HK, Mahan CM, Lee KY, Magee CA, Murphy FM. 2000. Illnesses among United States veterans of the Gulf War: A population-based survey of 30,000 veterans. *Journal of Occupational and Environmental Medicine* 42(5):491-501.

Kelsall HL, Sim MR, Forbes AB, Glass DC, McKenzie DP, Ikin JF, Abramson MJ, Blizzard L, Ittak P. 2004. Symptoms and medical conditions in Australian veterans of the 1991 Gulf War: Relation to immunisations and other Gulf War exposures. *Occupational and Environmental Medicine* 61(12):1006-1013.

Kulka RA, Schlenger WE, Fairbank JA, Hough RL, Jordan BK, Marmar CR, Weiss DS. 1990. *Trauma and the Vietnam War Generation: Report of Findings from the National Vietnam Veterans Readjustment Study*. New York: Brunner/Mazel Publishers.

INDEX

A

D

E

H

I

K

L

M

N

O

P

R

S

T

U

V